THOSE WHO COME TO BLESS

Loretta Greiner

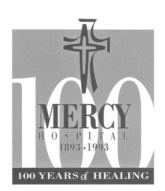

Mercy Hospital Medical Center
Des Moines, Iowa
1993

THOSE WHO COME TO BLESS

Sister Mary Seraphia McMahon, RSM
Mercy Hospital Medical Center
Project Administrator
Editor in Chief

Loretta Greiner
Mercy Hospital Medical Center
Author

Nancy A. Fandel
Allied Business Consultants, Inc.
Editor

Chris Conyers
Designgroup, Inc.
Creative Director

ACKNOWLEDGMENTS

Special thanks to all the Sisters of Mercy, staff, friends, and family of Mercy Hospital in Des Moines, who answered questions, read text, offered smiles, encouragement and prayers, to make this history possible. Special thanks to:

❧ Sister Mary Seraphia McMahon and Nancy Fandel, editors extraordinnaire, who brought a unique articulation to this history.

❧ Chris Conyers, who eased the blending of words and visuals into the volume design.

❧ Sister Patricia Clare Sullivan who encouraged this project from the beginning and to the end.

Printed in the United States of America by
Watt/Peterson,Inc., Plymouth, MN
First Edition 1993
Library of Congress Catalog Card Number 92-085293
ISBN: 0-96-34611-0-9

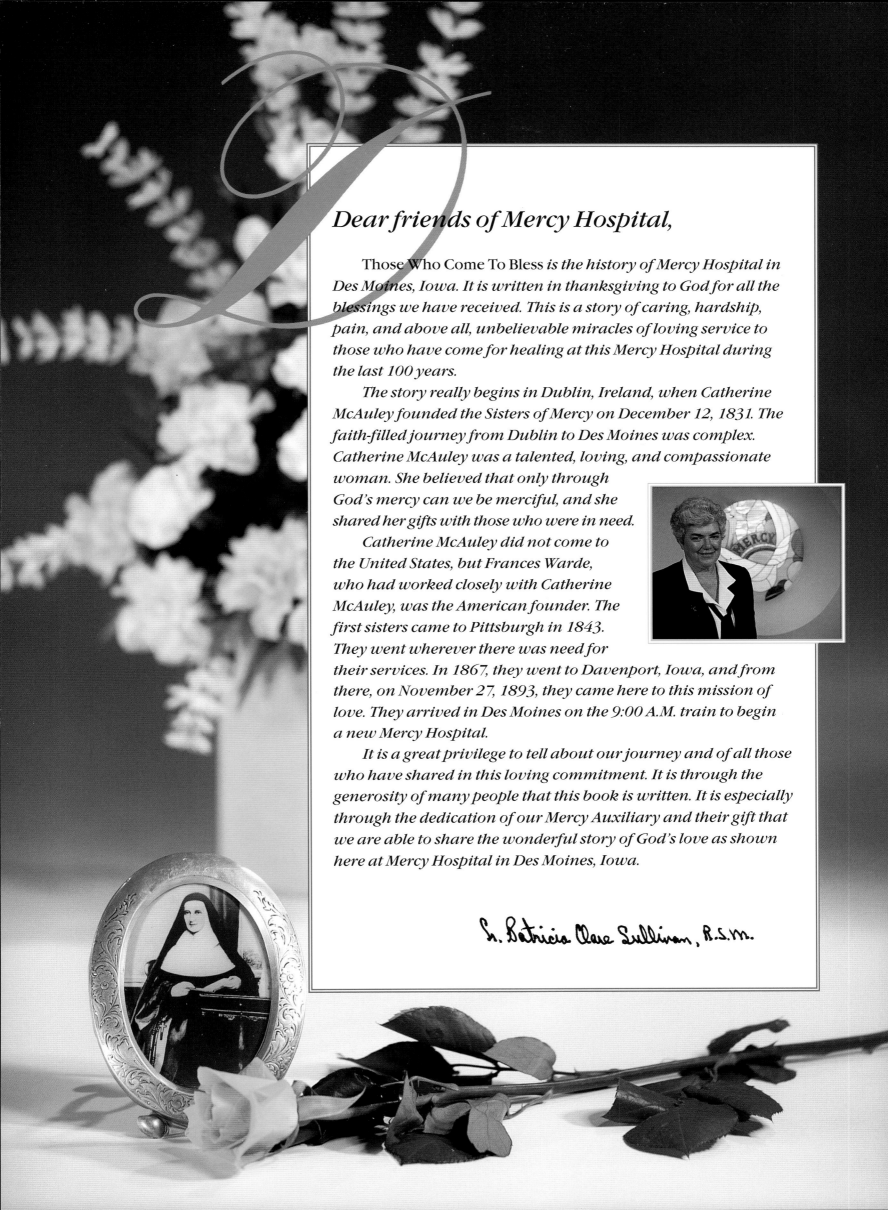

Dear friends of Mercy Hospital,

Those Who Come To Bless *is the history of Mercy Hospital in Des Moines, Iowa. It is written in thanksgiving to God for all the blessings we have received. This is a story of caring, hardship, pain, and above all, unbelievable miracles of loving service to those who have come for healing at this Mercy Hospital during the last 100 years.*

The story really begins in Dublin, Ireland, when Catherine McAuley founded the Sisters of Mercy on December 12, 1831. The faith-filled journey from Dublin to Des Moines was complex. Catherine McAuley was a talented, loving, and compassionate woman. She believed that only through God's mercy can we be merciful, and she shared her gifts with those who were in need.

Catherine McAuley did not come to the United States, but Frances Warde, who had worked closely with Catherine McAuley, was the American founder. The first sisters came to Pittsburgh in 1843. They went wherever there was need for their services. In 1867, they went to Davenport, Iowa, and from there, on November 27, 1893, they came here to this mission of love. They arrived in Des Moines on the 9:00 A.M. train to begin a new Mercy Hospital.

It is a great privilege to tell about our journey and of all those who have shared in this loving commitment. It is through the generosity of many people that this book is written. It is especially through the dedication of our Mercy Auxiliary and their gift that we are able to share the wonderful story of God's love as shown here at Mercy Hospital in Des Moines, Iowa.

Sr. Patricia Clare Sullivan, R.S.M.

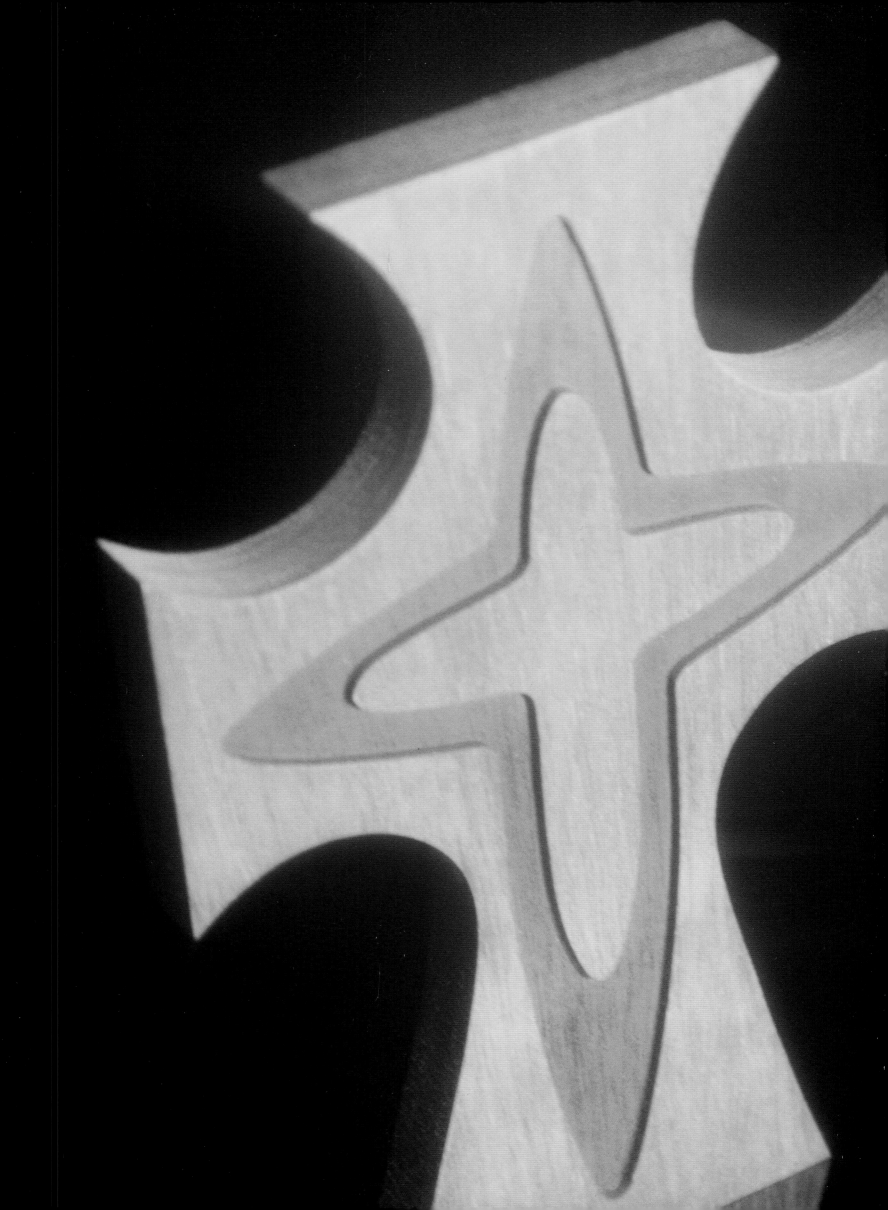

THE PHILOSOPHY OF MERCY HOSPITAL

The philosophy of Mercy Health Center of Central Iowa is derived from the Gospel, the philosophy of the Sisters of Mercy, and the philosophy of the Catholic Health Corporation.

We believe that our primary concern is to spread God's love in the community through a spirit of ecumenism by enabling its members to strive for wholeness in the healing ministry of sharing, helping, and forgiving.

We believe in the inherent dignity and right of all people to be treated with respect and genuine personal concern.

We believe that love, justice, mercy, and compassion are integral components in caring for the ill and in providing services that promote the concept of wellness.

We believe that we must provide quality care, offering our professional skills and knowledge in a supportive and warmly human manner.

We believe that the foundation of our corporate strength rests on the concept of combining individual strengths through partnerships in caring so that our leadership, ingenuity, energy, and resources may be fully dedicated to the task of meeting the healthcare needs of those we serve.

TABLE OF CONTENTS

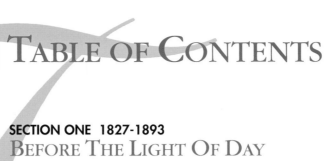

SECTION ONE 1827-1893

BEFORE THE LIGHT OF DAY

12 A SUN-KISSED HILL: THE LAND

The "sun-kissed hill" that Mercy Hospital sits atop held earlier lives that also were close to God.

18 PRIESTLY PIONEERS: THE CLERGY

One priest's farsighted dream paved the way for acquiring land on which to build Mercy Hospital.

23 MERCIFUL PIONEERS: THE SISTERS OF MERCY

Early Sisters of Mercy set the tone for compassionate care of the poor and suffering at Mercy Hospital.

26 MEDICAL PIONEERS: EARLY HEALING

The beginnings of health care in Polk County give historical reference to Mercy's longstanding tradition of high-quality medical care.

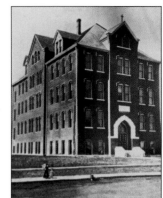

SECTION TWO 1893-1922

IN THE HEALING HANDS OF GOD

32 A CITADEL AGAINST SUFFERING: MERCY HOSPITAL

Papers bannered the news on front pages: "A Catholic Hospital...a Big One to be established in Des Moines." Hoyt Sherman Place was the first home.

38 ON THE SUN-KISSED HILL: FOURTH AND ASCENSION

In 1894, Mercy Hospital's first building, the East Wing, was lovingly built on the sun-kissed hill, the present campus.

50 THE TURN OF THE CENTURY

The Sisters of Mercy greeted the dawning new century with seven years of experience ministering to the healthcare needs of Des Moines.

57 CHANGING TIMES

Changes occurred at a rapid pace as Iowa's population grew, and as the first decade of the 20th century came to an end.

66 A NEW BEGINNING

Light shined brightly on new horizons for the Sisters of Mercy as they added additions to the hospital and gained independence.

70 THE END OF AN ERA

The brief but influential life of the Sisters of Mercy Motherhouse in Des Moines marked the way for the Council Bluffs sisters to begin anew.

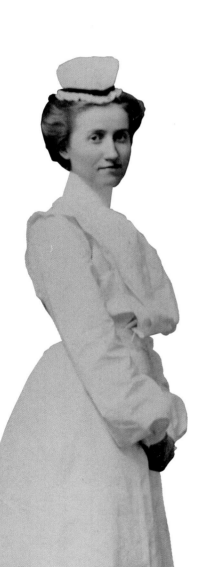

SECTION THREE 1922-1947

ON THE WINGS OF ANGELS

76 FURTHER GROWTH: NEW LEADERSHIP

New management came to Mercy Hospital fresh on the heels of World War I and a weakened farm economy. Hard work and wisdom guided the way.

84 A TEST OF STRENGTH: THE GREAT DEPRESSION

The Great Depression of 1929 to 1941 affected all classes of people and spawned suffering among those who once knew great wealth and good health.

96   UNITING FOR FREEDOM

As World War II clouds burst in Europe, Mercy's physicians boldly met
enemies abroad and at home, aided as always by Mercy sisters and nurses.

104   SCHOOL OF NURSING: 1922-1947

Tireless efforts of the sisters and nursing management helped Mercy
Hospital and its school of nursing reorganize in the 1920s.

118   MERCIFUL ANGELS: THE COUNCIL BLUFFS SISTERS

Mercy Hospital has been blessed with the talents of strong and comforting
"angels of Mercy" since its beginning. This amalgamation with Council Bluffs
brought a new spirit and dedication that never wavered.

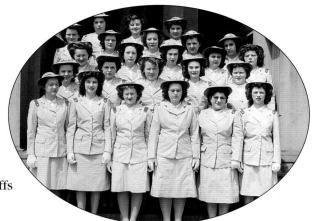

SECTION FOUR   1947-1969

TO THE GLORY OF THE LORD

124   PATHS NOT YET TAKEN: A NEW DIRECTION

Mercy Hospital met a changed world after the ravages of war and
depression, and it undauntingly took a new direction, promising continued
excellence in medical care for Des Moines.

134   TOMORROW'S HOPE: STRUCTURAL GROWTH

The years from 1947 to 1969 saw massive structural changes at Mercy
Hospital which proved to strengthen it from the inside out.

148   SCHOOL OF NURSING: 1947-1969

By the end of World War II, the status of nursing had undergone changes
and growth that permanently altered the image and duties of the profession.

156   MILESTONES: CARING FOR ALL

As Des Moines approached the end of the 1950s, "urban renewal" became
the watchword for all, including Mercy Hospital.

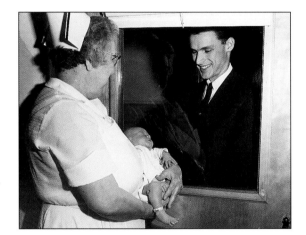

SECTION FIVE   1969-1993

THE TOUCH OF MERCY

170   A BRIGHTER VISTA: STRENGTHENING THE FOUNDATION

Mercy's sun-kissed hill had changed completely by the 1970s, reflecting
a strong institution untethered by tradition.

184   MERCY: LEADERS IN CARDIAC CARE

The roots of Mercy's cardiac care were planted and nurtured early in the 20th
century. As time passed, a strong program grew astride healthcare advances.

192   COMFORTING ARMS: CANCER CARE

Mercy's involvement with cancer care reaches back to 1917, when a Mercy
physician experimentally treated his own cancer in hopes of finding a cure.

196   GROWTH THROUGH THE CENTURY: THE BUILDINGS

206   FOR MERCY'S SAKE: THE GUILD

Shortly after World War II, Mercy Hospital began an organized volunteer
service known as the Mercy Guild. Their ongoing support makes it possible
to believe in miracles.

216   BOUNTIFUL CARE: MOVING TOWARD THE FUTURE

Incredible technological growth occurred in the 1980s and early 1990s. Mercy
Hospital expanded to meet the times, moving easily into the next 100 years.

234   FOOTNOTES

236   INDEX

238   CREDITS

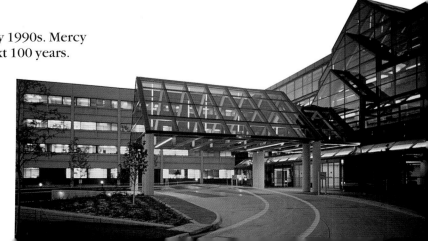

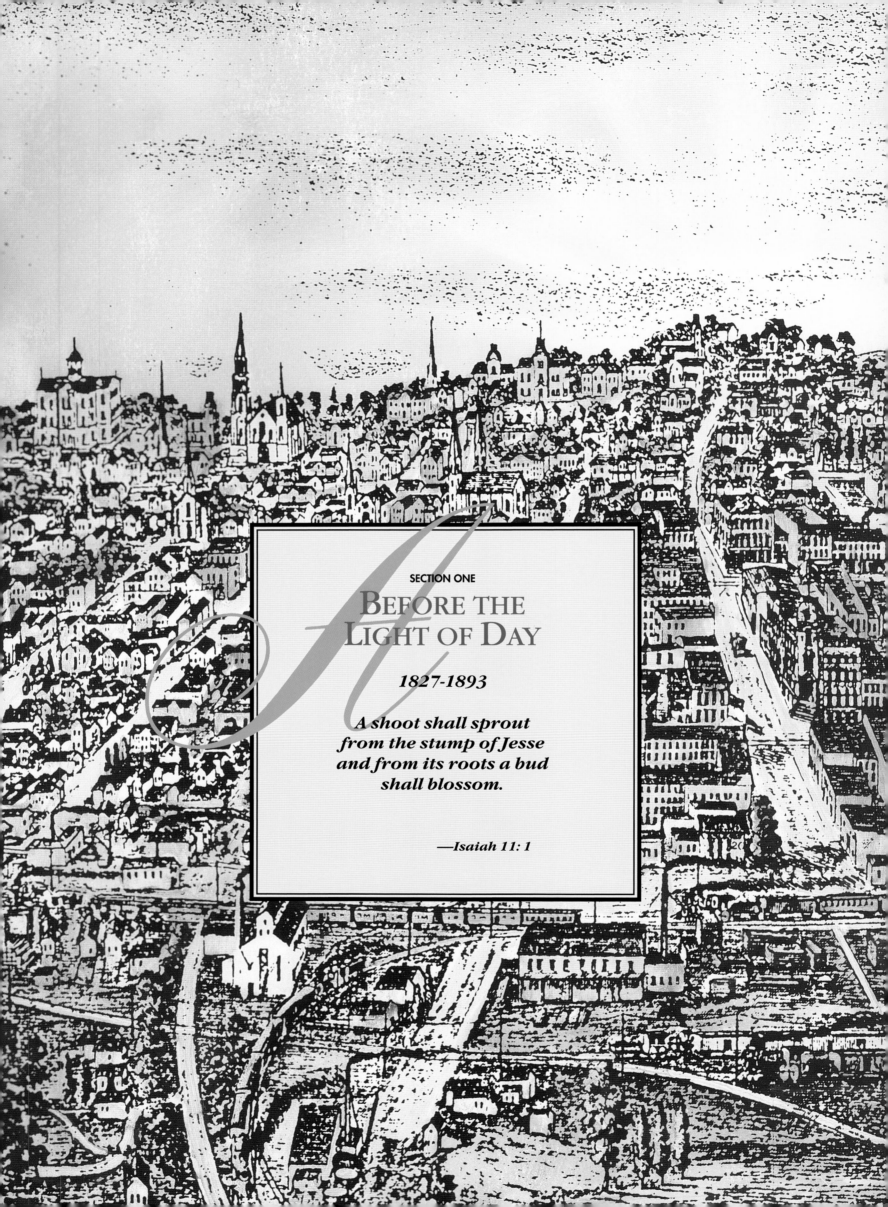

SECTION ONE

BEFORE THE LIGHT OF DAY

1827-1893

*A shoot shall sprout
from the stump of Jesse
and from its roots a bud
shall blossom.*

—*Isaiah 11: 1*

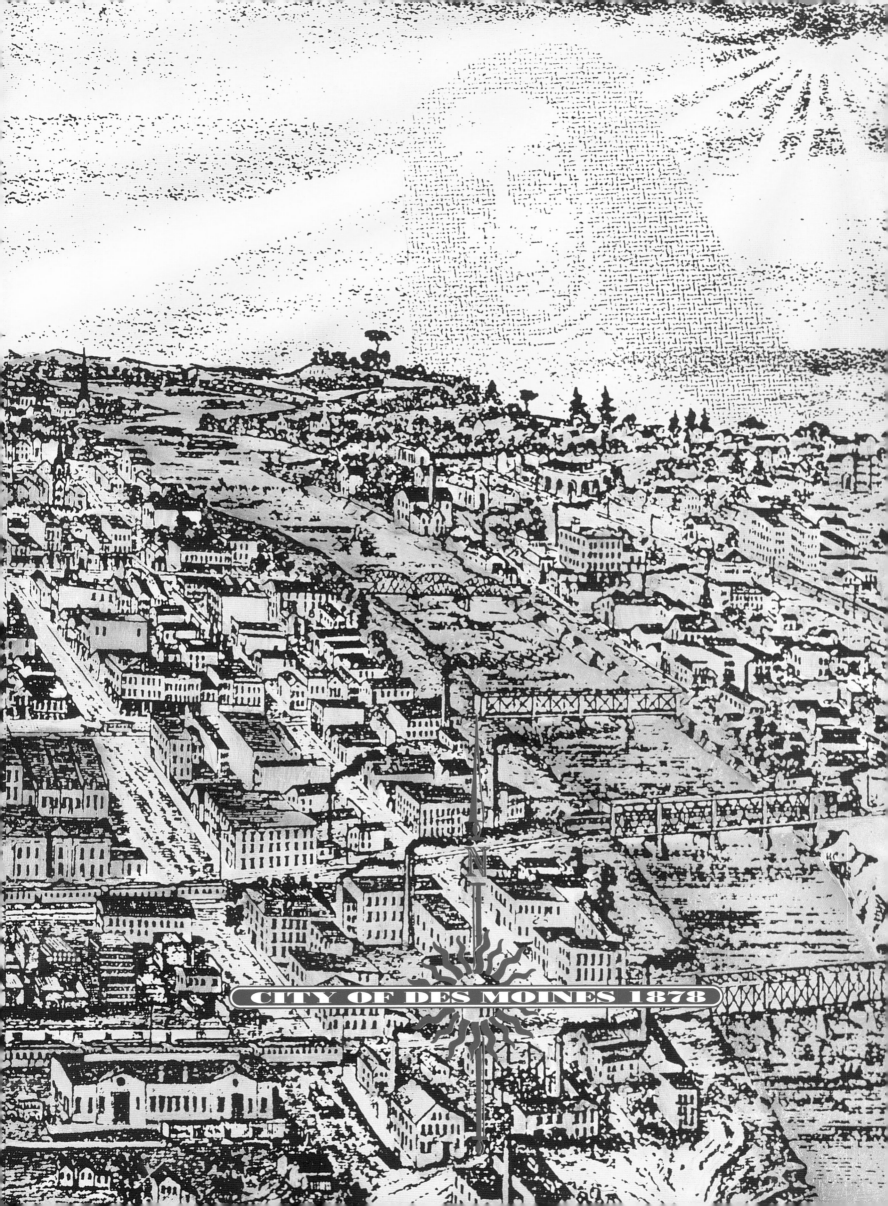

CITY OF DES MOINES 1878

CHAPTER ONE

A Sun-Kissed Hill: The Land

The sun-kissed hill that Mercy Hospital sits atop held earlier lives that were close to God. Religion and healing services played important roles in these lives: The site once held an Episcopal chapel; stories endure about an Irish priest who used an endowment to purchase the land to build a Catholic hospital; and the property was home for an earlier hospital in Des Moines.

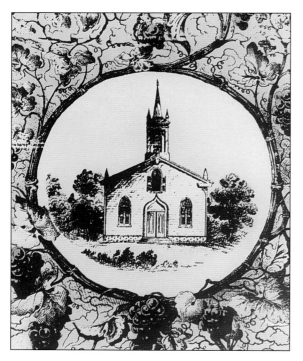

In 1856, members of St. Paul's Episcopal Church built Rutherford Chapel on the sun-kissed hill where Mercy Hospital dwells today. *A warranty deed drawn in 1881, opposite backdrop, transferred ownership of this property to Father John F. Brazill. The plat map, opposite inset, positions the site on Lot 4 of Block 18 in an area known then as Hall's Addition.*

Rutherford Chapel

In October 1848, two years after the opening of Polk County to settlers, Edwin Hall and his brother, Edward, laid claim to 150 acres of land on the north side of Des Moines Township. The plat that divided the land into blocks and lots was approved on February 20, 1856, and filed for record in March of that same year. This newly platted section was named appropriately Hall's Addition.[1] Later, when the Sisters of Mercy built on this site, it was dubbed "the sun-kissed hill."

In April, a deed in fee (or guardian deed) was given by the Hall family to St. Paul's Episcopal Church in Des Moines for Lot 4 in Block 18 of Hall's Addition. The terms of the deed read that "unless a chapel is erected upon said lot in 1856, for church and religious purposes, then this conveyance is to be null and void."[2]

St. Paul's rector, Edward Peet, chose to erect a mission chapel on the lot. Reverend Peet gathered together approximately $2,600 from a fund-raising campaign. He put $1,900 into St. Paul's building fund and used the remainder to build Rutherford Chapel on the Hall property.

The front of this chapel faced onto Sherman Street, later renamed Fourth Street.[3] What it looked like, how long it existed, and in what way it was used is not known fully. Records from St. Paul's Church show that marriages were performed at the chapel through July 1861. They also indicate that the chapel may have doubled as the rector's residence.

In September 1864, Edwin Hall died without leaving a will. At that time, a man named Ballinger was appointed guardian for minors of the Hall family, and another deed was issued to St. Paul's Vestry for the continuing operation of Rutherford Chapel. Four years later, on September 10, 1868, the Vestry sold the lot to Thomas D. Jewett for $500.[4]

A Mysterious Endowment

The land changed hands again in 1881 when Father John F. Brazill, an Irish priest and pastor of St. Ambrose Catholic Church in Des Moines, purchased the old Rutherford Chapel site from Jewett. Father Brazill intended to build a Catholic hospital on the land. The site was part of five lots he bought in Hall's Addition for $3,000. One frequently quoted story about the beginning life of Mercy Hospital concerns the priest and his purchase of this property.

According to tradition, an endowment left to Father Brazill enabled him to buy the land where Mercy Hospital now stands. This story is only partially true:

Maria M. Jewell & Hus.

Filed for Record and entered for record the 20th
day of *Aug.* A.D. 188_ at ____

J. J. Raynet ____

John F. Bragill

Know all Men by these Presents:

That *Maria M. Jewell and Thomas D. Jewell, husband and wife*

of *Pol____*

in hand paid by *Polk*

the following described pro____

Lots ____
eighteen (18) ____
included in ____
Iowa.

This deed ____
if_____ ____

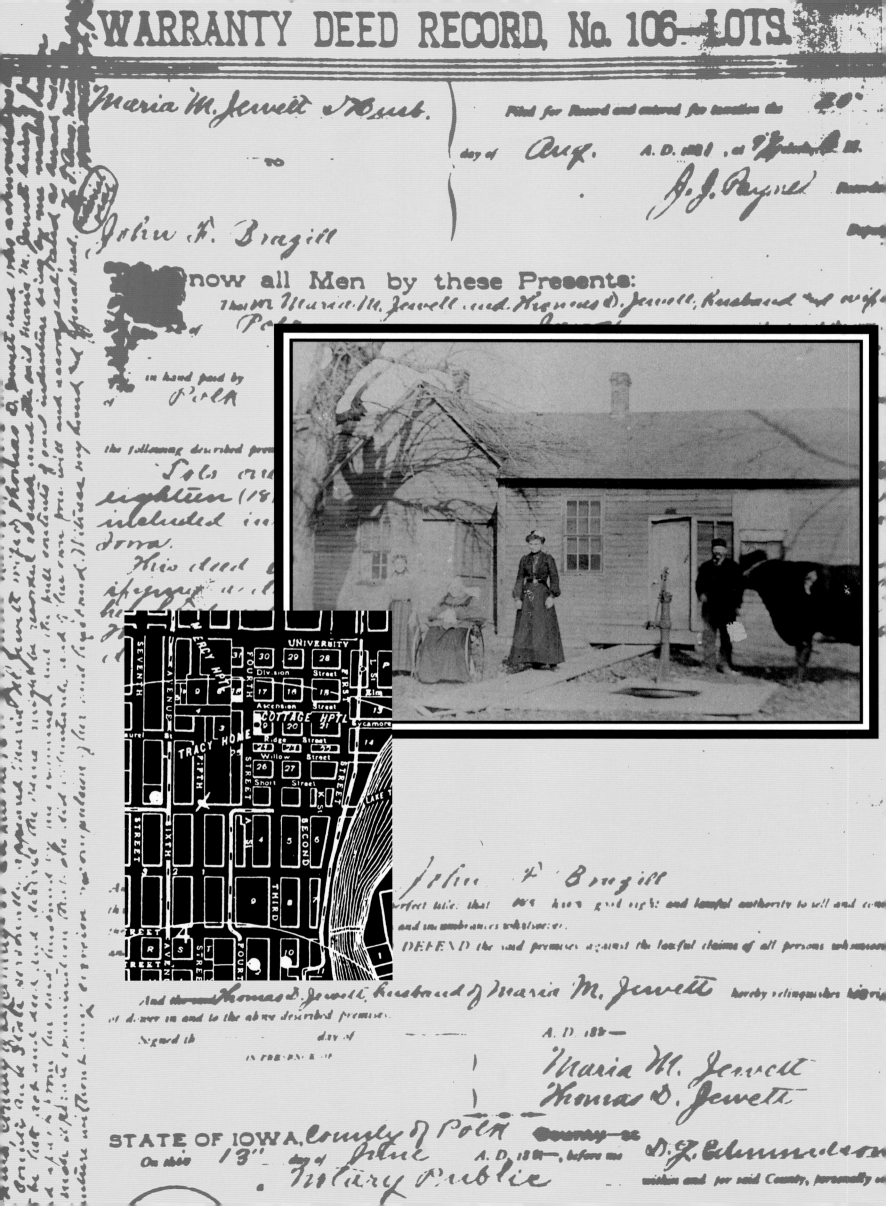

John F. Bragill

____ perfect title; that ____ has good right and lawful authority to sell and con___
and incumbrances whatsoever.

DEFEND the said premises against the lawful claims of all persons whomsoever

And the said *Thomas D. Jewell, husband of Maria M. Jewett* hereby relinquishes her ___
of dower in and to the above described premises.

Signed the ____ day of ____ A.D. 188—

IN PRESENCE OF

Maria M. Jewett
Thomas D. Jewett

STATE OF IOWA, *County of Polk*
On this *13"* day of *June* A.D. 188_, before me *D. J. Edmundson*
Notary Public within and for said County, personally

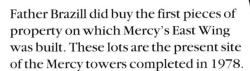

Father Brazill did buy the first pieces of property on which Mercy's East Wing was built. These lots are the present site of the Mercy towers completed in 1978.

No one knows for sure about the $3,000, however. Did it really come from an endowment? The question is shrouded in a mystery that began late in 1880 when a man named Myles Collins died.

A wealthy landowner, Myles Collins left part of his Cass County farmland to Father Brazill in a will he had executed in March 1880. His intentions for doing this were good: He wanted the land to be for the "use and benefit of St. Ambrose Catholic Church in Des Moines."[5] Father Brazill was more than likely aware of this will. In anticipation of receiving funds from the sale of the farmland, he promised to purchase the five lots in Hall's Addition.

What Father Brazill did not know at the time he made this promise was that another will had been drawn by Myles Collins in July 1880. This will designated Collins' daughter, Kate, and her husband, Peter Toner, as executors for her father's property.

Kate did not share her father's wishes for the land, and she made sure that Father Brazill received nothing from the estate. This forced the priest into reneging on his original promise to purchase the lots in Hall's Addition. Father Brazill did, however, find $3,000 somewhere, and in August of 1881, he officially purchased the property for that amount.[6]

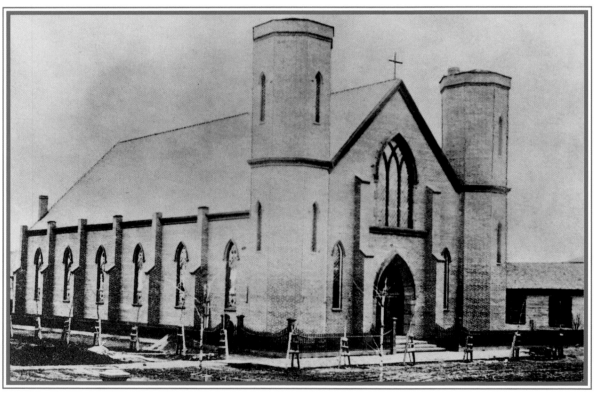

During the early Collins-Brazill dispute, Myles Collins' other daughter, Lizzie, a printer for the *State Journal,* was ill with consumption. Because she was a member of St. Ambrose Parish, Lizzie was comforted during her illness by Father Brazill. When she died on January 19, 1882, he was present.

In her will, Lizzie named Father Brazill administrator of her estate and left him property. According to the terms of Myles Collins' last will, however, Kate and Peter Toner, as executors, controlled the family real estate until Myles Collins' heirs married. Because Lizzie was unmarried when she died, the Toners disputed her right to leave the inheritance to Father Brazill. A drawn-out case ensued that was heard first in the Polk County Circuit Court, then settled in the Iowa Supreme Court.

As the estate trial went through appeal after appeal, everyone involved in the case received a great deal of attention in the local newspapers. The Collins family questioned the circumstances of Lizzie's will, which was hastily drawn just two hours before her death. Plus, Father Brazill's presence at Lizzie's death heightened their suspicions that he did not act in good faith. Father Brazill wanted control of at least Lizzie's portion of the Collins' estate, especially since he had been denied any claim to the land left him by her father.

During the trials, a witness testified that Lizzie Collins was very bitter toward her family. Lizzie believed that her sister had cheated Father Brazill out of the property her father had left "for the good of his soul."[7] The lawsuit continued even after Father Brazill died unexpectedly on August 25, 1885.

Three months before his death, Father Brazill deeded all of his claims to the Collins' properties to a group of trustees—J. S. Clarkson, M. H. King, J. C. Regan, John Hughes, J. B. McGorrisk, and W. H. Welch. In the will, Father Brazill's plans for the land became very clear. It read:

> *"The said property to be by them managed and used for the express purpose of erecting, maintaining, and sustaining an [sic] hospital, to be in the City of Des Moines. Hospital shall be conducted by some order of Sisters belonging to the Roman Catholic Church, said order or society of Sisters to be designated by the grantor herein, said hospital to be called Ascension Hospital..."* [8]

Father Brazill had appointed Bishop Henry Cosgrove, Regan, McGorrisk, and Hughes as administrators of his estate. The will was probated, another administrator was appointed to handle the Collins case, and the complicated and notorious legal actions continued for two more years. Finally, in December 1887, the Collins real estate was sold, netting $1,178.96. Father Michael Flavin, who succeeded Father Brazill as pastor of St. Ambrose, was the beneficiary of both Lizzie Collins' and Father Brazill's estates. Father Flavin petitioned for claims to be settled, and by the time all monies were dispersed, he received a total of $249.33 in March 1888. When the dust finally cleared from the Lizzie Collins lawsuit, Father Brazill's dream of a Catholic hospital on the Hall's Addition property began to see daylight.

Father Flavin successfully kept the property from being sold to settle debts Father Brazill had in excess of the money in his estate. No one questioned Father Brazill's intentions for the land, and Lots 1-5 on Block 18 of Hall's Addition—the old Rutherford Chapel site—eventually became the permanent home for a Catholic hospital—Mercy Hospital.

One mystery remained, however: Where *did* Father Brazill find $3,000 to purchase the lots in Hall's Addition?

After the conclusion of the Collins' case in 1883, before it was appealed to the Iowa Supreme Court, Bishop John McMullen of Davenport sued Father Brazill for control of certain property in Des Moines that he believed belonged to the Church. The suit was necessary because Father Brazill's land purchases were in his name.

This lawsuit was notorious enough to make for more interesting reading about Father Brazill in newspapers in Davenport, Des Moines, and Dubuque. Father Brazill tried to quiet things down by writing a letter to Des Moines' *Daily Iowa State Leader*. He wrote: "I regret having to appear in print on such matters. Necessity is my excuse. I regret it, moreover, for the whole matter has been honorably and fairly arranged between Bishop McMullen and myself." He further wrote that he had paid for certain mortgages, "by my own earnings. I never got a dollar for the purpose from anyone. I had five or six missions, and the salary I got from them was principally used for the benefit of St. Ambrose." [9]

More than likely, Father Brazill used some of this income to purchase Mercy's land in 1881.

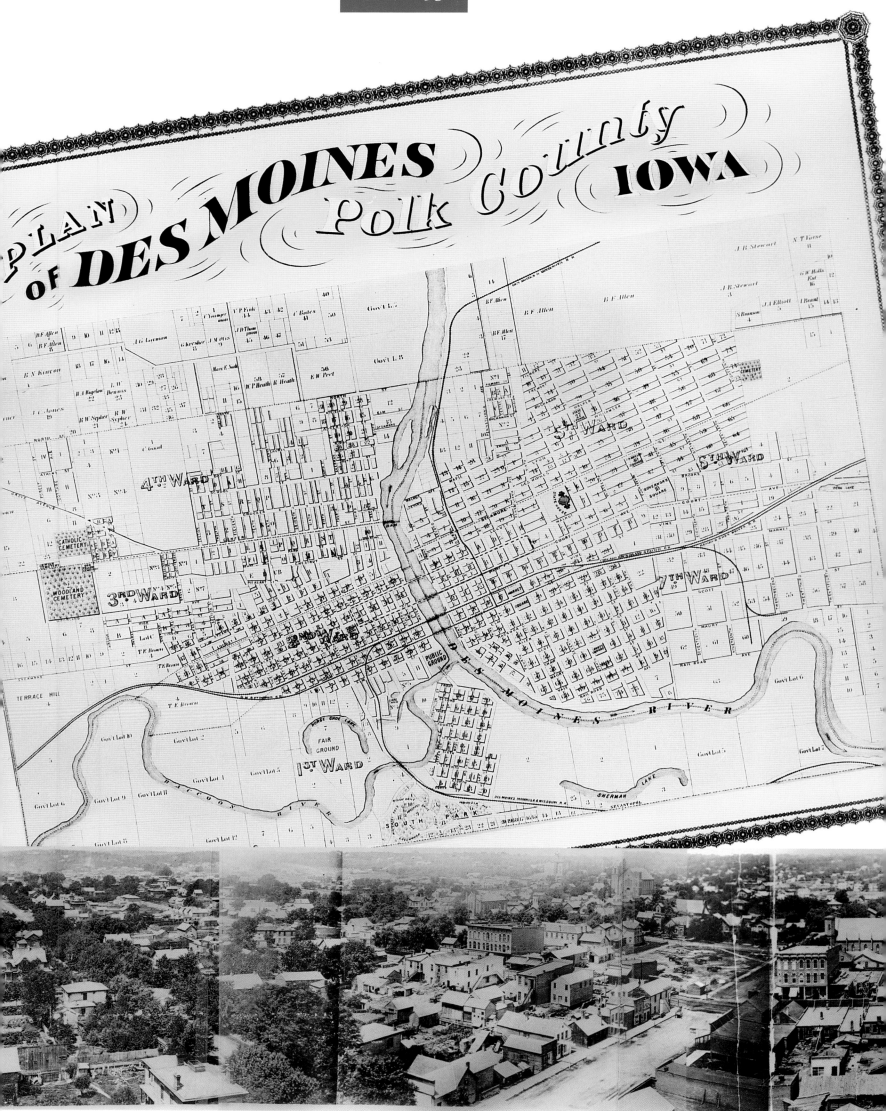

Des Moines' Second Hospital

A nearby tract of land in Hall's Addition is now part of the Mercy Hospital campus, as well. This site saw life as the second hospital in Des Moines.

On December 14, 1875, the ladies of the Helping Hand Society of St. Paul's Episcopal Church opened a hospital at 923 Seventh Street. They called it the Seventh Street Hospital at first, then later, Cottage Hospital. With the support of their rector and parish, these women gathered resources to equip the hospital.

Soon after the hospital opened, however, it became apparent that not everyone saw the creation of this new hospital as good for Des Moines. According to a letter to the editor in *The Daily Iowa State Register* on August 16, 1876, the Seventh Street Hospital was seen as "a disgrace to the good intentions of the founders of the enterprise." Written by one of the adjoining property owners, the letter claimed that the hospital was overcrowded and that the smell was intolerable.

About 10 days before this letter appeared, a lot was purchased by Annie B. Tracy, a hospital board member and one of the original members of the hospital's founding committee. This lot was located on Fourth Street between Ascension and Ridge Streets—Lot 7 on Block 19 of Hall's Addition, one block south and east of the old Rutherford Chapel site. The board of directors of the Seventh Street Hospital had been concerned with conditions there for some time. In reaction to this concern, they renamed the hospital Cottage Hospital and moved it to Mrs. Tracy's lot. Mrs. Tracy sold the land to the Cottage Hospital Board in 1882, and with the expansion of Cottage Hospital in the 1880s, the Board purchased Lot 6 to the north. Cottage Hospital operated on this site until 1899.

Eventually, these pieces of land also became the property of Mercy Hospital. Today, the old Cottage Hospital site is in the approximate location of Mercy's computer center and east parking ramp.

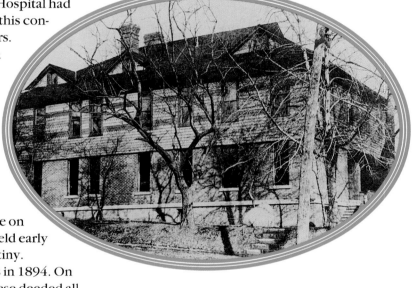

In The End

The quest to provide compassionate service and religious solace on Mercy's sun-kissed hill did not always come easily. Most who held early claims or deeds to the property worked hard to create this destiny.

Mercy began building on the first Hall's Addition properties in 1894. On July 24, 1894, Bishop Henry Cosgrove of the Davenport Diocese deeded all of the Hall's Addition properties held by the Church, including the old Rutherford Chapel site, to Mercy Hospital in Davenport.

In 1916, Mercy Davenport and Mercy Des Moines became separate entities. At that time, all of the Des Moines properties were transferred by Mercy Davenport to Mercy Des Moines. And in July 1922, all of the Mercy Des Moines properties were transferred to the Sisters of Mercy in Council Bluffs.[10]

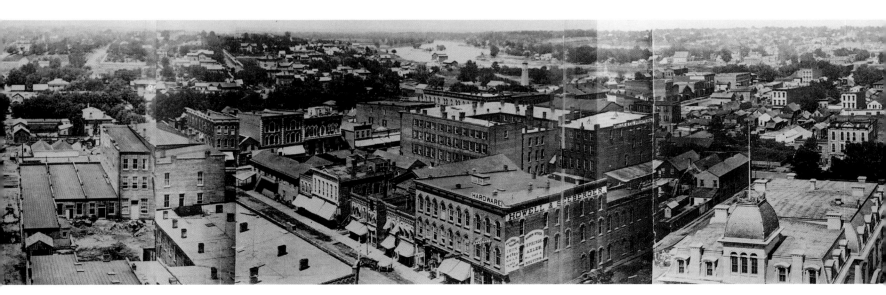

CHAPTER TWO
PRIESTLY PIONEERS: THE CLERGY

Father Brazill's farsighted dream paved the way for acquiring the land on which Mercy Hospital was built. His dream included the hope that the Sisters of Mercy would bring their healing ministry to Des Moines.

Although the sisters' reputation for loving Mercy care was well-known, their role in society was not prominent. It was up to local clergy, such as Father Brazill, to ensure community support for the sisters. These priestly pioneers had witnessed the effect of the sisters' work in other cities, and they encouraged the establishment of a Mercy hospital in Des Moines.

Countless clergy members made connections with influential citizens, offered advice, and, when they could, money, to aid in Mercy's progress. Father Brazill began it all with the land. Bishop Henry Cosgrove of the Davenport Diocese supported the Sisters of Mercy in coming to Des Moines. And, Father Michael Flavin helped make the dream a reality.

Very quickly, the skills of the Mercy sisters gained the respect and support of all with whom they came in contact. The Des Moines Catholic clergy acted as powerful supporters of the sisters' mission to provide much needed health care to the city. Later clergy benefited from the hospitality of the good sisters as they worked together to build the strong foundation of Catholic ideals that continues today at Mercy Hospital.

Father Brazill, *opposite,* **bought land at Sixth and High for today's St. Ambrose Cathedral, part of Piety Hill. The post-card,** *opposite center,* **details Piety Hill, looking north on Eighth Street.** *Below left* **to** *right,* **the first bishop of Iowa, Mathias Loras, 1837-1857; John McMullen the first bishop of Davenport, 1881-1883. Henry Cosgrove, bishop of the Davenport Diocese, 1903-1906.**

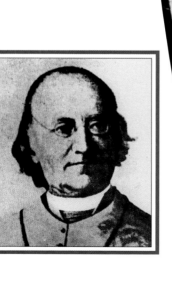

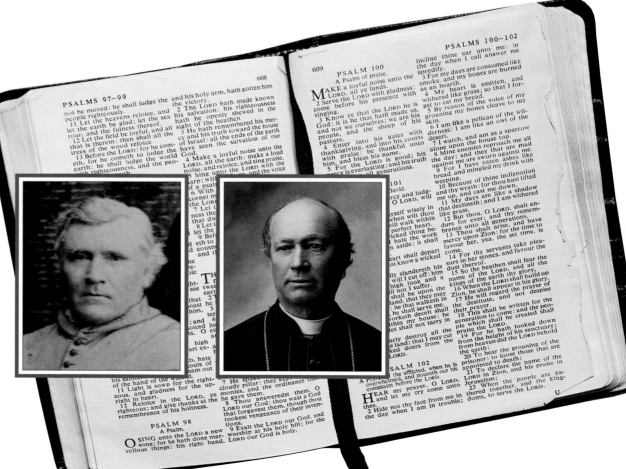

One of the brightest pioneer stars in Des Moines—influential in many aspects of the community and the history of Mercy Hospital—was Father John F. Brazill.

Father Brazill was the second pastor of St. Ambrose Catholic Church in Des Moines, appointed in 1860. An early biographer wrote that he was "kind, courteous, affable, energetic, public-spirited, and always diligent in advancing the welfare of his church, his schools, and the city." [1]

Many older priests still reminisce about this intriguing Catholic clergyman. One story they tell concerns Father Brazill's role in the erection of the Iowa State Capitol building. Father Brazill is given credit for securing the tie-breaking vote that ensured funds to build the Capitol in Des Moines.

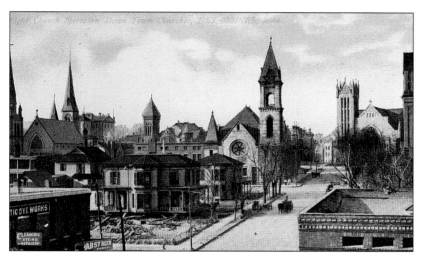

Opposition to building the Capitol advanced the issue to a third and final reading. Spirited vote-polling promised a close race, with the tie-breaking vote held by a known "fence sitter." On the morning of the vote, the man was absent from the House chambers. Knowing that he was a friend of Father Brazill, members of the House asked the priest to try to find him in time for the vote.

Father Brazill found the man, inebriated, "down by the 'Coon River." It seems that on the night before, members of the opposition party had "entertained" this important voter and left him in his own misery. Father Brazill hustled the fellow to the House floor in time to cast his important "Aye" vote, bringing an end to the question of the location of the Capitol building. [2]

Father Brazill realized the importance of securing property for the advancement of his goals for the Catholic Church, as well. During his tenure as pastor of St. Ambrose, he obtained title to lots on Sixth Avenue at Locust, Grand, and High to build a school, rectory, convent, and the present-day St. Ambrose Church.

Father Brazill also recognized the need for a good hospital in Des Moines. A diphtheria epidemic caused considerable concern in Des Moines during the mid-1870s. An influx of new inhabitants to the county—lured by the railroad and coal mining industries—brought myriad problems. Many of these immigrants were extremely poor,

uneducated, and susceptible to all forms of sickness. There were frequent accidents, both in the mines and on the railroad.

Des Moines' physicians were taxed to the limits to find suitable quarters for the recovery of these victims. St. Paul's Episcopal Church founded Cottage Hospital late in 1875, and another benevolent group tried to start a nonsectarian hospital called Union Hospital.

In his dreams, Father Brazill had always envisioned a Catholic hospital. Catholics were excluded from early endeavors to found a Des Moines hospital, but Father Brazill did not remain quietly in the background. He knew that Des Moines needed the kind of nurturing and merciful health care provided by a religious order of sisters. As Vicar General of the Dubuque Diocese, Father Brazill became aware of the activities of the Sisters of Mercy, who had already established hospitals in the eastern part of Iowa. He planned to find a place in Des Moines for the sisters to fulfill his dream of a Catholic hospital.

As a pastor, Father Brazill was in a position to receive gifts from benefactors to the Catholic Church in Des Moines. On one occasion, a dying woman, Lizzie Collins, named Father Brazill administrator of her estate, giving him control of all of her property and her rights to her wealthy father's estate. This bequest became the object of a much-publicized lawsuit instigated by Lizzie's family. The case was brought before the Iowa Supreme Court, where the family's lawyers questioned Lizzie's right, as a single woman, to hold property. Eventually, the issue was resolved in favor of Father Brazill. [3]

All of Father Brazill's land purchases were in his name. In his will, the priest "devised unto Right Reverend Henry Cosgrove, Bishop of the Diocese of Davenport, Iowa, for the use and benefit of the Roman Catholic church all my real estate situated in the city of Des Moines, Polk County, Iowa." [4] Father Brazill also chose his will to announce plans to erect a Catholic hospital. The document further read that the hospital "shall be erected as contemplated in a certain deed of trust by me to J. S. Clarkson and others..." [5]

Father Brazill's vision for a Catholic hospital in Des Moines began long before its doors opened, and he systematically set the wheels in motion. In 1876, he appointed the first board of trustees to plan for a Catholic hospital; in 1881, he purchased the lots in Hall's Addition. These lots were the former location of the old Rutherford Chapel. They sat to the west, catty-cornered from Cottage Hospital.

In 1893, eight years after his death, Father Brazill's hopes were fulfilled when Mercy Hospital opened. The land he purchased formed the cornerstone for the present Mercy campus in Des Moines, and his successor, Father Michael Flavin, invited the Sisters of Mercy to come to Des Moines.

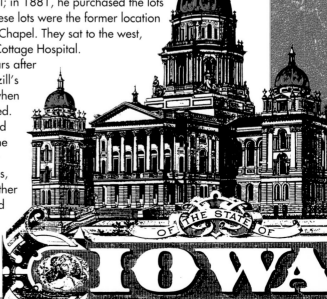

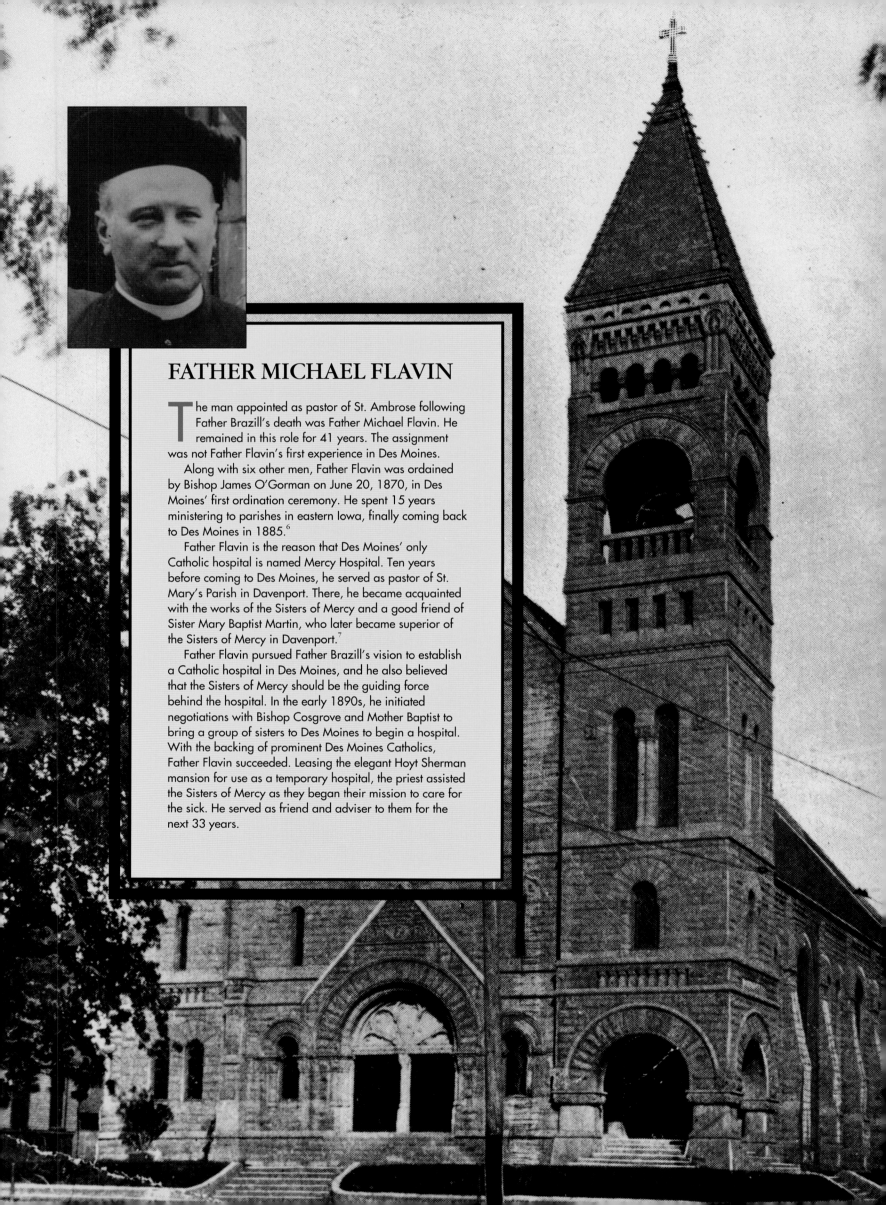

FATHER MICHAEL FLAVIN

The man appointed as pastor of St. Ambrose following Father Brazill's death was Father Michael Flavin. He remained in this role for 41 years. The assignment was not Father Flavin's first experience in Des Moines.

Along with six other men, Father Flavin was ordained by Bishop James O'Gorman on June 20, 1870, in Des Moines' first ordination ceremony. He spent 15 years ministering to parishes in eastern Iowa, finally coming back to Des Moines in 1885.[6]

Father Flavin is the reason that Des Moines' only Catholic hospital is named Mercy Hospital. Ten years before coming to Des Moines, he served as pastor of St. Mary's Parish in Davenport. There, he became acquainted with the works of the Sisters of Mercy and a good friend of Sister Mary Baptist Martin, who later became superior of the Sisters of Mercy in Davenport.[7]

Father Flavin pursued Father Brazill's vision to establish a Catholic hospital in Des Moines, and he also believed that the Sisters of Mercy should be the guiding force behind the hospital. In the early 1890s, he initiated negotiations with Bishop Cosgrove and Mother Baptist to bring a group of sisters to Des Moines to begin a hospital. With the backing of prominent Des Moines Catholics, Father Flavin succeeded. Leasing the elegant Hoyt Sherman mansion for use as a temporary hospital, the priest assisted the Sisters of Mercy as they began their mission to care for the sick. He served as friend and adviser to them for the next 33 years.

As the first light of day was awakening on the Mercy site, people unafraid to dream created events which led to the hospital's presence on this sun-kissed hill.

Each section of this book will record People of Vision who dedicated themselves to perpetuating the compassionate and unique care given by the Sisters of Mercy at Mercy Hospital in Des Moines.

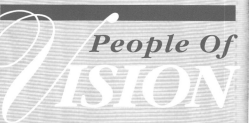

People Of VISION

1827-1893

Venerable Mother Catherine McAuley, RSM
· *Founder, Sisters of Mercy, 1827*
· *Effected the creation of Mercy Hospitals worldwide*

Sister Mary Frances Warde, RSM, left
· *American Founder, Sisters of Mercy Pittsburgh, 1843; Chicago, 1849*
· *Began numerous Mercy Foundations in Ireland and the U.S.*

Bishop Clement Smyth
· *Second Catholic Bishop of Iowa, 1857-1865*
· *Appointed Father John F. Brazill to St. Ambrose in Des Moines*

Father John F. Brazill
· *Pastor, St. Ambrose Catholic Church, 1860-1885*
· *Purchased land on which to build Mercy Hospital*

Bishop John Hennessy
· *Third Catholic Bishop of Dubuque Diocese and first Archbishop, 1866-1900*

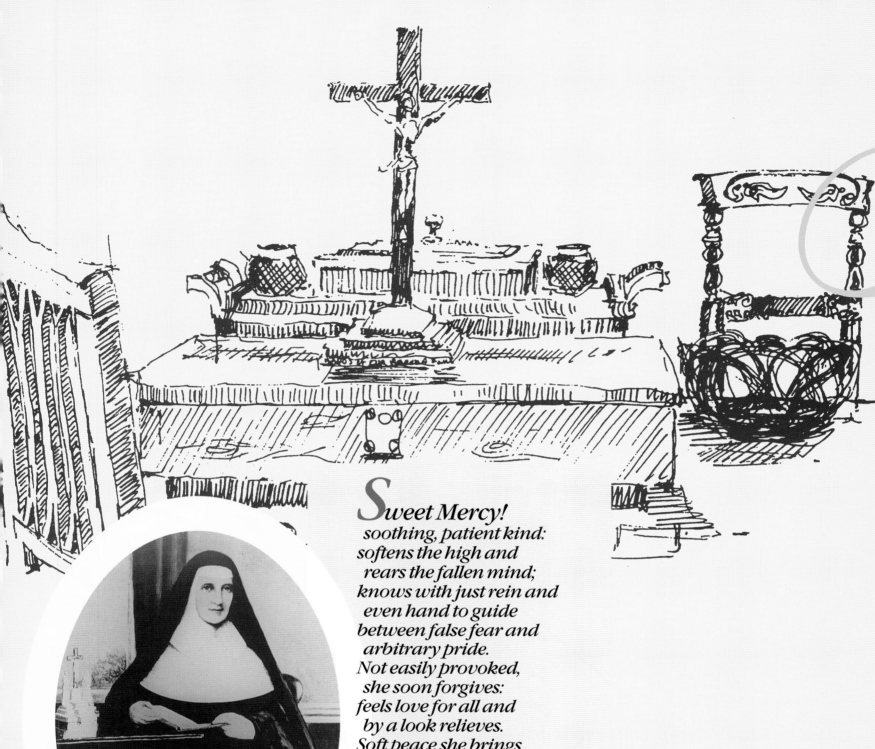

*S*weet Mercy!
soothing, patient kind:
softens the high and
 rears the fallen mind;
knows with just rein and
 even hand to guide
between false fear and
 arbitrary pride.
Not easily provoked,
 she soon forgives:
feels love for all and
 by a look relieves.
Soft peace she brings
 wherever she arrives,
removes our anguish
 and transforms our lives;
lays the rough paths
 of peevish nature even—
and opens in each heart
 a little Heaven.

M. C. McAuley

Magnificat of Mercy written for
the Feast of Our Lady of Mercy in
1828 by the Venerable Mother
Catherine McAuley, RSM

The Venerable Mother Catherine McAuley, RSM, *opposite,* founded the order of the Sisters of Mercy in Ireland in 1827. Her Irish convent, Baggot Street, *below,* became home to many poor and suffering women of Victorian Ireland. Catherine's compassionate nature fostered a religious order that today ministers the world with comforting arms and superior hospital care.

CHAPTER THREE

MERCIFUL PIONEERS: THE SISTERS OF MERCY

Behind the growth and development of Mercy Hospital lies the vital mission of the Religious Sisters of Mercy (RSM)—to provide compassionate care for poor and suffering humanity. This mission was the legacy envisioned by the founder of the Sisters of Mercy, the Venerable Mother Catherine McAuley, RSM. The history of Mercy Hospital really began with her in 1827 in Dublin, Ireland.

CATHERINE MCAULEY

Dublin's wealthy segment of population contrasted sharply to the extreme poverty of the majority of its citizens in 1827.

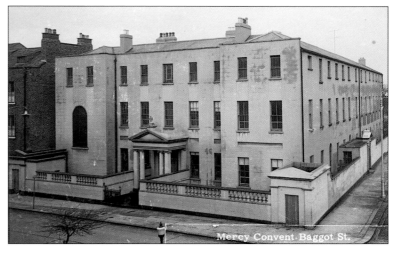

Mercy Convent. Baggot St.

Catherine McAuley's childhood was "chequered by transitions from wealth to poverty, to orphanhood and to reliance on charity."[1] She learned firsthand that "there are things which the poor prize more highly than gold, though they cost the donor nothing. Among these are the kind word, the gentle compassionate look and the patient hearing of sorrows."[2] This experience and belief were the forces that led Catherine to choose a life of ministering to the poor and sick who flooded the streets of Dublin.

Catherine inherited $1 million from William Callaghan, a wealthy friend who provided a home for her during her early adult life. Ultimately, she decided to use this inheritance to build a shelter for homeless women and children—a House of Mercy.

In the mid-1820s, Catherine boldly situated this shelter on Baggot Street in the middle of one of the wealthiest sections of the city. The house became the talk of the neighborhood, for her wealthy neighbors felt it was one thing to meet the poor on the street where they could step aside; meeting them on the doorstep was another matter.[3] Catherine cared more about the needs of the poor than she did about the wagging tongues of her affluent neighbors. "Her concern to promote, as she said, 'the ease, comfort and cleanliness' of the sick poor was integral to her conception of mercy."[4]

Catherine attracted all manner of the poor to Baggot Street—servant girls, orphans, and old women. Her godlike charisma also drew single women easily into the fold to share in her passion for charity and mercy. Imitating Catherine, these women "adopted a similar form of dress and [became] known as 'The Ladies of Mercy' or 'The Baggot Street Ladies.' "[5]

It was never Catherine's intent to create a religious order or to start a convent. She simply wanted to serve God by taking care of His poor. Her work seemed to have a life of its own, however, and the Church wanted that life to be surrounded by a defined structure. At the insistent urging of the Dublin clergy, Catherine entered a Presentation convent for a year's training in a religious community. After her return, she established the women of the House of Mercy as the Religious Sisters of Mercy (RSM) and Baggot Street as a convent in December 1831.

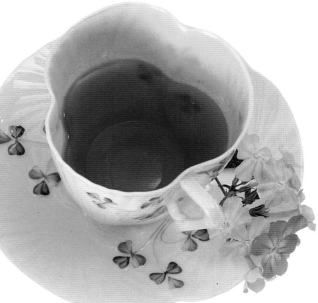

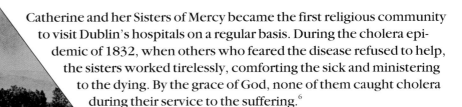

Catherine and her Sisters of Mercy became the first religious community to visit Dublin's hospitals on a regular basis. During the cholera epidemic of 1832, when others who feared the disease refused to help, the sisters worked tirelessly, comforting the sick and ministering to the dying. By the grace of God, none of them caught cholera during their service to the suffering.[6]

FROM DUBLIN TO IOWA

Possessed with the Irish missionary spirit, the Sisters of Mercy formed new convents throughout Ireland and the world. Sixteen years after Catherine opened the doors of Baggot Street, the order established its first foundation in the United States. The small band of sisters opened the first U.S. Mercy hospital in Pittsburgh on January 1, 1847.[7] In 1849, Sister Mary Frances Warde, RSM—who had brought Mercy to Pittsburgh—founded Mercy Hospital in Chicago.[8] This facility became one of the first stepping-stones to Mercy health care in Iowa. Bishop Loras attempted to begin a hospital in Dubuque in 1849 with the help of another religious order of sisters. This effort was short-lived, however. Three hospitals were started successfully in Iowa before the first Mercy hospital: a general hospital in Keokuk, 1850; a mental hospital in Mt. Pleasant, 1855; and a military hospital in Keokuk, 1862. The Sisters of Mercy played an important role in the opening of the military hospital.

In 1861, several Chicago Sisters of Mercy traveled to Jefferson City, Missouri, to care for wounded Civil War soldiers at a hospital there.[9] In mid-April 1862, at the height of the war, several steamboats loaded with convalescent and disabled soldiers arrived in Keokuk, Iowa. One of those steamboats, the *Empress,* also carried the Mercy sisters. They arrived on Holy Saturday after spending five weeks caring for the men on the steamboat.

The Medical College hospital, established in Keokuk in 1850, was full of patients. In desperation, the community turned every available large building into a hospital, with the majority of soldiers cared for at Estes House, a local hotel.

Keokuk's proximity to the waterways prompted the military to begin Iowa's third hospital there in 1862. This Army hospital remained in operation until September 1865.[10] The first monthly report of the United States General Hospital stated that 599 patients were received. The Sisters of Mercy who came to Keokuk on the *Empress* played a prominent role in health care there. They were proficient in pharmacy, as well as in nursing, and because of a lack of expertise in this area among the local nursing staff, their help was accepted gratefully.[11]

DAVENPORT SISTERS OF MERCY

The first Mercy hospital in Iowa began as an outgrowth of a school started by the Sisters of Mercy in 1867. On a mission to raise funds for their school in De Witt, Iowa, the sisters toured the Davenport poorhouse and were moved by the inmates' neglected condition. After receiving permission from her Chicago motherhouse and setting up stringent terms of agreement, Mother Mary Borromeo Johnson opened Mercy Hospital in Davenport on December 8, 1869.[12]

Mother Borromeo, Mother Mary Baptist Martin, and Mother Mary Francis Monholland were the first Sisters of Mercy—all Irish born—whose extraordinary talents and dedication formed the initial roots of Mercy health care in Iowa.[13] All three sisters came well qualified, for they had nursing experience during cholera epidemics and the U.S. Civil War. Mother Borromeo received recognition for her service as one of 92 Civil War "Nuns of the Battlefield."[14]

The new Mercy hospital in Davenport soon established a reputation as an "admirable place of retreat for the sick,"[15] and the Davenport Sisters of Mercy

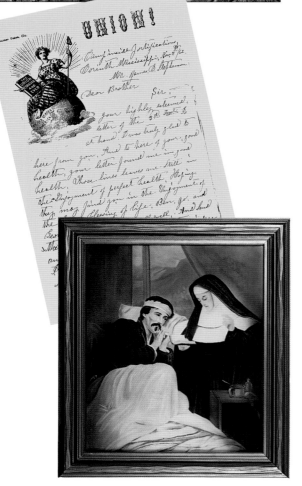

expanded their mission of health care to other areas in Iowa, directly affecting the establishment of 15 additional hospitals in the state.

On September 27, 1873, the sisters opened Mercy Hospital in Iowa City to fulfill the clinical needs of the Medical Department at the University of Iowa. Within five months, they had treated more than 300 cases.[16]

Mercy Hospital in Iowa City, sometimes referred to as the "Sisters' Hospital," served as the only clinical practice facility for the Medical School for more than a decade, until demands exceeded its capacity. In 1885, Mother Isidore O'Connor purchased a nearby property and began the move to eventually separate Mercy Hospital from the University Hospital. Articles of Incorporation, limiting board membership to Sisters of Mercy and changing the name of the hospital from Mercy Hospital to Mater Misericordia Hospital, were filed on December 5, 1885.[17]

The Davenport Sisters of Mercy expanded to Dubuque in 1879 and opened a hospital there in 1880. In 1893, the Davenport sisters, under the leadership of their superior, Mother Mary Baptist Martin, opened Mercy Hospital in Des Moines. In 1900, they began Mercy Hospital in Cedar Rapids, and in 1903, Mercy Hospital in Marshalltown.

Because the Davenport Sisters of Mercy went to Dubuque, created Mercy Hospital there, and started a foundation of Sisters of Mercy, other Iowa hospitals can trace their roots back to the Davenport sisters, even though they actually were founded by the Dubuque Sisters of Mercy. They are: Sioux City, 1890; Clinton, 1892; Waverly, 1904; Webster City, 1905; Fort Dodge, 1908; Cresco, 1910; Mason City, 1916; and Algona, 1949.

Anamosa and Oelwein Mercy hospitals can be connected indirectly to Davenport, although they were founded in the early 1900s by the sisters from Cedar Rapids.

COUNCIL BLUFFS SISTERS OF MERCY
The Sisters of Mercy came to Council Bluffs from Anoka, Minnesota, in September 1887, establishing another strong link in Mercy health care on Iowa's western border.

The Council Bluffs sisters immediately opened a small hospital in a two-story house on Fourth Street and Ninth Avenue. This became St. Bernard's Hospital. St. Bernard's established a reputation for skillful care of the mentally ill until Mercy Hospital in Council Bluffs opened. The sisters at St. Bernard's also cared for the physically ill from the area. They built Mercy Hospital within one block of St. Bernard's and began accepting patients in January 1903.[18] The Council Bluffs sisters also expanded their healing ministry into Centerville, Iowa, in 1910. They used an existing hospital facility to establish St. Joseph's Mercy Hospital.

The Sisters of Mercy in Council Bluffs became the administrators at Mercy Des Moines in 1922. And finally, in 1986, St. Joseph's Mercy Hospital became a sister corporation with Mercy Des Moines.

THE LEGACY CONTINUES
In the early days, it had been up to local clergy such as Father Brazill and Father Flavin to "grease the community wheel" to get Mercy Hospital built in Des Moines. As time passed, however, the role of the clergy diminished, and the sisters' profile in the community grew.

In the 1890s, awareness of the sisters' merciful health care grew in the United States as quickly as the new frontier. Responding to religious and social needs, the Sisters of Mercy founded a chain of more than 30 Mercy hospitals from coast to coast.[19] Mercy Hospital in Des Moines is a vital link in that chain, providing one of the finest reflections of Catherine McAuley's legacy of comforting and unique Mercy care.

Des Moines, Iowa

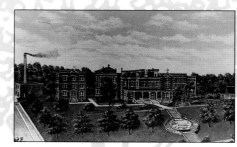

Council Bluffs, Iowa

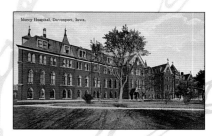

Davenport, Iowa

Chicago, Illinois

Pittsburgh, Pennsylvania

The Irish Sisters of Mercy formed new convents throughout Ireland and the world in the 1800s. They opened Mercy Pittsburgh in 1847, Mercy Hospital in Chicago in 1849, and Mercy Hospital in Davenport in 1869. Mercy Hospital in Council Bluffs was begun by Minnesota Sisters of Mercy who migrated to Iowa in 1887. Both the Davenport and Council Bluffs sisters played key roles in the history of Mercy Hospital in Des Moines.

CHAPTER FOUR
Medical Pioneers: Early Healing

Mercy is the oldest continuously operating hospital in Des Moines. A look at the beginnings of health care in Polk County helps to understand how Mercy's longstanding tradition of high-quality, compassionate health care fits into the history of Des Moines.

As the Sisters of Mercy were arriving in Pittsburgh in 1843, the first settlers were coming to Des Moines. Those settlers were soldiers who inhabited a military post at Fort Des Moines. Accompanying them was Assistant Surgeon John S. Griffin, who later became post surgeon.[1]

The area opened officially to white settlers on October 11, 1845. In 1846, the Act of Territorial Legislature created Polk County. The population of the area began to grow, and by 1847, Polk County had 1,792 residents.[2]

The first civilian doctor in Polk County was Dr. Thomas K. Brooks, *opposite left*. He arrived in the fall of 1845, and practiced medicine until about 1851. After that time, his interests turned to other activities.[3] Like most early physicians, Dr. Brooks needed a second source of income. He also more than likely grew weary of exhausting and discouraging work performed in primitive and unsanitary conditions.

These early doctors prepared and dispensed their own medicines, performed surgeries in family bedrooms—or sometimes on kitchen tables—and most of the time, received help only from the patient's family. Deadly outbreaks of cholera, yellow fever, diphtheria, influenza, typhoid, scarlet fever, and small pox were frequent. Payment for services sometimes came in the form of farm produce, including chickens, cows, and other livestock. It was a dangerous job that yielded little cash to pay the bills.

Early Hospitals
In May of 1865, a farm situated about five miles north of Des Moines was purchased for $4,000 by Polk County. This became the poorhouse. County physicians were invited to submit bids for providing medical care to its residents.

The spirit that built a strong America came to Des Moines on wagon-trains with the first settlers in the mid-1840s. Dr. Thomas K. Brooks, *opposite left,* arrived in 1845 to tend to growing medical needs. Dr. Archelaus G. Field, *opposite right,* influenced the establishment of a hospital to care for immigrants with typhoid fever, *opposite above.*

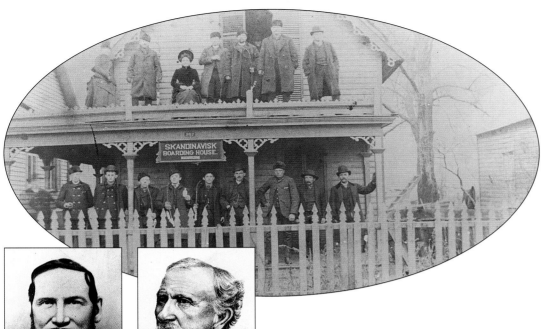

Dr. Archelaus G. Field
· *County Physician, 1860s*
· *Instrumental in beginning
the first hospital in Des Moines*

**Mother Mary Vincent
McDermott; Mother
Mary Magdalen Bennett**
· *Founders, St. Bernard's
Hospital, Council Bluffs, 1887*
· *The sisters of Council Bluffs
became Mercy Des Moines
administrators in 1922*

Father Michael Flavin
· *Pastor, St. Ambrose Catholic
Church, 1885-1926*
· *Petitioned to bring Sisters of
Mercy to Des Moines*

**Mother Mary Borromeo
Johnson, RSM**, left
· *Founder, Mercy Hospital,
Davenport, 1869*
· *Her healing vision
brought 16 Mercy Hospitals
to Iowa*

Mercy Hospital
· *First Board of Directors,
1876*
· *Father John F. Brazill
chose prominent Des Moines
citizens for the first Catholic
hospital board of directors.*

Michael H. King
Public Servant

John W. Geneser
Brick Contractor

J. B. McGorrisk
Builder and Contractor

J. S. (Ret) Clarkson
*Editor and Publisher,
The Iowa State Register*

John C. Regan
Businessman

Dr. Archelaus G. Field, *near left,* presented the most reasonable bid and became the first county physician. Two years later, a report praised the success of the county farm and wished that "some specific provision be made as to quarters for that class of paupers afflicted with infectious diseases."[4]

In 1868, the need for a hospital of this sort in Des Moines became apparent to Dr. Field. One day, he found a group of Swedish immigrants crowded into a single room in East Des Moines. Many were suffering from typhoid fever. Moved by what he saw, the good doctor wrote an impassioned plea for the establishment of a hospital. The request appeared on the front page of *The Daily Iowa State Register* on September 2, 1868. Dr. Field indicated that the county poorhouse was available, but added that the "confusion and noise of overcrowded rooms is always injurious to the sick."

As a result of Dr. Field's letter, the newspaper supported his desire for a hospital and reported events surrounding that cause for weeks. The Polk County Board of Supervisors appointed Michael H. King, a public servant, to work with Dr. Field to secure a place for the diseased immigrants.

TYPHOID HOSPITAL

Within two weeks, Dr. Field and Mr. King convinced several citizens to join in their endeavor. A brick building on Market Street on the east side of the river bank in Des Moines was chosen to be used as a "typhoid hospital." Members of various churches and charitable institutions whitewashed the building and contributed food and bedding in order to make the hospital ready for occupation. Thirty ailing immigrants received help through this effort; 18 at the hospital and 12 in apartments because they were too sick to be moved.[5] Only two immigrants died.

A contemporary map of Des Moines suggests the location of this hospital probably was on the State Capitol side of the Des Moines River, one block south of the Court Avenue district.[6] A later account of the founding of this first hospital reported that it began in the vicinity of Mercy Hospital. This 1921 report was made by Dr. Field in the Journal of the Iowa State Medical Society. Dr. Field said that Father Brazill eventually secured the property, and that it was to become the location of Mercy Hospital.[7] There is no evidence to support this particular Father Brazill story, however.

Five weeks after the first article appeared in the paper, the "typhoid hospital" was dissolved. The paper tried again to arouse interest within the community, this time with the idea that a permanent public hospital be established. This vision failed to become a reality, and no more attempts to begin a permanent hospital took place for eight years.

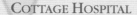

COTTAGE HOSPITAL

During 1875, Des Moines suffered a diphtheria outbreak. Every month of that year, Iowa weathered below-normal temperatures, with the months of January and February being two of the coldest on record.[8] Anticipating another cold winter, and realizing Des Moines was ill-equipped to take care of its sick and homeless, several humanitarian groups began looking at their resources.

On December 14, 1875, the Helping Hand Society of St. Paul's Episcopal Church and Rector Reed began discussing the possibility of establishing a hospital. The women present at that first meeting were "Mesdames Crocker, Tracy, Monroe, Myers, Jewett, Porter, and Savery, and Misses Abbie Mitchell and Sallie Griffith."[9]

Guided by Rector Reed, these ladies leased the Klipstein property at 1322 Locust Street. They planned to open a hospital there on February 1, 1876. However, shortly before the opening of this hospital, several of the neighbors began to protest, fearing the outbreak of contagion and the devaluation of their property. This caused a split among hospital supporters.

The Society already had named a hospital board of directors. The board secretary, Mrs. J. C. Savery, left to join a newly formed group of concerned citizens attempting to garner support for another facility named "Union Hospital." Their bases for creating this new hospital were to make it nonsectarian and to locate the hospital where it would not endanger citizens.[10]

No evidence suggests that the proposed Union Hospital ever existed, but its incorporation title was "Des Moines Union Hospital and Home for the Friendless." Funds from this endeavor ultimately may have assisted a later Des Moines organization known as the "Home for Friendless Children."

Rector Reed invited the citizens of Des Moines to help him find a more suitable location for his hospital, which he also said would be nonsectarian. His intention was to begin like "Abraham, who went out, not knowing whither he went."[11] A building at 923 Seventh Street became the home for the Seventh Street Hospital on February 15, 1876. Later, the hospital was renamed Cottage Hospital.

The hospital admitted all patients except those with contagious diseases, and it promised there would be no discrimination based on religion or nationality.[12] The first patient recorded at Cottage Hospital was a young man suffering from pneumonia. Two other patients were accepted at the same time.

Neighbors immediately began complaining about crowded conditions and unpleasant odors at the hospital. Board members already were in the process of purchasing land to relocate the hospital because they, too, were dissatisfied with conditions there.

Late in the summer of 1876, the hospital moved to the Annie B. Tracy property at 1105 Sherman Street between Ascension and Ridge Streets.[13] In time, the hospital expanded, and the board purchased this property. In the 1880s, the lot to the north also was acquired.[14] Cottage Hospital operated on this site until 1899.

Like any new endeavor during the first few years, Cottage struggled financially to remain open. However, aid for the hospital came from a surprising source in 1877.

On August 29, a severe summer storm caused a train accident known as the "Four-Mile Railroad Wreck." Eighteen persons were killed, including members of an advance car for the P. T. Barnum Circus. Most of the injured were taken into Des Moines. Five circus people were treated at Cottage Hospital. To show his appreciation, Barnum gave a lecture to benefit Cottage Hospital, netting more than $300.[15]

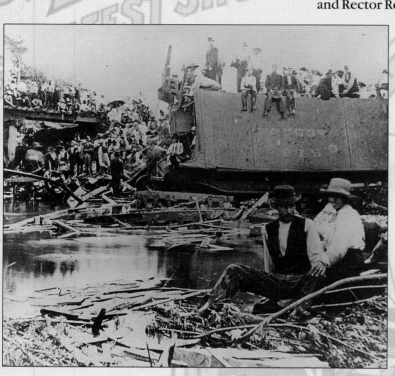

Accidents plagued the community of Des Moines during the late 1800s. None proved quite as notorious as the "Four-mile Railroad Wreck" in the summer of 1877. Among the injured were members of P.T. Barnum's circus. Cottage Hospital in Des Moines treated the disabled performers, and Barnum expressed his gratitude by giving temperance lectures to benefit the hospital.

Amusements.

COTTAGE HOSPITAL BENEFIT.
MOORE'S OPERA HOUSE!
Sunday Evening, Sept. 9th.

Hon. P. T. BARNUM,
THE GREAT SHOWMAN,

Will deliver a Temperance Lecture for the Benefit of Cottage Hospital next Sunday Evening.

PRICE OF ADMISSION.

Reserved Seats..........75 Cents
General Admission........50 Cents

Tickets will be on Sale at the different Book Stores on Thursday morning at nine o'clock.

A special circus performance the following day brought total donations to more than $12,000.[16]

St. Paul's Episcopal Parish provided a major source of support for Cottage Hospital over the years. Thanksgiving collections between 1878 and 1885 were made on behalf of the hospital. Items such as cotton, coal, and surplus stovepipe from building a new church also were donated.[17] After many years of planning and actual operation, the Articles of Incorporation were filed by the hospital on May 16, 1881.[18]

About six years later in May of 1887, managers of Cottage Hospital approached the Vestry of St. Paul's to act as a hospital advisory board. By-laws were written, appointing the Vestry as the board of trustees for the hospital, with the power to audit the finances and to oversee funds and legacies. A separate "Good Samaritan Fund" was established from which only the interest could be spent.

The board of trustees proved to be a valuable aid to Cottage Hospital. They assisted in the reorganization of the medical staff with an eye toward developing a medical program at Drake University in the 1890s. After the Medical School opened at Drake, Cottage Hospital was the only facility in the city that could provide a place for clinical practice. Medical education at that time consisted primarily of lectures. Cadavers were hard to obtain, so clinical laboratory experience was sporadic.[19]

When Mercy opened the doors on its present location, Cottage Hospital was "catty-cornered" to the southeast. Cottage Hospital, and the more complete Mercy Hospital, supplied Drake students with clinical facilities for laboratory and dissection studies.[20]

Cottage Hospital continued to operate until late in the summer of 1899 when a lack of funds caused it to close. About this same time, plans were in the works for the establishment of a Methodist Hospital in Des Moines. The managers of Cottage Hospital felt that with two major hospital facilities—Mercy and the planned Methodist facility—their hospital could not thrive.[21]

TRACY HOME HOSPITAL

Annie B. Tracy served on the Cottage Hospital board for many years. Sometime in 1888, she started an institution known as Tracy Home Hospital. After severing her connections with Cottage Hospital, Mrs. Tracy opened the new facility on two adjoining lots south of Cottage Hospital. This "home" was equipped with galvanic, Faradic, and static processes used primarily for the treatment of invalids. It is not known how long the facility stayed open. However, the hospital is not listed in Des Moines City directories after 1900.

The property was used again in the early 1900s by the city of Des Moines as a "pest house" to quarantine contagious diseases, such as small pox.[22] It was reported in *The Des Moines Daily News* on March 30, 1901, that the city employed a guard for the home because they feared the neighbors would dynamite the house. The property was sold by Mrs. Tracy's estate in 1903, and it has been said that Des Moines later used the building as a detention hospital for incorrigible juveniles.[23]

THE TIME HAD COME

By the early 1890s, only two hospitals served Des Moines: Cottage and Tracy. There were several specialized homes, such as the Des Moines Home for Friendless Children, Polk County Insane Asylum, Polk County Poor Farm, and the State Medical and Surgical Institute.[24] Catholics were excluded from early attempts to provide health care. It became clear that Des Moines needed the kind of dedicated hospital services and loving care offered by the Sisters of Mercy in Davenport.

The time had come for the comforting arms of Mercy Hospital.

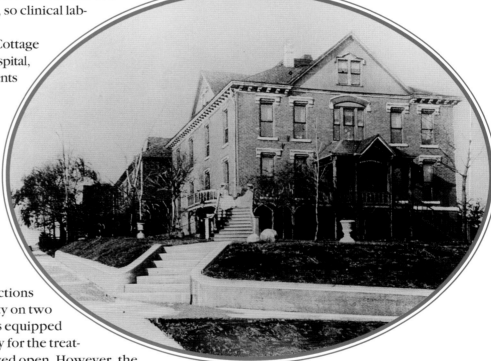

Tracy Home Hospital, above, was begun by Des Moines citizen, Annie B. Tracy, in 1888. A longtime director of Cottage Hospital, Mrs. Tracy realized that Des Moines needed an institution to care for invalids. Treatment rooms, top, were well-equipped. Tracy Home Hospital sat on land later acquired by Mercy Hospital.

IN THE HEALING HANDS OF GOD

1893-1922

The location is a good one,
outside the bustle of the city
on a sun-kissed hill
overlooking the river.
The air is pure,
the sunshine is warm,
and they who administer,
trained and faithful in
Mercy Hospital . . . .
The noble Catholic Sisters of Mercy
have belted the globe and
blessed all lands with their mercy.
All that other women consider worth
so much in life have they given up
to do good, to administer, and to heal;
to smooth the pathways of the world
and to soothe its sufferings
and its sorrows.
To their devotion they have added
all the science of the sick room.
None are better trained for the
care of the sick, and
none are more firmly consecrated.
Mercy Hospital will bless many,
and may heaven bless
them who are come to bless.

The Iowa State Register
April 24, 1895

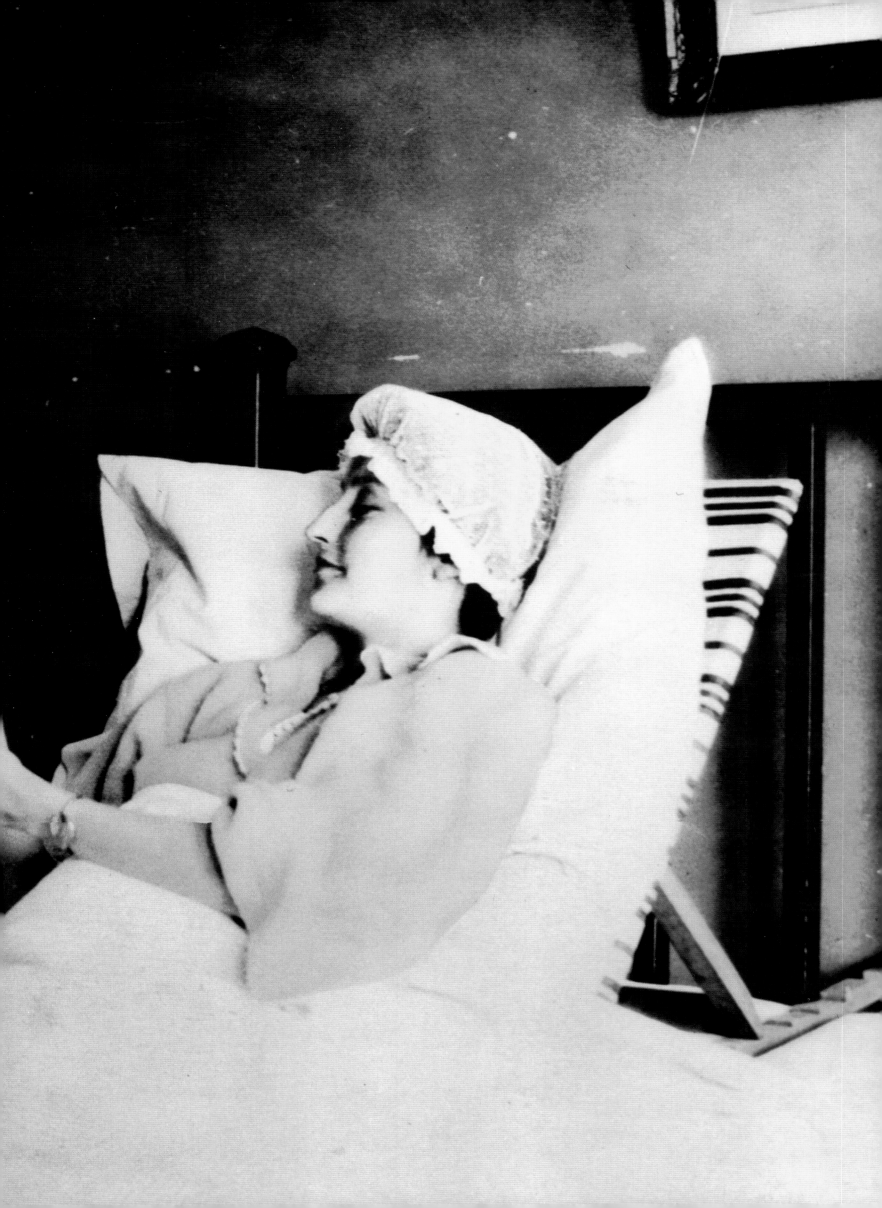

CHAPTER ONE
A CITADEL AGAINST SUFFERING: MERCY HOSPITAL

Seventeen years after Father Brazill appointed the first board of directors to establish a Catholic hospital in Des Moines, it finally was happening. The papers bannered the news on their front pages: "a Catholic Hospital...a Big One to Be Established in Des Moines." [1]

Mother Mary Baptist Martin, superior of Mercy Davenport, came to Des Moines to look for a suitable location for the new Mercy Hospital. She and Father Michael Flavin were given the opportunity to survey the home and property of prominent citizen, Hoyt Sherman, situated at Fifteenth and Woodland Streets in Des Moines.

Hoyt Sherman was the youngest of 11 children. His father had been a member of the Ohio Supreme Court. His brother was Civil War General, William Tecumseh Sherman, who marched through Georgia during the last days of the war. Hoyt Sherman was postmaster for Des Moines in 1850 and a member of the Iowa State Legislature in 1861. Sherman hosted many politicians and presidents in his elegant mansion which, by 1893, encompassed four city blocks. [2]

After touring Hoyt Sherman Place, Mother Baptist and Father Flavin agreed that the residence would function well as a temporary location for Mercy Hospital. Mr. Sherman leased Hoyt Sherman Place to the Sisters of Mercy for 18 months, with a six-month extension possible.

While Father Flavin handled the press and the ensuing fervor about a Mercy hospital locating in the city, Mother Baptist returned to Davenport to make arrangements for a group of sisters to come to Des Moines to staff the facility. Early accounts say she planned to bring eight sisters back with her, and that she would continue to supervise both Mercy Davenport and Mercy Des Moines. Long-range plans called for a permanent brick-and-stone structure to be erected within two years on Catholic Church property at Fourth and Ascension Streets. This was the land purchased 12 years earlier by Father John Brazill.

HOYT SHERMAN PLACE
The location of Hoyt Sherman Place was familiar to Des Moines residents. One attractive feature was its proximity to the Des Moines City Railway Company's Walnut Street and Kingman Avenue streetcar line. The car passed directly in front of Hoyt Sherman Place on Woodland Avenue, providing convenient access to the hospital.

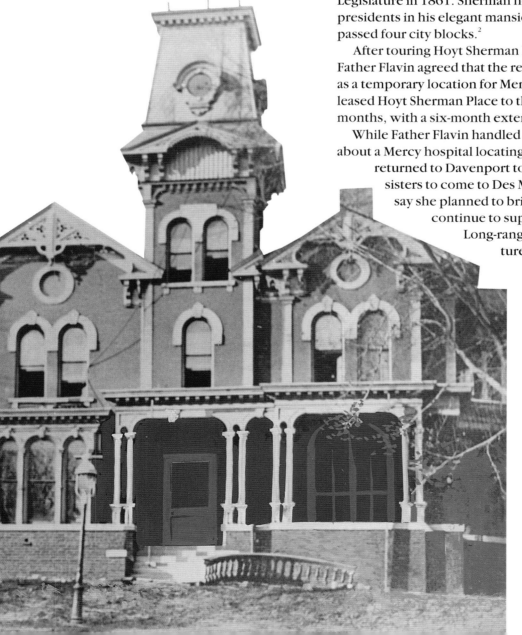

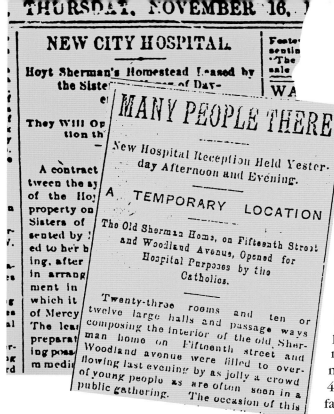

THURSDAY, NOVEMBER 16,

NEW CITY HOSPITAL

Hoyt Sherman's Homestead Leased by
the Sister

They Will Op
tion th

A contract
tween the a
of the Hoy
property on
Sisters of
sented by
ed to her b
ing, after
in arrang
ment in
which it
of Mercy
The lea
preparat
ing pos
m medi

MANY PEOPLE THERE

New Hospital Reception Held Yesterday Afternoon and Evening.

A TEMPORARY LOCATION

The Old Sherman Home, on Fifteenth Street and Woodland Avenue, Opened for Hospital Purposes by the Catholics.

Twenty-three rooms and ten or twelve large halls and passage ways composing the interior of the old Sherman home on Fifteenth street and Woodland avenue were filled to overflowing last evening by as jolly a crowd of young people as are often seen in a public gathering. The occasion of this

The first sisters arrived in Des Moines on the 9:00 A.M. train from Davenport on Monday, November 27, 1893.[3] The Catholic community held a social the following afternoon, welcoming them to Hoyt Sherman Place. St. Ambrose Church's Literary and Dramatic Society entertained with a program of readings, string music, and vocal soloists. The newspapers reported more than 400 persons toured the new facility which had 23 rooms and several large halls. Visitors were told that most of the larger rooms would be used to accommodate two patients. The temporary hospital had bathrooms, steam heat, and gas lights throughout.

A BRIGHTER PROMISE

Friday, December 8, 1893, dawned dark and foggy. In the early morning hours, the fog was so dense that one could only presume daylight had arrived. By 9:00 A.M., however, the fog lifted and the day held promise of brighter things to come.[4]

The date had special meaning. Traditionally on December 8, Catholics celebrate the Feast of the Immaculate Conception in honor of Mary, the Mother of God. On that day in 1869, the Sisters of Mercy opened the doors of Mercy Hospital in Davenport for the first time. On this date in 1893, the first patient was admitted to the new Mercy Hospital in Des Moines. Patient records from that time have long since disappeared, so, it is not known who that lucky patient was. It is known, however, that the comforting arms of the Sisters of Mercy were there to welcome—to ease the suffering.

HUMANITY'S CAUSE

On the day following the opening of Mercy, physicians who were interested in providing services to the hospital were asked to meet for the first medical staff meeting. Those present included: Drs. James W. Cokenower, William VanWerden, F.E.V. Shore, N.C. Schiltz, and F.L. Wells.

Dr. Cokenower, as temporary chairman, called the meeting to order and the physicians elected officers. Dr. T.F. Kelleher was chosen president, and Dr. Wells was elected secretary. Drs. Kelleher, VanWerden, and Cokenower comprised a committee that would confer with the sisters regarding drugs and dressings. The group came to a consensus about rotating physician services, each deciding to take a two-month shift. The final order of business provided for officers to meet with Father Flavin to draft by-laws for the medical staff.[5] Early medical staff meetings were infrequent, sometimes only once a year. Regular meetings began to occur in 1898.

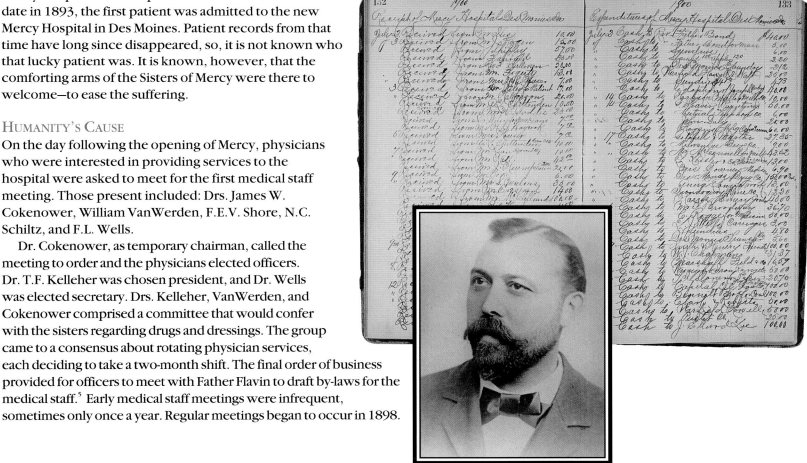

B LESS THOSE WHO COME TO BLESS: THE FOUNDERS

Obscured by time and incomplete records, answers remain unclear to questions asked about who founded Mercy Des Moines and what were the names of the sisters who first came to Des Moines.

Mercy Hospital in Des Moines was a daughter foundation of Mercy Davenport. As a result, a pattern prevailed that had been established for many of the preceding Mercy hospitals. Usually, the sister in charge of the mother institution laid the groundwork and traveled to the site of a proposed Mercy Hospital to make preliminary plans. She normally stayed for a short period of time until the daughter institution was functioning. Based on this precedent, it can be stated that Mother Mary Baptist Martin founded Mercy Hospital in Des Moines.

MOTHER MARY BAPTIST MARTIN

Mother Mary Baptist Martin was born Catherine Martin in Wexford County, Enniscorthy, Ireland, in 1833. Her parents were Thomas and Anne Martin. Catherine became a Sister of Mercy at the age of 21.

Two of Mother Baptist's sisters, Mary Ann and Ellen, also entered the Mercy order in Chicago at St. Xavier's Convent. Mary Ann became Sister Mary Evangelist Martin and later worked with Mother Baptist in Iowa. Ellen became ill and returned to Ireland shortly after being received into the order.

Sisters Baptist and Evangelist received their nurses' training in Chicago. There, they became acquainted with caring for cholera patients during the many epidemics of the mid-1800s. Sister Baptist also served as a Civil War nurse.

These blood sisters were cousins to Mother Mary Borromeo Johnson who founded Mercy Davenport.[6] At Mother Borromeo's invitation, Sisters Baptist and Evangelist migrated to De Witt in 1867. In 1869, Sister Baptist was appointed superior/principal of St. Mary's School in Davenport. At that time, the teaching sisters lived at Mercy Hospital and helped care for the patients there before and after their work at the school.

Father Maurice Flavin and his brother, Michael, were at different times in the 1800s, pastors of St. Mary's Catholic Church in Davenport. Sister Baptist's appointment as principal of St. Mary's School began a close and longtime association between Father Michael Flavin and the Sisters of Mercy.[7]

After Mother Borromeo's death in 1874, Mother Baptist became superior of the Davenport sisters and served two separate terms. It was during her second term, 1888–1895, that negotiations began for the establishment of a Catholic hospital in

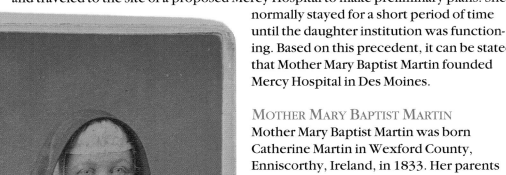

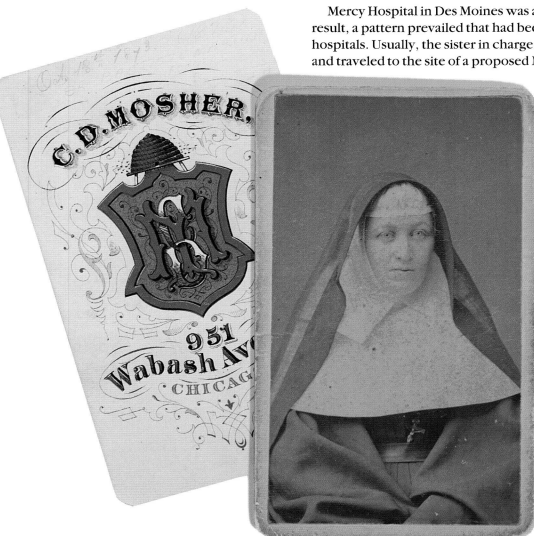

Mother Mary Baptist Martin, *above,* founded Mercy Hospital in Des Moines. She served as administrator for both Mercy Davenport and Mercy Des Moines until she gave the responsibility to Mother Mary Xavier Malloy in 1894.

Des Moines.[8] Sometime in the early 1890s, Father Michael Flavin, who was pastor of St. Ambrose in Des Moines, requested that the Davenport sisters come to Des Moines to establish a Mercy hospital.[9]

The Sisters of Mercy were welcomed to Des Moines formally on November 28, 1893.[10] There are differing accounts as to which sisters accompanied Mother Baptist to Des Moines. One record states that the community of sisters in Des Moines was: Sisters Mary Mechtildes Hogan, Adelaide Lynch, Gabriel Mulcrone, Elizabeth Butler, and Scholastica Kerns.[11]

THE FOUNDING SISTERS

Sister Mary Mechtildes Hogan: Born in Carlow, Ireland, Sister Mary Mechtildes Hogan entered the Sisters of Mercy in Davenport in 1889, and for most of the time from the 1890s until 1914, served in Des Moines.[12]

In 1943, Sister Mechtildes wrote a letter to Sister Mary Anita Paul, administrator of Mercy Hospital in Des Moines at the time, relating a little of the early history of the Des Moines hospital. A postscript on the bottom of the letter indicates that Sister Mechtildes was in Des Moines at the time Mercy Hospital was founded.[13] A Des Moines nursing school graduate of 1916, Mabel Trumm, remembers Sister Mechtildes as her nursing superintendent there.[14] Sister Mechtildes' service at Mercy Des Moines was primarily in education of nurses.[15]

In 1907 when a bill was introduced into the Iowa legislature for the registration of nurses, Sister Mechtildes worked diligently for its passage. According to Mercy Davenport historian, Sister Mary Magdalene Stransky, Sister Mechtildes personally drafted the questions for the first nursing board exam.[16] On July 18, 1907, she was chosen to be a member of the Nurses' Examining Committee. She was reappointed for four successive terms.[17] In 1914, Sister Mechtildes was transferred to St. Thomas Mercy Hospital in Marshalltown where she stayed until 1922. She died in Davenport in September 1956.[18]

Sister Mary Adelaide Lynch: Convent records for Irish-born Sister Mary Adelaide Lynch reveal that she was involved in novitiate duties in Des Moines as early as 1892. Indications are that she did not stay in Des Moines for long, but spent the majority of her life in Davenport at Mercy Hospital. She died there in 1959.[19]

Sister Mary Gabriel Mulcrone: It is not definite that Sister Mary Gabriel Mulcrone ever spent time in Des Moines. However, a Sister Gabriel was included on a list of sisters sealed in the 1897 cornerstone for Mercy Hospital. According to convent records, Sister Gabriel was born in Ireland and entered the order in Davenport in 1890. It is said that she was the first in Davenport to be trained in the new x-ray process. Sister Gabriel became the first x-ray technician in the department at Mercy Davenport and stayed in that position for 20 years. She died in 1930 after suffering a long illness due to overexposure to x-rays.[20]

Sister Mary Elizabeth Butler: Born in Syracuse, New York, Sister Mary Elizabeth Butler entered the Sisters of Mercy in Davenport in 1877. Her service records indicate that she was a housekeeper at Mercy Des Moines in 1895.[21]

Sister Mary Scholastica Kerns: Very little is known about Sister Mary Scholastica Kerns. Records indicate she entered the convent in Davenport in 1875 and became a Sister of Mercy in early 1879. She died in Davenport on January 1, 1923.[22]

MOTHER MARY PHILOMENA KEATING

Sister Mary Catherine Slattery has written another account of the founding of Mercy Hospital in Des Moines that includes Mother Mary Philomena Keating among the first sisters to arrive.[23]

Mother Philomena was born Sara Keating in Davenport early in 1860. She entered the Sisters of Mercy in November 1886. Whether Mother Philomena was among the first group of sisters to come to Des Moines is not definitely known. She was mother superior in Davenport for a time before coming to Des Moines.[24]

Actual dates regarding Mother Philomena's service in Des Moines are not known, but it is clear that she was one of the most influential members of the early history of Mercy Hospital. Her administrative career in Des Moines spanned more than 25 years. She died in Des Moines on December 28, 1921.

A NEW MOTHER SUPERIOR: MOTHER MARY XAVIER MALLOY

Shortly after the opening of Mercy Hospital at Hoyt Sherman Place, Mother Baptist appointed Davenport's Sister Mary Xavier Malloy to administer the new hospital. Mother Xavier arrived in Des Moines on February 11, 1894.

The newspaper account of this arrival does not list her by name, but Mother Xavier is listed as president of the Mercy Corporation in the Articles of Incorporation filed in July 1894. [25]

Mother Mary Xavier Malloy was born as Mary Malloy in New York in 1854. She moved with her parents to the Dubuque area, and in 1875, she entered the Davenport novitiate. In 1888, Mother Xavier was elected to the position of mistress of novices in Davenport. Mother Philomena was in the novitiate at this time.[26]

It has been written that Mother Xavier had a strong personality and some control over Mother Philomena.[27] Both sisters appeared to possess strong executive abilities, and since Mother Xavier was 16 years older than Mother Philomena, it might have been natural for the older sister to become a mentor to the younger.

Mother Xavier's powerful individuality and independent spirit proved to be a source of later problems at Mercy Hospital in Des Moines. For most of the 23 years that Mercy Des Moines and Mercy Davenport were allied, Mothers Xavier and Philomena served alternately as superior/administrator. However, it is believed that they were not among the first group of sisters to come to Des Moines in November 1893.

PIONEERING SPIRITS

Early ministering to the sick at Hoyt Sherman Place saw days of sacrifice and trials; times of progress and blessed events for the Sisters of Mercy. Mother Baptist brought dynamic souls to Mercy Hospital by appointing sisters such as Mothers Xavier and Philomena to lead these efforts. Time has hidden many other names and faces of the Sisters of Mercy who served in Des Moines during this time. Mercy Hospital stands today as a proud memorial to their unselfish service. It bears witness to their pioneering spirits forever etched in the mind of God.

For most of the years between 1893 and 1922, Mothers Philomena Keating, *top,* and Xavier Malloy, *above,* alternated as superior/administrator at Mercy Des Moines.

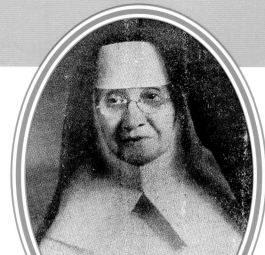

SISTER MARY ANTHONY

Sister Mary Anthony Reilly often is added to the list of founders of Mercy Des Moines. There is no mention of Sister Anthony in the earliest minutes or 1897 cornerstone artifacts at the hospital. According to her obituary, Sister Anthony did not come to Mercy until 1901.

Sister Anthony was one of three Davenport sisters who chose to remain in Des Moines at the time the hospital became a separate facility from Mercy Davenport. As a result, it appears that some have mistaken her as one of the founding sisters. She was referred to often as one of the "original founders of Mercy."

Sister Anthony was born as Margaret Reilly in New York City in 1859. She entered the Sisters of Mercy in Davenport in 1879 and became a Sister of Mercy in 1883.

Sister Anthony holds the distinction of being the first professionally licensed nurse in Iowa from a religious order. In 1907, Sister Mechtildes Hogan finished working on the legislation for registering nurses, and she encouraged several sisters to become licensed. The Iowa Board of Nursing lists Sister Anthony as the 19th licensed nurse, with no other religious licensed before

fashioned a pocket, sized to her needs and pinned discreetly at the waist level on the inside of the habit. In addition to holding her necessities, Sister Anthony's pocket carried a flask of whiskey—an old "Irish" remedy she used to soothe her patients and ease them into a restful night's sleep.

One patient has a childhood memory of the "beautiful trays" Sister Anthony fixed to brighten patients' days. Another remembered: "She was always doing something in the room. If the drapes were closed, she would open them a little. If open, she would close them a little." [29]

Sister Anthony was much loved. When she celebrated her golden jubilee as a Sister of Mercy in 1930, Bishop Thomas W. Drumm said: "Sister Anthony was a symbol of Mercy Hospital. Those who spoke of Mercy Hospital thought of Sister Anthony. Those who spoke of Sister Anthony thought of Mercy Hospital." [30] Ten years later, as Sister Anthony was about to celebrate her sixtieth year as a Sister of Mercy, she died. More than 400 people from all walks of life attended her funeral. Rich and poor came to pay a last tribute to Sister Anthony for her 39 years of unselfish service to the sick. [31]

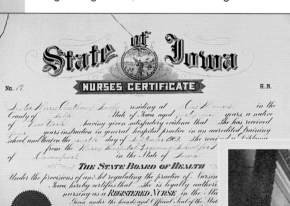

her. Sister Mechtildes held license number 25.

Many stories are told about Sister Anthony. She spent 39 years ministering at Mercy Hospital, developing a reputation for special care. As supervisor of the first floor, Sister Anthony lavished her patients with loving attention. Many of the wealthier ones responded by furnishing her rooms with beautiful treasures. The first floor became known as the "Gold Coast." Reminiscences tell of rooms with oriental carpets and brass beds that beckoned patients to request Sister Anthony and the Gold Coast for their place of quiet respite. [28]

Another often repeated story about Sister Anthony centers around the pocket of her religious habit. The Sisters of Mercy were not allowed to wear items on the outside of their habit, except for their rosaries and crucifixes, which were worn at their waists. Each sister

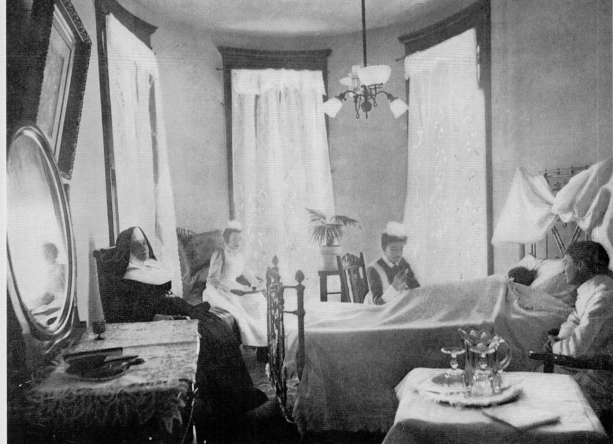

Although she was not among the first to come to Mercy Des Moines, Sister Anthony's stewardship and comforting arms in the early days of Mercy's history are remembered with enduring love.

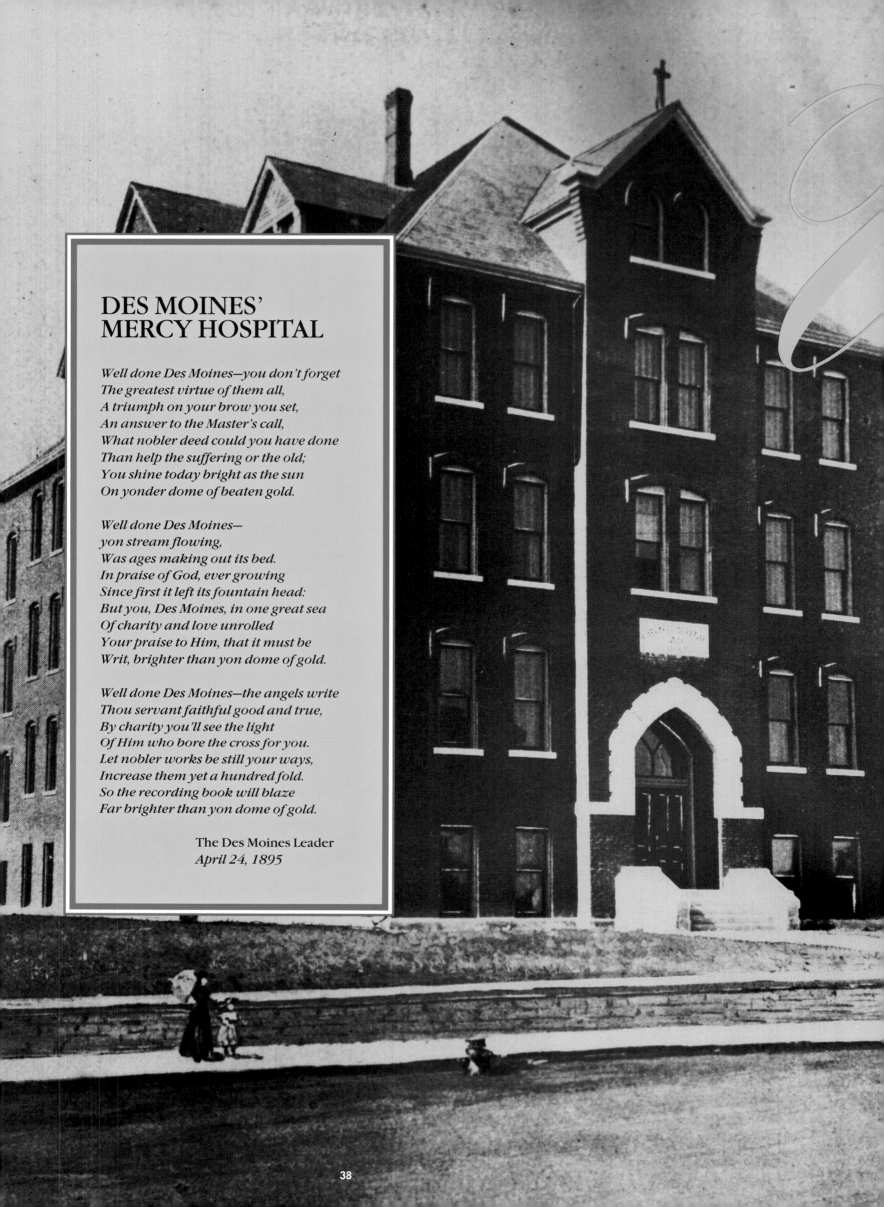

DES MOINES' MERCY HOSPITAL

Well done Des Moines—you don't forget
The greatest virtue of them all,
A triumph on your brow you set,
An answer to the Master's call,
What nobler deed could you have done
Than help the suffering or the old;
You shine today bright as the sun
On yonder dome of beaten gold.

Well done Des Moines—
yon stream flowing,
Was ages making out its bed.
In praise of God, ever growing
Since first it left its fountain head:
But you, Des Moines, in one great sea
Of charity and love unrolled
Your praise to Him, that it must be
Writ, brighter than yon dome of gold.

Well done Des Moines—the angels write
Thou servant faithful good and true,
By charity you'll see the light
Of Him who bore the cross for you.
Let nobler works be still your ways,
Increase them yet a hundred fold.
So the recording book will blaze
Far brighter than yon dome of gold.

The Des Moines Leader
April 24, 1895

CHAPTER TWO
ON THE SUN-KISSED HILL: FOURTH AND ASCENSION

Within three months of Mother Xavier's arrival in Des Moines, Mercy announced that the permanent hospital was to be built on the property at Fourth and Ascension Streets. In a public meeting at Hoyt Sherman Place, the Sisters of Mercy invited Des Moines' citizens to view their plans for a multi-story, brick-and-stone structure. The completed size of the hospital was to be 50x100 feet, and the building would face east onto Fourth Street. The sisters hoped to accommodate at least 60 patients in the new facility.[1]

The Sisters of Mercy opened the first permanent building of Mercy Hospital, opposite, in 1895. Located at Fourth and Ascension Streets, the facility was heralded as "a great institution of charity to stay with the city for all time."

THE EAST WING
The first of many official groundbreakings in Mercy's long history occurred on July 3, 1894, on Lot 18 in Hall's Addition. The new building became the East Wing in later years and was in precisely the same location as the old Rutherford Chapel on the sun-kissed hill.

One day after the groundbreaking, Articles of Incorporation were filed in Polk County, establishing the corporation known as Mercy Hospital in Des Moines, Iowa. Mother Xavier signed the documents as president, Sister Mary Joseph as vice-president, and Mother Philomena as treasurer.[2]

A few days earlier, a contract had been drawn between the Sisters of Mercy in Davenport and the Sisters of Mercy in Des Moines to formalize the relationship between the two communities. The 10-year contract provided for the following: Mercy Hospital in Des Moines would be under the jurisdiction of the Davenport hospital, and the sister superior in Davenport would appoint the local superior in Des Moines. Money for building and staffing the new hospital in Des Moines would be loaned by the Davenport hospital. This contract would become null and void only if the Davenport Diocese was divided and a new bishop was appointed over Des Moines. If that happened, the jurisdiction of Mercy Hospital in Des Moines then would fall under the new bishop. When and if this occurred, Mercy Des Moines would have 10 years to pay off the Davenport loan at 6% interest. If they were unable to repay the loan, Mercy Des Moines would be given an additional 10 years to do so.[3]

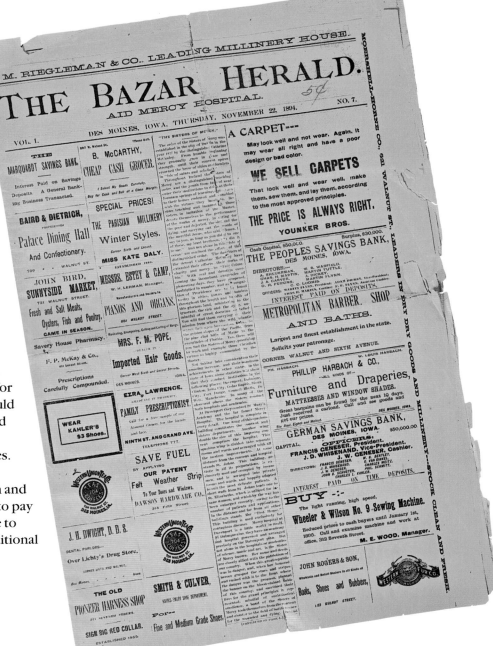

AN INSTITUTION OF CHARITY

Work proceeded rapidly on the new hospital. By February 20, 1895, enough of the building was finished to begin the move from Hoyt Sherman Place.

The formal dedication of the permanent Mercy Hospital was held on April 23, 1895. In memory of Mother Catherine McAuley, who always encouraged her sisters to be merry and put "a piano in every community room," the Sisters of Mercy

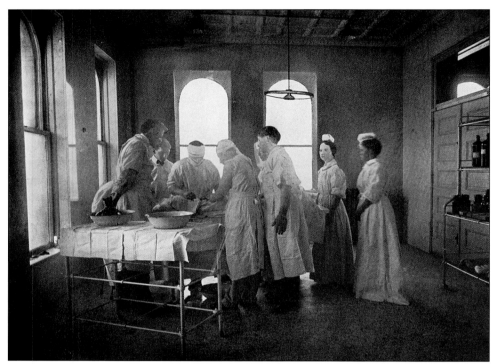

extended the first of many Irish welcomes during this dedication. At noon they hosted a formal dinner for 65 leading citizens from Des Moines and Davenport. A long, unfinished hall on the fourth floor held a flower-trimmed banquet table, where an elaborate 14-course meal took more than two hours to serve. After the meal, dedication exercises were held in the corridor.

Mayor Isaac Hillis of Des Moines made the opening remarks. Hillis welcomed the visitors and praised the Sisters of Mercy for their works of charity throughout the years. He wished the sisters heartiest congratulations on their bright future in Des Moines.[4]

Other speakers on that day included Mayor Henry Vollmer of Davenport; Drs. R. A. Patchin and J. W. Cokenower of Des Moines; E. M. Sharon; Drs. A. W. Cantwell and J. B. Crawford from Davenport; and Henry Wallace. Governor Frank Jackson had planned to attend, but his schedule kept him from doing so.

The final address of the day was given by Father Joseph Nugent. He predicted that this dedication marked "the opening of a great institution of charity to stay with the city for all time."[5] Visitors were greeted that day by Messers Geneser and Enright. Frank Flynn and Ed McGuire assisted as tour guides, while the Des Moines Mandolin Club performed.

Tours of the new facility showcased the "sun-kissed hill" and a panorama of Des Moines to the south. The top floor also unveiled a commanding view of the city to the east. Many comments were made about the sight of the gold dome of the Capitol on the eastern horizon.

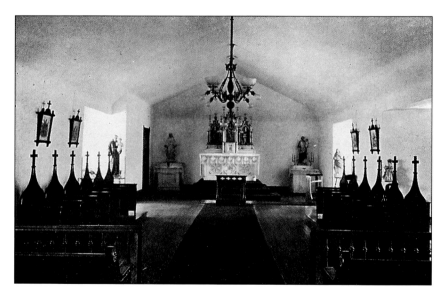

The first floor of the new hospital contained a sewing room, dining room, laundry, reception room, kitchen, two staff rooms, and a boiler room. The second floor housed a parlor, operating rooms, dispensary, reception room, and several rooms for female patients. Male patients were cared for on the third floor in wards and single rooms. The fourth floor was not completed at the time. There were baths, toilet rooms, and closets on all floors, as well as a dumb-waiter to ease the distribution of supplies. One newspaper account said the hospital had a capacity of 50 beds, 14 of which were private.[6]

The new Mercy Hospital featured a chapel, *above,* and an operating room, *top,* with an abundance of natural light.

Many individuals, organizations, and businesses donated furnishings for the new rooms. The list included: Dr. Cokenower, Mr. and Mrs. E. C. Firestone, Dr. McGorrisk, the National Daughters of Isabella, Chicago & Great Western Railroad, Des Moines Insurance Company, Mrs. M. Kenney, Bishop Henry Cosgrove, Father Michael Flavin, Younker Brothers, Younker Brothers' employees, Des Moines & Kansas City Railroad, and Mrs. McConnell. Two full wards were furnished by the Ancient Order of Hibernians of Polk County.[7]

Conflicting reports exist as to the number of stories the building had in the beginning. Some say there were three; others say four. The oldest pictures and illustrations show four stories above a full underground basement. Long-time members of the Mercy Hospital building maintenance department say that the building never had less than four above-ground stories. Perhaps there is confusion because the top floor was not completed until later. Around 1902, the attic above the fourth story was converted into a chapel and rooms for the sisters. Previously, the chapel was located on the first floor.[8]

The newspapers were full of good things to say about the new facility. All complimented its location—far enough away from the noisy streetcar, but only one block from the Sixth Avenue line. They encouraged everyone to patronize Mercy Hospital regardless of faith or circumstances. Readers were assured that the question asked of patients was not one of "religion, but what is needed to make them well."[9]

Once the dedication was over, the Sisters of Mercy began building a reputation for compassionate care in what was to become the most enduring medical facility in Des Moines' history. During that first year of operation in the new hospital 221 patients received some form of treatment. There were 90 different diagnoses with an overall mortality of 6.2 percent.[10]

When the East Wing opened, the sisters who staffed the hospital were: Mother Xavier, superior; and Sisters Philomena, Joseph, Josephine, Gertrude, and Elizabeth.[11] Father J. H. Renihan lived at Mercy as the resident chaplain.[12]

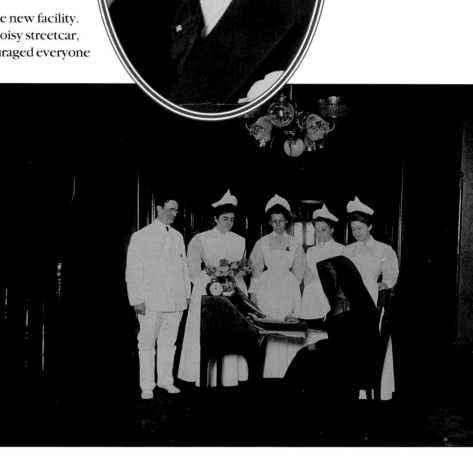

EARLY CARE

Very few reminiscences remain from these early days. There were no tape recorders or video cameras to capture moments in time. Long days of hard work did not leave time for keeping journals or diaries. However, one pioneer physician with a long Mercy association provided delightful glimpses into those younger Mercy Hospital days during the school of nursing's 50th anniversary celebration in 1949. Dr. Edwin B. Walston recalled performing surgeries in patients' rooms. The operating table was brought into the room and the patient placed on it. When surgery was finished, the patient was moved back into bed, and the operating equipment removed from the room.

Dr. Walston remembered that early sterilization consisted of boiling instruments on a gas stove in a carbolized solution. Eventually, they upgraded to what was considered the "height of cleanliness:" The instruments were sterilized in a steam bath procedure, using a copper boiler.

The surgical team consisted of three people: a surgeon, anesthetist, and one surgical assistant. "Today," Dr. Walston said in 1949, "when we go into an operating room and see the number taking part, it is difficult to find the patient." Ether and chloroform were the only types of anesthetics during those days, and they were administered "by most anybody who happened to be available."

Dr. Edwin B. Walston, *top,* recalled early care when primitive instruments and surgical techniques were used. In those days, physicians wrote orders in a book kept on a hall table as shown *above.*

Other equipment that doctors relied upon seems primitive when compared to today's technology. Laboratory testing devices consisted of "a little alcohol lamp, some test tubes...[and] a microscope used for counting red and white blood cells." X-ray equipment was hand-operated, and eight glass discs generated the power for the tubes.

According to Dr. Walston, things became "very high hat" when one change in procedure occurred. While making his rounds on a particular day, Dr. Walston found a little table, chair, book, and pencil in the center of the hall. Upon examination, he discovered that physicians were recording their nursing orders in the book. Until this time, doctors' orders had been verbal. Dr. Walston decided to try this new procedure in a rather unique way.

An elderly patient was not responding to treatment. Dr. Walston thought a dose of whiskey might perk her up, and he entered the following instructions to the nurses in the book: "Eggnog to be served to my patient in 101." The next morning upon visiting the patient, Dr. Walston found the eggnog sitting untouched on the woman's bedside table. She had refused to drink it because it contained whiskey. To prove a point to the patient, Dr. Walston drank the eggnog, and found it so good that he immediately proceeded to the hall table where he wrote: "Give Dr. Walston an eggnog at 10:00 A.M. tomorrow." The next day, he found the eggnog as ordered. Years later he added: "I have often thought that would make a nice standing order, possibly with [one] little change. Instead of putting the egg and milk in with the whiskey, we might change the order to whiskey and white soda!" [13]

Compared to today, medical expenses in the late 1800s appear quite reasonable. In 1896, three weeks of Mercy care cost $30.

MERCY EXPANSION

From the beginning, plans were in the works for an addition to the East Wing. Early designs called for the hospital to continue building north on Fourth Street on Father Brazill's purchases. This addition would contain a better operating room and an amphitheater for students. [14] Plans changed, however, and the new addition called for an entrance on the south side, facing the city of Des Moines. Property was purchased and by late summer 1897, the basement was finished.

On September 8, 1897, a small religious ceremony was held to lay the cornerstone for the new wing. Father Michael Flavin officiated. He complimented the sisters on their excellent management skills and predicted that Mercy Hospital would develop into one of the leading and most popular hospitals in the west. A few small artifacts were sealed in the cornerstone for posterity. In 1974 when the Central Wing was demolished, the contents of this cornerstone yielded: three daily newspapers, religious medals, bills, handwritten lists of the resident Sisters of Mercy and contemporary state and local officials. After the cornerstone was in place, it was hoped that the building could be shelled in before winter. Delays with plans and bids kept the project from entering this stage until the spring of 1898.

THE CENTRAL WING: ANOTHER JEWEL

Mother Xavier hired local architect, Oliver O. Smith, to direct the building of the Central Wing. When she presented the plans to the Mercy Davenport Corporation, however, Mother Xavier was told they were "too elaborate." Modifications were made. [15]

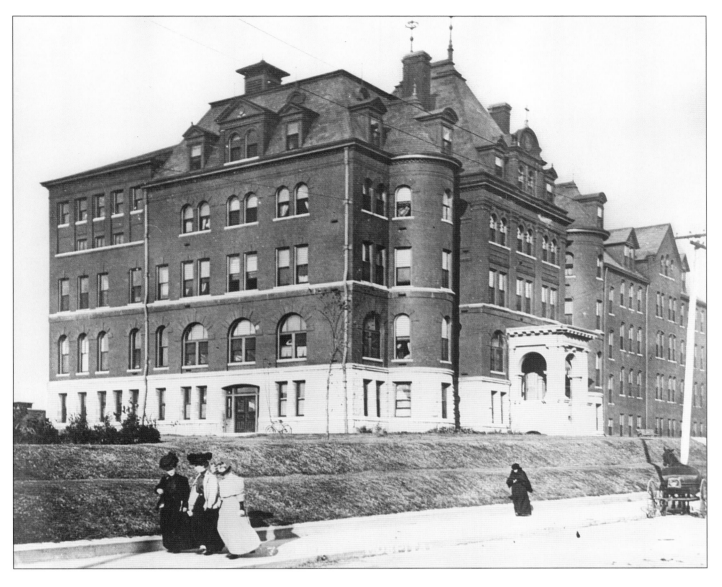

A contract drawn with Capital City Brick and Pipe Company listed omissions such as special outside finishing touches and inside plastering and finishing. Plans did include an amphitheater and accommodations for student nurses. Two support beams used in the top floor were provided by Eagle Iron Works, a Des Moines company still in business today.[16] The finish date for phase one of the Central Wing was set for October 1, 1898.

The Central Wing dedication came with the sisters' usual warm Irish welcome on November 15, 1899, several months after its completion. A ceremony was held in the new amphitheater where music, flowers, food, and speeches greeted hundreds from Des Moines and Davenport who came to view the new facility. Tours were given, and once again, newspapers heralded the growth and reported that beds were full.

This new addition became the main building of the hospital. Seventy-five "spacious and eloquently appointed" rooms could now accommodate up to 150 patients. A private operating room contained the latest provisions for surgical cleanliness—marble walls, steel ceilings, and white tile floors. A series of spacious corridors and stairways connected the floors, providing easy access to all parts of the building.[17]

Even as this day of celebration drew to a close, plans were underway for another addition on the west side of the Central Wing. Years later, those who remembered visiting Mercy Hospital, as patients or visitors, recalled the Central Wing most vividly. They reminisced that it looked like an old castle with long steps to the front door that opened into a beautiful hallway with a graceful stairway. The Sisters of Mercy had added another jewel to their crown of successes in Des Moines.

The Central Wing of Mercy Hospital was designed and built by Des Moines architect, Oliver O. Smith, in 1898. Pedestrians passed this addition on their way to catch the Sixth Avenue Streetcar Line.

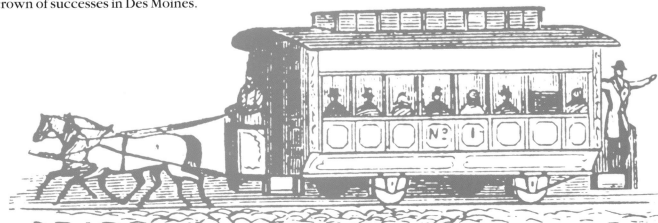

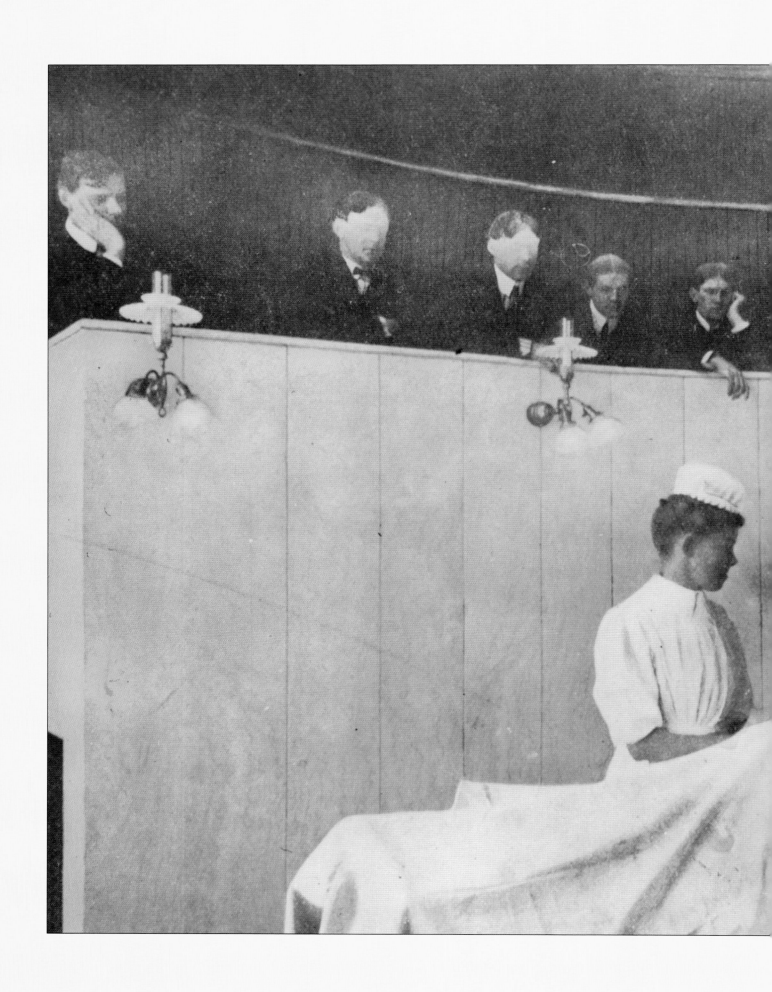

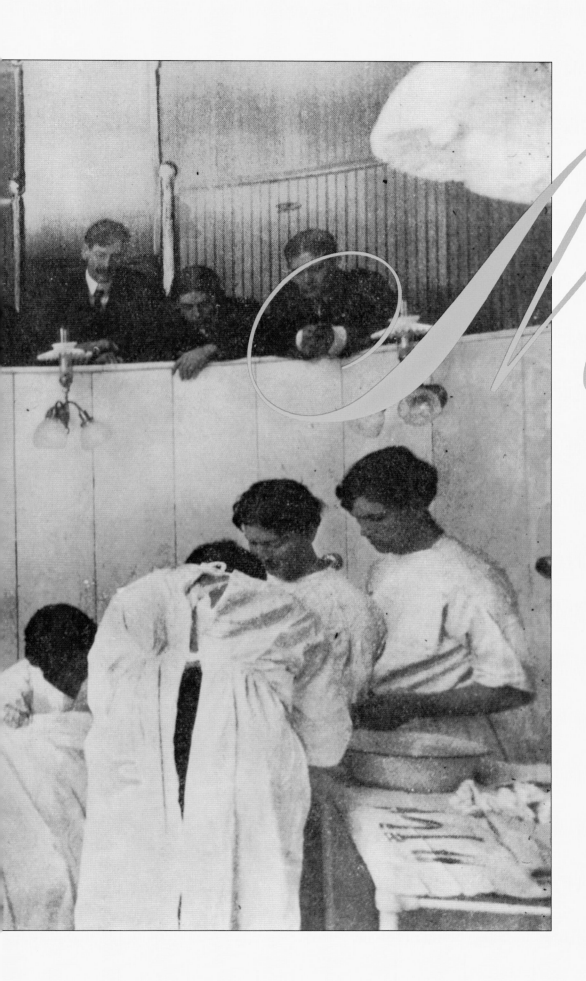

Mercy's Central Wing was constructed in 1898. One of the most impressive features of this addition was an amphitheater located in the large operating room. This arena functioned as a first-class clinical setting for students from Drake's medical school.

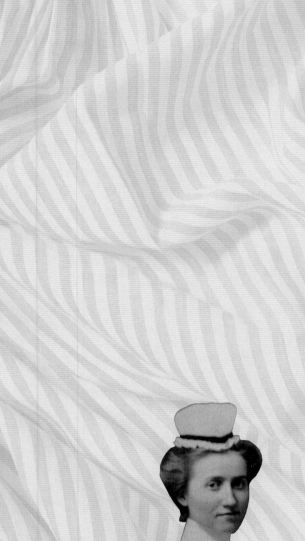

SCHOOL OF NURSING

The Mercy Des Moines School of Nursing formally opened in 1899. Today, the school is the oldest in Des Moines and the only one operated by the Sisters of Mercy in what is now the Regional Community of Omaha.

The education of women has always been a primary mission of the Sisters of Mercy. From the beginning of their healthcare ministry, the sisters were the key care-givers, and they were responsible for equipment maintenance, housekeeping chores, education of staff, and more.

As demands for advanced medical knowledge increased along with hospital usage in the late 1800s, a need for professionally trained nursing personnel presented itself. The sisters at Mercy Des Moines first responded to this need in October 1897, when they planned a lecture curriculum. Physicians were assigned to a series of eight lectures, which were scheduled from 8:00 P.M. until 9:00 P.M. on Friday evenings.[18] They began on the first of November and continued for six months. This made long days for the students because, at that time, nursing personnel were working 12-hour shifts, usually from 7:00 A.M. until 7:00 P.M.

When the first written medical staff by-laws were finalized in April 1898, Article IX established this lecture series as part of the staff schedule.[19] In October of the same year, physicians planned another schedule that would take place on Monday, Wednesday, and Friday.

Evidently, these first attempts to establish lecture services outside of a formal educational curriculum lacked continuity. With nursing schools springing up all over the nation, Mercy decided to formally organize its own school.

ANOTHER BEGINNING

In a special meeting of the medical staff on April 7, 1899, the first item of business was the opening of a training school for nurses. It was agreed that this effort would benefit Mercy Hospital greatly, and a plan for lectures was adapted from the St. Joseph's Training School for Nurses in Chicago.

Twelve categories of instruction were prepared, and physicians cast lots to decide who should lecture on which subject. On April 14, 1899, at the quarterly meeting of the Mercy staff, plans were formalized for the nurses' training school. Lectures would be held on Mondays and Fridays from 8:00 P.M. until 9:00 P.M., beginning on April 17, 1899. Graduation exercises for the first two-year program were held on June 17, 1901.[20] Seven students graduated in that first Mercy Hospital Training School class. They had entered the school between January and November of 1899.

SOOTHING HANDS

For the first few years after the school opened, students spent their first month as probationers or "probies," as they were commonly called. By 1904, a two-month probationary period became mandatory.

During the probie period, the new nursing students wore colored dresses with an apron that covered their skirts. They each were assigned to an older, capped student who acted as mentor. The probies' primary duty was to provide water or bedpans in response to patient call-lights. This probationary time gave them a chance to find out whether or not they really wanted to pursue a career in nursing. Once this period was over, they decided to finish their nurses training at Mercy or leave. If they stayed, they were issued a cap and a bib to go with their apron, and they began receiving formal nursing instruction.

While in school, the students wore a long-sleeved, blue and white pin-striped, floor-length uniform that was covered by a white apron. The usual nursing day ran from 7:00 A.M. until 7:00 P.M. with a two-hour break about 2:00 in the afternoon. When the work-shift ended, the students would have supper, and then, go to class. Everyone took turns with night duty.

Students learned to give bed-baths while on floor duty. One older nurse was the head or "medicine nurse." She responded to physicians' orders and administered

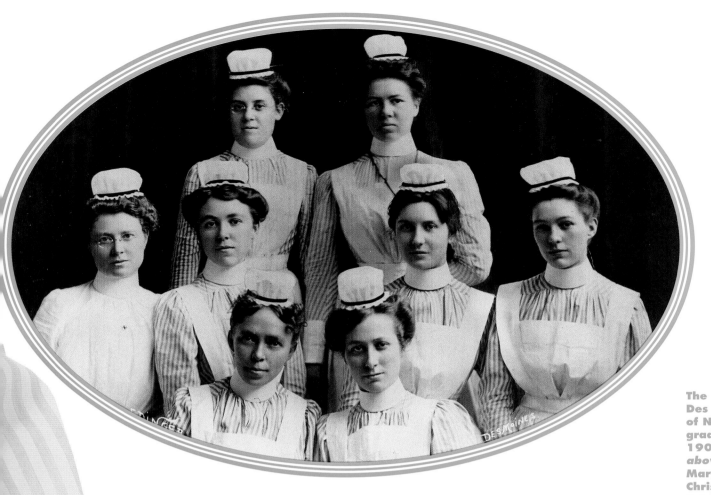

medications. She assigned students to six patients on each floor. Male orderlies took care of the male patients in wards with six beds to a room. Nursing students did not take care of male patients unless they were assigned to special duty.

Female patients were given private rooms that were quite common in appearance. All were furnished identically, with a single bed and washstand. During these early times, there was no carpeting on the floors. It was the duty of one of the students to scrub floors daily. Eventually, some rooms were carpeted with beautiful oriental rugs and furnished with brass beds.

Students' training time was counted in eight sections: general, special medical and surgical, obstetrical, night, operating room, dressing room, vacation, and time lost. These early nurses ministered their healing skills with a hands-on approach. Soothing hands provided backrubs. Supporting arms positioned the patients, fluffed pillows, and adjusted wooden backrests.

Early pain medications consisted of morphine and codeine. Mustard plasters mixed with a large wooden spoon and applied hot were used to treat pneumonia. Woolen blankets warmed with bricks soothed aching joints. Antibiotics, urinalysis, respiratory therapy, and other medical advances waited on tomorrow's horizon.

Mercy did not accept contagious cases, but occasional cases of typhoid, tuberculosis, and scarlet fever merited isolation care. Frequently, physicians would request follow-up home care for patients, and a nursing student would be sent to administer that care. On these home visits each nurse carried the following: clinical thermometer, fever charts, hypodermic syringe, fountain syringe, and tablets of strychnine, nitroglycerin, morphine, digitalis, and bichloride.[21]

GOLDEN RULE DAYS

Young Daisie Barclay entered Mercy's School of Nursing on December 1, 1901. When she arrived, there was no Fifth Avenue along the hospital's west side. The unpaved, dirt road simply was called Fifth Street. A small ditch with a footbridge ran along the side of the street. After a good rain, the only way of crossing the road was to return to Fourth Street and walk on the south side of Ascension Street.

Daisie recalled that for a long time there were only eight nurses staffing the hospital—two day nurses and one night nurse for each floor. The students were given a half-day off every two weeks on Sunday, whenever the operating room or dressing room nurse could relieve them. Their half-day lasted from 2:00 P.M. until 9:00 P.M., and they had to be in by the 9:00 P.M. curfew. Nine students graduated in Daisie's class of 1904.[22]

By the year 1901, the Mercy Nurses Training School program had expanded to two-and-a-half years. Lecturers no longer were decided by physicians casting lots but were scheduled by the sisters.[23] These and other changes at Mercy were prompted by the presence of Sister Mechtildes Hogan who was very active in early nursing education and professionalism in Iowa. Sister Mechtildes served on the first Iowa Nursing Board of Certification. She helped to shape the direction of professional nurses' training.

Prior to 1907, prospective nursing students were not required to have a formal education before applying for training. Sister Mechtildes and a committee outlined new minimum requirements, and a certificate of grammar school or a passing grade on an equivalent examination became mandatory.[24] Prospective students also were expected to present credentials that reflected good moral character.[25]

MERCY ALUMNI ASSOCIATION

Mercy's School of Nursing Alumni Association began in 1907.[26] No records exist regarding a first meeting, but several notices announcing dates for Mercy Alumni Association meetings appeared in local newspapers throughout the years. In 1914, the annual meeting was held in the Chamberlain Hotel. Forty alumni attended the banquet where Nellie McCarthy was toastmistress. At that time elected officers were: Rose Mahoney, president; Mrs. J. Hart, vice president; Veronica Stapleton, treasurer; and Lucretia Hayes, secretary. Five women were from out of town; one from Colorado.[27]

IN RESPONSE TO WAR

As World War I became an increasing threat, Iowa launched a drive to register 400 graduate nurses in the Red Cross. Fourteen women from Des Moines responded immediately in 1914 and were prepared to leave at a moment's notice. Anna C. Kelly became Mercy's representative to recruit nurses.[28] She asked Dr. Robert O. Matthews, who had visited hospitals in the war zone, to speak to Mercy nurses, encouraging them to help in the war effort.[29] Four Mercy nurses were the first to sign up: Louise Gaass, Sarah Murray, Margaret Mulroney, and Christine Hoffman.[30] Lucille Dulin joined her fellow nurses later.[31]

The first nurses to sail from the U.S. to Europe left in early September 1914. One Mercy nurse, Mary White, went overseas in 1918.[32] She was followed a

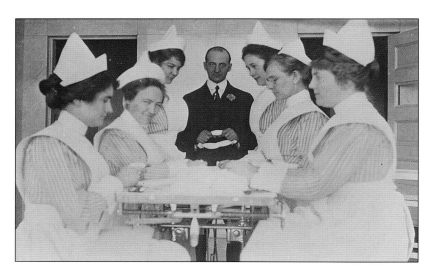

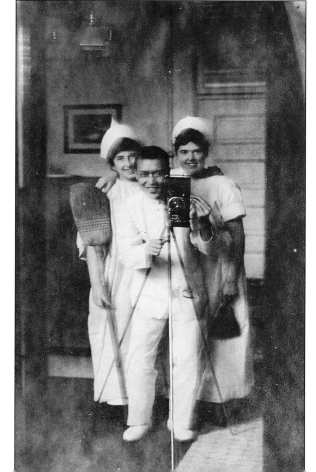

Daisie Barclay, *top*, remembered her Mercy nurse's training as a time when hard work was expected and playfulness thrived, in spite of the requisite 9:00 P.M. curfew. ❧ Dr. Paul Tang, *right*, who interned at Mercy in 1915, left a photographic legacy which brings a smile today.

few months later by Gertrude Portel, another Mercy School of Nursing graduate.[33]

By the time World War I ended in 1919, Iowa almost had reached its quota—325 had enlisted in the Red Cross. Many honors were paid to doctors and nurses who served in this capacity, and once a year, roses were handed out to these medical professionals as a token of gratitude.

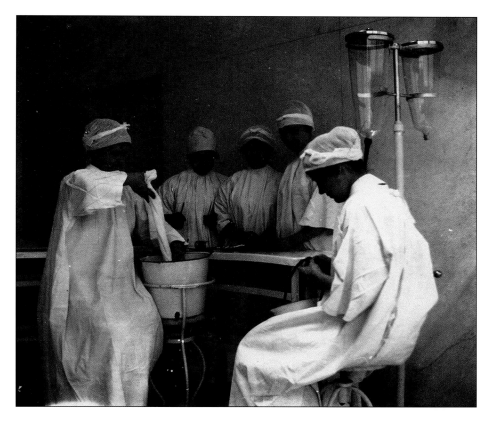

RIGOROUS TRAINING

The beginning of the 1920s saw a change in nursing professionalism. Enrollment in nursing schools had declined sharply and first among the reasons given was the intense training. Graduate nurses spoke of tough disciplines: long hours with unpredictable time off; lectures and study squeezed in during recreation time; and an early curfew time of 9:30 P.M. unless special permission was granted. Whenever there was an epidemic or shortage of help, these young nurses were expected to put in longer days than the usual 10 hours. Low pay was said to be one of the major reasons for the lack of interest in nurses' training at any hospital.[34]

Graduate nurses could look forward to receiving about $50 per week. However, only healthy young women could be expected to work enough to receive that amount. The average pay turned out to be about $1,700 a year, which was comparable to the wage of a stenographer at that time.

Most graduate nurses felt that unless the pay and liberty during school was changed, it would be hard to entice young women from positions as stenographers or clerks, which required only a few months of much less rigorous training and paid well from the start.[35] After the war, many blamed the trend away from nursing on increasing opportunities for young women in business.

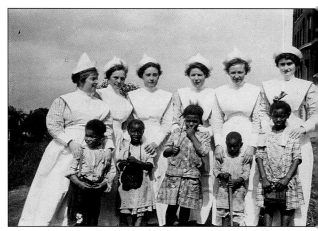

Long hours of rigorous training fostered firm and life-long friendships among Mercy's nursing students.

PROFESSIONAL NURSES' TRAINING

In 1921, Iowa's registered nurses began planning for legislation to change the nursing profession. They endorsed several changes: a board of nursing that would be separate from the health department, a shorter training curriculum with stronger supporting high school work, and a new minimum daily wage of $6 for an 18-hour work day.[36]

Late in the summer of 1921 after these changes were put into effect by professional nurses' associations, there still was a shortage of students in Des Moines. Methodist Hospital had six probationers to start its fall class. Mercy had a total enrollment of about 60 students, compared to its normal 80 students. Sister Augustine said the shortage at Mercy was not as bad as it was in 1920, however.[37] Mercy's first advertisement for its nursing school appeared in Des Moines newspapers in September 1921.

A PROMISING FUTURE

With the Central Wing and a school of nursing added to the hospital by 1899, the sisters in Des Moines were better prepared to meet future challenges. Continuing their quest to provide the best hospital care, they improved their facility and graduated nurses who practiced with competence, warmth, and common sense. These pioneer caregivers succeeded in promoting compassionate healing in a world where hospitals were looked upon as places of death. The Sisters of Mercy counted many successes as they looked with pride toward a promising new century.

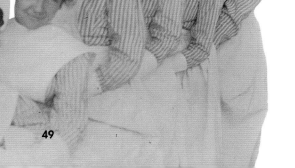

CHAPTER THREE
THE TURN OF THE CENTURY

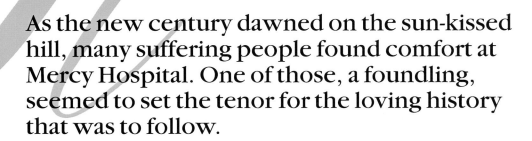

As the new century dawned on the sun-kissed hill, many suffering people found comfort at Mercy Hospital. One of those, a foundling, seemed to set the tenor for the loving history that was to follow.

In 1900, an orphaned baby boy was left with the sisters. No one knows who the child was, but a ledger reference indicates a charge for the travel of the nurse accompanying him to Chicago as: "Cash for the adoption of 'Joseph.' " [1] The foundling was welcomed with open arms and quickly endeared himself to the sisters. Early statistics for Mercy have long ago disappeared, but the U.S. Census of June 13, 1900, includes this baby boy and provides some interesting details about Mercy Hospital. Eleven Sisters of Mercy were in residence. The patient census for the day was 28, including one baby, one foundling, and five roomers. The hospital had 13 nurses, one elevator boy, one intern, one telephone girl, and 12 servants. Father George H. Schumacher was the chaplain. [2]

CARE FOR THE SUFFERING AND POOR

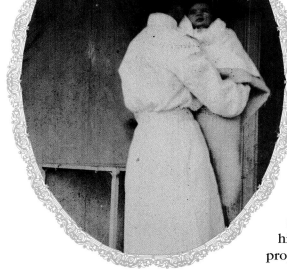

At the turn of the century, Mercy Hospital was always there when a great need arose. Victims from coal mining accidents, boiler explosions, attempted murders, and vehicular mishaps were rushed to Mercy for care. [3]

On Thanksgiving Day 1902, a streetcar careened out of control because a brake-rod snapped. The vehicle raced downtown on Sixth Avenue from School Street, throwing passengers from the car before it smashed on the sidewalk of Locust Street. The tragic accident sent several patients to Mercy Hospital via police ambulance.

The youngest patient, 8-year-old Helen Ray Frawley, had been traveling with her mother to Thanksgiving services at St. Ambrose. Helen was rushed to Mercy where she underwent several hours of brain surgery, but she died early the following morning. Witnesses at the scene of the wreck told of seeing "the prayer book clutched tightly in [Helen's] almost lifeless fingers. She met grim death on her way to worship God." [4]

Shortly before Christmas of 1903, Mercy's charity to the poor and homeless touched the hearts of the Des Moines community. A 60-year-old man was found alone in a poorly heated room on Ninth Street. He was suffering from hunger and cold "without friend or neighbor to look in on him." The city humane officers took him to Mercy because "he will receive proper care, the only hope to save the small amount of life that remains." [5]

PREPARED FOR DISASTER

Mercy Hospital became the major trauma center for Des Moines at the turn of the century. Many of the best Des Moines surgeons used Mercy's facilities almost exclusively. Drs. Wilton McCarthy, W. S. Conkling, Granville Ryan, and John C. Rockafellow had large practices, including many of the local railroad companies. When two train accidents occurred two years apart, Mercy was prepared.

The first accident happened on February 9, 1905. The Milwaukee Overland Limited No. 1 derailed while crossing a bridge west of Marshalltown. One person was killed and 18 were taken more than 25 miles, by another train, to Mercy. Buses, ambulances, and cabs met the injured at the train station in Des Moines and transported them to Mercy. Reports at the time said the hospital already was crowded, but arrangements were made quickly, on all three floors. Worried relatives of the victims besieged the hospital with telephone queries.

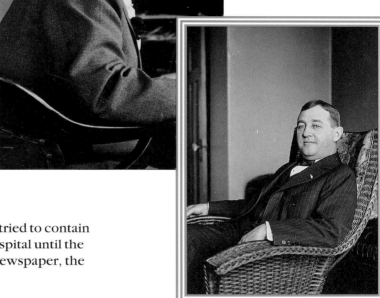

> *"The entire staff of physicians were pressed to the utmost with the additional duties thrust upon them. A dozen operations of a more or less intricate nature were made necessary by the bad wounds of the wreck victims and the operating room was never without its patient. Later in the night, after the physicians had completed their rounds for the evening, the nurses, attired in their white gowns, passed among the sufferers, giving a kind word here, a glass of water there, doing everything to ease the sufferings of all. Warm poultices on the weak and a drop of stimulant made all pleasant, and at last, quiet sleep visited the rooms of the sick."* [6]

The second train accident happened a little closer to home on February 6, 1907. A Chicago & Northwestern coal train derailed on the north edge of Des Moines in the early evening. The train carried miners who were returning home after a long day's work, as well as several other passengers. Seven of the train riders were killed as the train broke apart and fell over a 12-foot embankment. The coal stove in the caboose started a fire continuously fueled by the coal carried on the train.

Several nearby farmers and miners rushed to aid the injured and tried to contain the fire. They set up a nearby farmhouse to serve as a temporary hospital until the seriously injured could be transferred to Mercy. According to the newspaper, the scene at Mercy Hospital appeared this way:

> *"Mercy hospital came as near [to] being a place of excitement last night as a well regulated hospital ever becomes. Already full of sick and accident cases, room was quickly found for the suffering men who had been crushed and torn and crippled under the overturned cars of coal. The parlor was made a ward very quickly and three of the injured were placed there. Beds were prepared in some of the wards and eight of the nine were cared for. The other did not need a bed. The vacant place in the parlor was explained by the covered stretcher in the dead room in the basement."* [7]

Dr. McCarthy directed the surgery team at Mercy at that time, and he performed at least one delicate brain operation (trephining) to remove a piece of coal from an injured miner's skull. Of the injured treated at Mercy, two died and the rest recovered.[8] These accidents, combined with outbreaks of contagious diseases early in the century, kept Mercy full, constantly taxing its capacity.

Yearly outbreaks of typhoid concerned all healthcare institutions in Des Moines. With

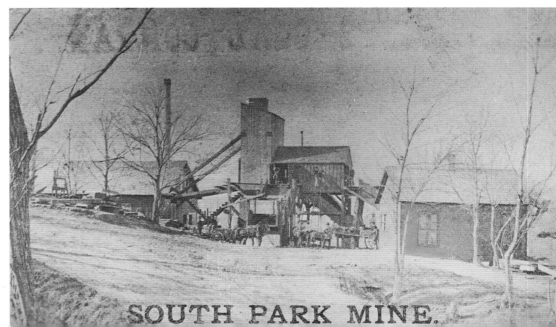

SOUTH PARK MINE.

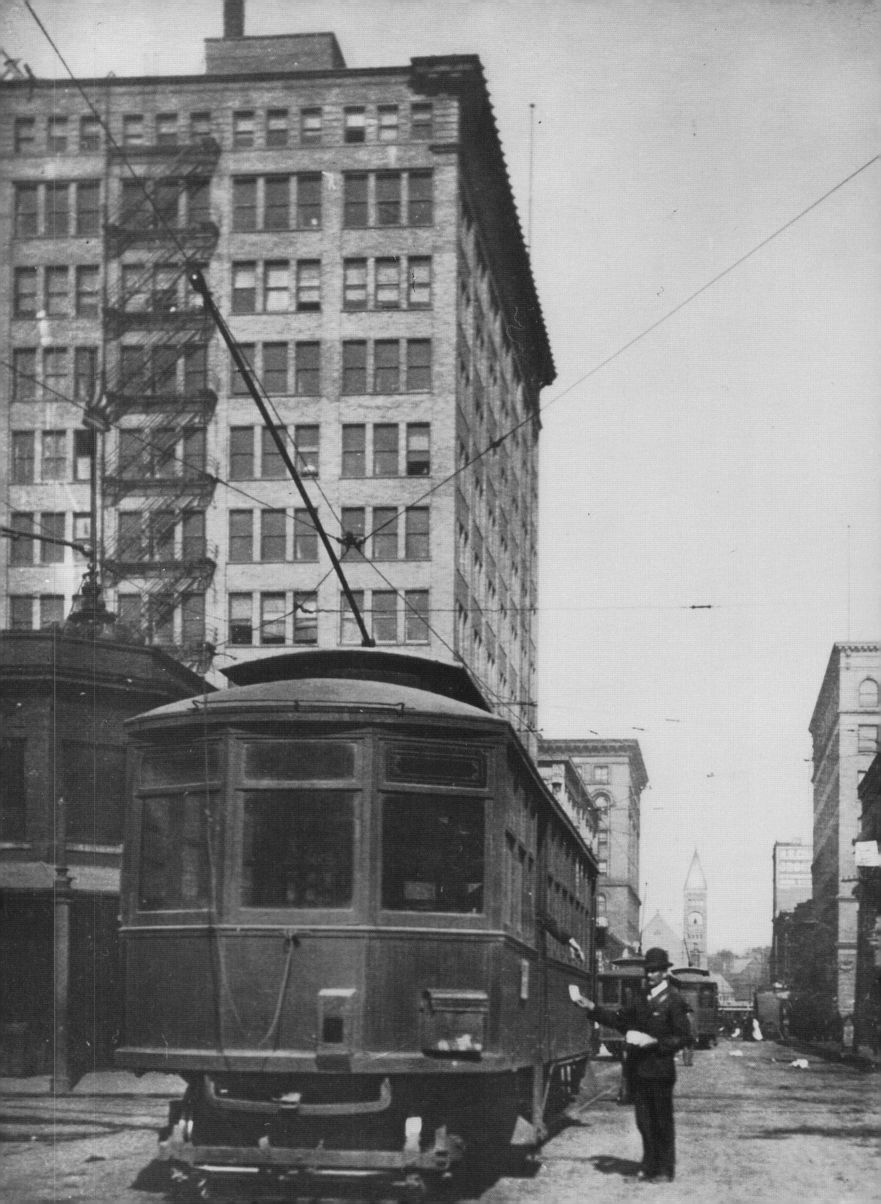

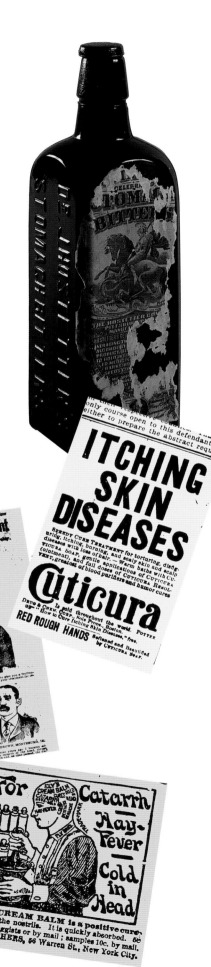

newly discovered "microbes" and effective methods for testing water, Dr. Losh, the city physician, periodically published warnings to the public to boil all drinking water. Autumn was a particularly susceptible time for germ growth, and Mercy treated more than 20 cases of typhoid each week for two months in 1907. Tons of ice were used to control fevers. It was a constant battle to fight this effect of the disease.[9]

TIMES OF TURMOIL

After seven happy and prosperous years, Mercy experienced unrest late in 1900 when Mother Xavier was removed as mother superior. Although ending her tenure in this capacity followed the rules of the order, Mother Xavier did not wish to step down.

The rules and customs of the Sisters of Mercy designated that the mother superior of a convent would hold office for three years, and that she could be re-elected by permission from the local bishop for an additional three years. The election for a new mother superior to replace Mother Xavier should have occurred at Mercy about May 27, 1900. No actual record exists to tell whether it did or what really happened during the election.

Mother Xavier had been in charge at Mercy Des Moines for all the years since Mother Baptist appointed her superior. She apparently possessed leadership qualities that went beyond that of most of the sisters in Des Moines at that time, with the exception perhaps of Mother Philomena. It appears that when it came time to elect the new superior, no clear-cut candidate emerged. It is thought that Mother Philomena was nursing her pleurisy in a drier climate, and she was not elected. Records are unclear as to whether she was appointed or voted in, but Sister Mary Visitation Faherty became the new superior/administrator of Mercy Hospital in Des Moines in 1900.

SISTER MARY VISITATION FAHERTY

Sister Mary Visitation Faherty was born Mary Faherty in Dubuque in 1861. She entered the Sisters of Mercy there in 1880. Her early years were spent teaching in Davenport and in the hospital office. Not much is known about Sister Visitation's tenure as Des Moines administrator.

In November 1900, Father Flavin wrote one of his regular letters to Bishop Cosgrove. The priest must have relayed complaints against the new superior because Bishop Cosgrove responded to the letter with surprise, stating that Sister Visitation was "always looked upon [in Davenport] as an excellent sister [who] filled every office she held with great credit to herself." The Bishop's letter also indicated that Mother Xavier was still in Des Moines, for it said: "when [she] is taken away from there I think there will be peace. She never yet held a position in which she did not give me an immense amount of trouble." [10]

Following close on the heels of this correspondence was a letter to Bishop Cosgrove from the Iowa State Traveling Men's Association. L.C. Kurtz, as secretary, relayed that a group of men representing the parishes in Des Moines had been meeting to discuss the future of Mercy Hospital. They wanted independence for the hospital from Davenport. He stated that the entire Des Moines medical fraternity supported the plan. He told of their concerns that a "Protestant hospital [was] to open soon" backed by some of "the best known public men in this state, and men resourceful in every particular." The men behind the move for independence felt that as long as the physicians as a unit supported Mercy, the new hospital would not thrive.[11]

It is thought that Sister Visitation did not favor separation because this proposal was not acted upon, and she fulfilled her three-year term as superior.

On December 21, 1900, one month after Sister Visitation's appointment, a special medical staff meeting was held at Mercy to discuss the resignations of members of the hospital's attending staff. A meeting had been held at the hospital four days earlier, and the physicians felt that their concerns had been ignored. After much discussion, Drs. Kelleher, Wells, VanWerden, Cokenower, and Rawson voted to dissolve their memberships as attending staff of Mercy Hospital. Minutes from that pre-Christmas meeting closed with a poignant "there being no other business the meeting adjourned to meet no more." [12]

Whether these resignations were prompted by lack of response to the move for independence or by dissatisfaction with Sister Visitation's negative support of this effort is not known. The sisters resolved the matter within a few days by appointing a new "advisory board" with Drs. Kelleher and Cokenower as members. [13]

Sister Visitation's three-year term of office was the only time until 1922 that either Mother Xavier or Mother Philomena were not in charge of Mercy Hospital in Des Moines.

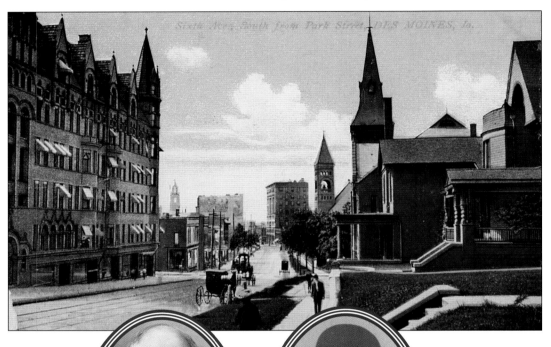

A HOSPITAL ON PLEASANT STREET
On January 16, 1901, Iowa Methodist Hospital opened. Methodist layman, Theodore Gatchel, asked ministers, interested laymen, and businessmen to build a hospital under the direction of the Iowa Methodist Church. The founding fathers considered erecting their hospital on the old Cottage Hospital site, across from Mercy. However, plans changed, and Iowa Methodist Hospital first opened in the old Callanan College building on Pleasant Street—the current site of Iowa Methodist Medical Center.

THE WEST WING
Faced with an ever-increasing patient load, Mercy continued its 1899 plans to add another addition onto the hospital. On October 26, 1907, Mother Philomena who was superior at that time, announced plans for a West Wing which would expand patient capacity by at least one-third. Mother Philomena and the other Sisters of Mercy invited a few friends of the hospital to view plans and to seek support for the proposed addition. The new wing would be attached to the west side of the Central Wing, running parallel to Ascension Street. Planners hoped to finish this addition by summer 1908. [14]

These were ambitious plans and delays kept the completion from occurring until Spring 1909. There is no record of a gala opening for this wing as there had been in the past. A mention in late January 1909 said the new wing would be ready about March 1. Several people wished to furnish rooms as soon as they were completed. One woman offered to provide furnishings for three rooms. [15]

When the addition was finished, Mercy continued to provide expanded clinical services to Drake's Medical School. [16] In 1909 during a reunion of the merged Keokuk Medical School and Drake alumni, experts from the medical field were called in to conduct special surgical clinics as part of continuing education for graduate students. Dr. Deaver from Philadelphia, an expert on appendicitis procedures, conducted one

Looking south from Mercy, the view of Sixth Avenue in Des Moines, *top,* shows the former Victoria Hotel. ❧ Dr. Lewis Schooler, *above left,* was Mercy's chief of staff in 1901. ❧ Dr. J.W. Cokenower, *above right,* served as secretary from 1903 to 1929.

of these clinics at Mercy. He demonstrated the use of ice packs on 14 appendicitis patients. Dr. Deaver performed at least one surgery, which took four times longer than his usual 15 minutes because it was the most "aggravated case of appendicitis he [had] ever been called to treat."[17]

Increased Competition

Not long after the opening of the West Wing, Mercy began to face more competition within the city. The Swedish Lutheran church began talking about building a hospital, although their dreams did not begin in earnest until 1912. At the same time, Iowa Methodist Hospital announced a new five-story east wing for their facility. The Still Osteopathic College purchased property on E. 12th, the site of the former Seventh Day Adventist sanatorium, as they planned for an osteopathic hospital.

Drake began operating a dispensary and outpatient department at its 406 Center Street building. Eventually, this became Broadlawns Hospital, after operating under the name of Samaritan, a city hospital that cared for contagious and social diseases during World War I and into the 1920s.[18] The Congregational Church began its plans for their hospital at Fourteenth and Clark Streets. Sixty years later, this facility would become part of Mercy Corporation after opening as Bishop Drumm Home in 1939, and finally, as the House of Mercy in 1987.

Tremendous Growth

The new century awakened on Mercy's hill to the open arms of the Sisters of Mercy. It was a time of tremendous growth and activity for the Des Moines community. Methods for treating the ill became more sophisticated as new cures for old diseases were researched and discovered. People looked to hospitals for care, and Mercy responded by moving toward the future with increased knowledge, expanded facilities, and renewed energy.

More change was in the wind.

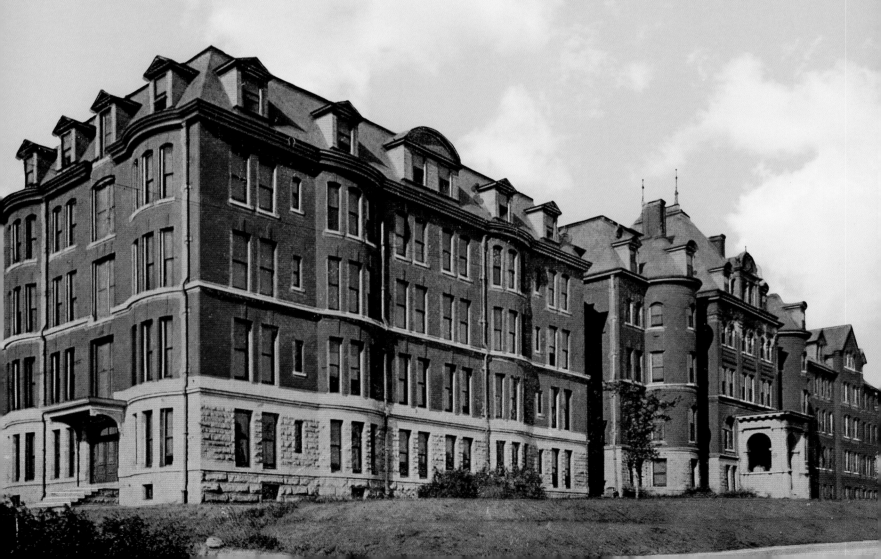

Mercy Hospital's West Wing, *below,* was completed in 1909. Attached to the west side of the Central Wing on Ascension Street, this third addition to the hospital increased Mercy's bed capacity by one-third.

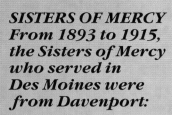

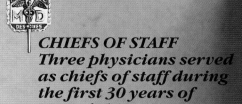

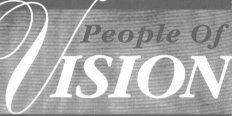

People Of VISION
1893-1922

SISTERS OF MERCY
From 1893 to 1915, the Sisters of Mercy who served in Des Moines were from Davenport:

Adelaide Lynch
Agatha
Alacoque Plunkett
Alphonsus Fox
Anthony Reilly
Baptist Martin
Berchmans Daly
Dorothy O'Brien
Elizabeth Butler
Francis Roche
Gabriel Mulcrone
Gertrude Walsh
Isabelle Connolly
Joseph Rogge
Josephine O'Loughlin
Loretta Hunter
Mechtildes Hogan
Philomena Keating
Scholastica Kerns
Thecla Roche
Vincent Conway
Visitation Faherty
Xavier Malloy

Mercy Des Moines was an independent convent from 1916 to 1922. The sisters who came to Des Moines or entered the novitate during that time were:

Agatha Endres
Alphonsus Kelly
Ancilla Cain
Angelita Senecal
Antoinette Hill
Augustine O'Flaherty
Baptist L'Estrange
Bertha O'Brien
Consilii Finn
Dorothy Flaherty
Eugene Dunleavy
Evangelist L'Estrange
Genevieve Reed
Joseph Byrne
Josephine Curran
Mercedes Reed
Perpetua McKeown
Theresa Marie McDermott

CHIEFS OF STAFF
Three physicians served as chiefs of staff during the first 30 years of Mercy's history:

T.F. Kelleher, 1893-1900; 1904-15
Lewis Schooler, 1901
J.T. Priestley, 1902-03; 1916-21

SCHOOL OF NURSING DIRECTORS
Miss Wheeler, 1899
C.C. Feeney, 1900-01; 1912-15
Miss Schooler, 1901
Miss Carey
Miss Long
Anna C. Kelley, 1916-20
E. Cleo Cavanaugh, 1921-22
Sister Mary Antoinette Hill, 1922

CHAPLAINS
James Renihan, 1895
Charles R. Waldron, 1896
Clement Lowery, 1897
John F. Kempker, 1898
Alban Rudroff, 1899
Gerhard Schumacher, 1900-05
Daniel Mulvihill, 1906
Albert M. Nodler, 1907-08
Bernard J. Sheridan, 1909
John Murphy, 1910-11
Bartholomew Kueppenbender, 1912
J. Denvir, 1913
H.C. Pouget, 1914-15
John J. Galligan, 1918
Vitus Stoll, 1921

CHAPTER FOUR
CHANGING TIMES

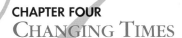

Fueled by a healthy farm market, Iowa settled into relative prosperity as the first decade of the new century came to an end and changes began to occur at a rapid pace.[1] Des Moines' population topped 100,000 by 1912.[2] Major concerns of the city fathers centered around providing help for the numerous sick and poor and improving overall conditions within the city.

Pneumonia was the number one killer, causing the death of 125 people in Des Moines in 1912. Cancer was the second biggest concern. Experiments using radium to control cancer were being investigated in Paris and local papers heralded successes with this venture. Severe outbreaks of typhoid and diphtheria still occurred every year, and frequent vehicular accidents added to a burgeoning patient load at Mercy Hospital. Patients were transported to Mercy by police ambulance, replacing the ever-faithful team of horses—"Peaches and Cream."[3]

In anticipation of the closing of Drake's Medical School, the sisters decided that Mercy's auditorium should be converted to a patient care area. The auditorium located in the northwest corner of the building was remodeled in 1912 to hold an additional 18 beds.[4] A new structure

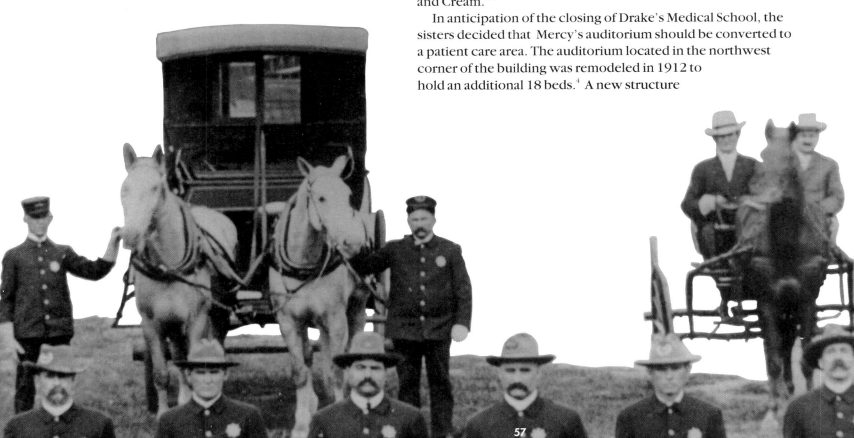

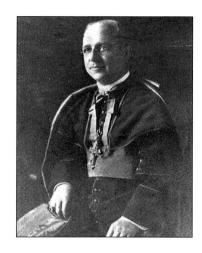

behind the Central Wing was being planned when news from Rome caused a flurry of activity in the Des Moines Catholic community. Ultimately, this news brought a windfall to Mercy.

A NEW CATHOLIC DIOCESE IN IOWA

In November 1911, after years of speculation and planning, Pope Pius X issued a Papal Bull which would form the fourth Iowa diocese, establish Des Moines as the See City, and provide a bishop located within the city. Catholics in southwestern Iowa had prayed devoutly for this event. The answer to their prayers forever altered the course of Mercy's history.

Austin Dowling, right, served as the first bishop of the Des Moines Diocese. Herndon Hall at 2000 Grand Avenue, bottom, became Dowling's home. ॐ The heirs of Jefferson and Julia Polk, below right, gave this home to the diocese, stipulating that an endowment should then be given to Mercy Hospital to build a wing for charity patients.

The first bishop of Des Moines, Austin Dowling, arrived in the city on May 2, 1912. More than 5,000 people welcomed the new bishop who faced the task of administering a diocese which had been directed from 170 miles away for more than 30 years.

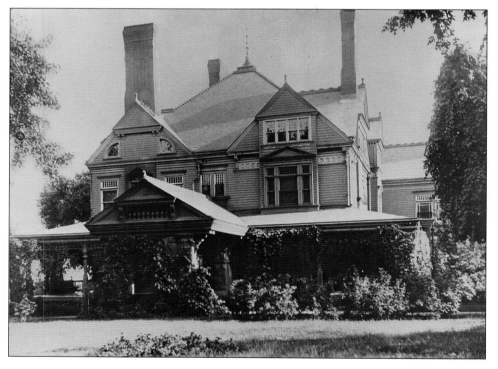

The day after Bishop Dowling arrived in Des Moines, Mrs. Julia H. Polk died. Along with her husband, the late Jefferson S. Polk, Julia Polk had been a prominent member of Des Moines business and society. The family lived in a palatial home, Herndon Hall, at 2000 Grand Avenue. Upon Julia's death, the Polk heirs decided to offer the residence to Bishop Dowling for his new home. There was, however, one catch. In return for the home, the Des Moines Diocese agreed to give Mercy Hospital $20,000 from money collected over the years in anticipation of the new diocese. The sisters planned to use this money to build a new wing. At this time, they entered into a contract with the Polk heirs.[5]

The contract specified that construction begin in 1912 and be completed by the end of 1913. In return, Mercy would maintain at least four beds for the exclusive care of patients who had no means to pay. The Polk heirs asked that two double-bed wards be created—one for men and one for women. A brass plaque with the name of each of their parents, Jefferson S. and Julia H. Polk, was to be inscribed and placed on the doors of each ward. Most importantly, the care of these patients was to be no different from those patients who could afford to pay. Mercy willingly complied because the stipulation did not differ from the compassionate care on which their reputation had always been based.[6] The contract was signed May 13, 1912, two weeks after Bishop Dowling's installation.

The sisters were delighted with the Polk endowment. Already in the middle of constructing a new building behind the Central Wing, they now were able to embark on another expansion that would not be equaled until the late 1960s.

NEW AND VAST IMPROVEMENTS

Mercy entered an ambitious building phase from 1910 through 1916, adding three new structures to the hospital: an area behind the Central Wing, the Red Wing, and the North Wing (Polk Endowment).

In December 1912, the addition behind the Central Wing was opened in a burst of "firsts" for the new Catholic diocese. Bishop Dowling blessed the new building in the first official blessing of this kind since his appointment to Des Moines. The Mass celebrated that happy day was the first Mass offered by Bishop Dowling at Mercy Des Moines.

The day chosen for the celebration was an important one for the Sisters of Mercy. December 12, 1912, was the 81st anniversary of the founding of the Order of Mercy in Dublin in 1831.[7] Those who visited the new building that day saw a structure located directly behind the Central Wing. This endeavor was a large part of improvements to Mercy which cost $50,000. A new kitchen area occupied more than half of the first floor. It was the sisters' pride and joy. With a special floor that prevented dirt from collecting, this new facility was said to be the most modern and sanitary kitchen in Des Moines. Walls were finished in white tile; the ceiling in steel. Windows were located high on the walls for good ventilation and protection from the dangers of the ground-level location. New steam tables, modern utensils, cold storage areas, and special vegetable- and meat-handling areas boosted this new dietary department into the most up-to-date and efficient kitchen available.

Diet kitchens for each of the hospital's four floors were located above this main kitchen. All were connected to the main kitchen by an electrically operated dumb waiter. Gone were the days of the hand-operated dumb waiter and the need to reheat food after it was prepared in the old main kitchen and carried to each floor.

The needs of each patient could be met easily, no matter what time of day, and with greater convenience to the staff. Food temperature control minimized the dangers of poisoning. Handling the food less often meant fewer germs were transferred between floors.

As soon as dedication day festivities for this expansion were over, the Sisters of Mercy intended to turn their attention toward construction of the North Wing as provided by the Polk family endowment. However, before the North Wing was completed, the sisters built the Red Wing, also behind the Central Wing.

THE RED WING: STATE OF THE ART
The Red Wing[8] was a two-story addition also located at the rear of the Central Wing. When it was completed in 1913, the building housed new operating rooms, and an electro-therapeutic department, and a laboratory.

The upper floor housed the operating rooms which featured windows and sky-lights that flooded theaters with a maximum amount of natural light from the north. White marble and tiling were used on the walls and floor. These rooms featured an up-to-date sterilizer, operated by foot levers to prevent anyone from touching even the lids of the boiling vats.[9]

The electro-therapeutic and laboratory departments were located below the operating rooms, connected by a stairway. Dr. N. O. Lier was in charge of the single

DR. & MRS. DANIEL J. GLOMSET

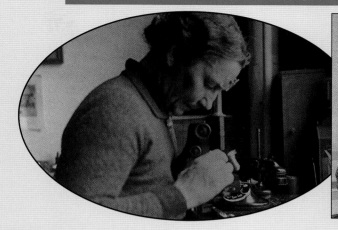

D r. and Mrs. Daniel J. Glomset were early instructors in Mercy's School of Nursing. Dr. Glomset was a graduate of Rush Medical School who came to Des Moines around 1910 to be the first and only professor of pathology at Drake University. After the school closed, he practiced for a time as pathologist for Dr. Fay. Drs. Rockafellow and McCarthy invited Dr. Glomset to take charge of Mercy's laboratory.

Mrs. Glomset was a bacteriologist and chemist. The husband and wife worked together as a team at Mercy. Mrs. Glomset cut and pre-pared frozen sections. Dr. Glomset used a microscope to identify diseases. They were the first to attack the purity of the Polk County milk supply. The pair proved that the

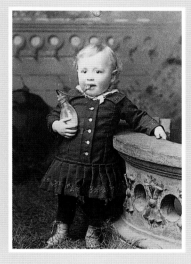

majority of milk used in the county was contaminated. They urged pasteurization as a means of solving the problem.[10]

Mercy's laboratory was equipped with a room where animals were kept as culture specimens. The Glomsets' son, Dr. Daniel A. Glomset, recalls his mother telling him that she kept the inoculated animals in cages under Mercy's warm smoke-stack which served the laundry, and, along with the boiler, was located in a small, separate building behind the Central Wing.

The Glomsets worked together at Mercy and taught laboratory techniques, bac-teriology, and chemistry to nursing students until Dr. Daniel J. Glomset left to serve in World War I.[11]

The "death-dealing long-tube nursing-bottle," *above*, was banned in Buffalo, New York, in 1906. It was difficult to sterilize, and the milk supply often was unpasteurized.

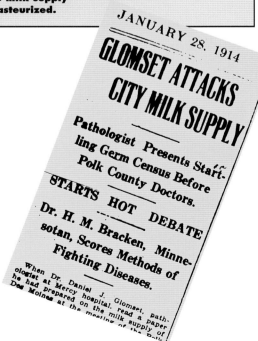

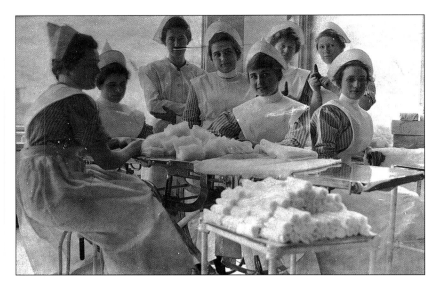

department which today would be the separate departments of radiology and physical therapy. Dr. Lier specialized in x-ray studies. The instruments he used sound peculiar and quaint—interrupterless machine, tracheoscope, radioscope, and stereoscope—but were nonetheless the latest in technology at the time. The electro-therapeutic department also utilized other electrical equipment for physical therapy.

The laboratory was conveniently located below the operating rooms, providing quick support for surgeons who needed immediate analysis of tissue, sputum, and blood and other special studies. The laboratory engaged in research under the guidance of Dr. Daniel J. Glomset.[12]

The Red Wing gave Mercy the best operating room and laboratory "west of the Alleghenies."[13] Now, the sisters could give full attention to finishing the Polk-endowed addition—the North Wing.

THE NORTH WING: A FAMILIAR SKYLINE

Mercy enthusiastically began its task of adding the North Wing onto the hospital. The three previous hospital wings were parallel to Ascension Street. The North Wing would be attached onto the back of the West Wing and would continue north along the Fifth Street side of Mercy's property. Although it was called the North Wing at that time, in later years it was known as the West Wing.

Work on this addition began in April 1913. J. B. McGorrisk of the Capital City Brick and Tile Company acted as contractor for the anticipated $57,000 addition.[14] The Polk rooms officially opened a year later on April 14, 1914. Mercy continued to provide this care for charity patients in the Polk rooms for 15 years. They ministered to more than 550 people and donated nearly $30,000 in services to charity patients.[15]

The opening of the North Wing merited another gala event sponsored by the Sisters of Mercy later that year. More than 200 guests were entertained on October 7, 1914, at Mercy Hospital. The evening banquet was reported to be the "most brilliant ever given in Iowa." Halls were decorated with multi-colored electric lights covered with autumn leaves. American Beauty roses graced the tables. Dr. James T. Priestley acted as toastmaster, as he had at the opening of the Central Wing 16 years earlier. Other speakers of the evening included Harry H. Polk, Dr. Thomas Duhigg, Harvey Ingham, Judge Marcus Kavanaugh, Monsignor Michael Flavin, Hal S. Ray, Pleas J. Mills, and F. W. Sargent.

This occasion also marked the 20th jubilee of Mother Mary Philomena's service to Mercy Hospital in Des Moines. A Pontifical High Mass was offered in her honor early in the morning. She and the work of the Sisters of Mercy were praised at the evening dinner.

Nursing students, *above*, roll bandages in the new surgical area of the Red Wing. ❧ The North Wing, *below*, was attached to the back of the West Wing. This addition housed the Polk Rooms for patients without means. The building was completed in April of 1914.

Dr. Priestley, on behalf of medical staff members and business leaders, presented Mother Philomena with a car.[16] Reminiscing years later, Sister Mary Dorothy Flaherty recalled: "[The car] was a two-seater, and we had a chauffeur."[17]

With the addition of the North Wing, Mercy Hospital now could accommodate 250 patients. For those seeking Mercy care in Des Moines, this familiar skyline of buildings remained unchanged in appearance until the mid 1950s.

WORLD WAR I: LEADEN RAIN

World War I erupted in the summer of 1914 with the murder of Serbian royalty. Although far removed from Des Moines, these events were watched with more than a little worry. By 1915, hostilities in Europe filled the front pages of Des Moines newspapers. They were enhanced by the drawings of the famous cartoonist, J. N. "Ding" Darling. Prejudice and rage abounded.

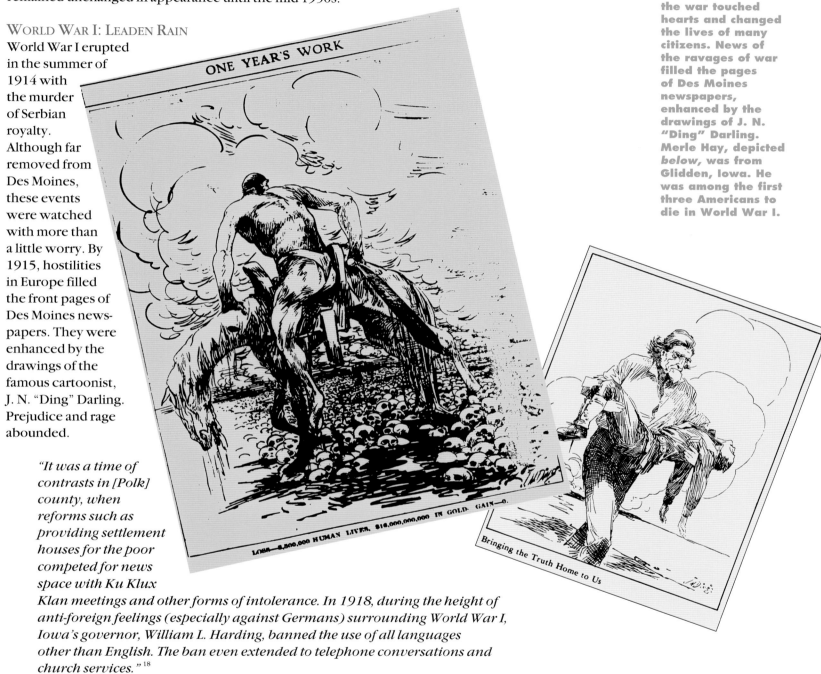

"It was a time of contrasts in [Polk] county, when reforms such as providing settlement houses for the poor competed for news space with Ku Klux Klan meetings and other forms of intolerance. In 1918, during the height of anti-foreign feelings (especially against Germans) surrounding World War I, Iowa's governor, William L. Harding, banned the use of all languages other than English. The ban even extended to telephone conversations and church services."[18]

Sister Sebastian Geneser, growing up in the shadow of Mercy, remembers vividly the German prejudice during World War I:

"I was in grade school during World War I. They were teaching German at St. Mary's when I was [there] because that was a German parish. All the parents wanted their kids to learn German. All at once, the sisters were told that they should burn all the books, all the German books, and stop teaching German."[19]

Amid this prejudice and uncertainty, Iowa prepared for the possibility of war. One of 16 national recruiting centers was built north of Des Moines at Camp Dodge in the suburb which is now known as Johnston. A National Guard camp was prepared to care for thousands of soldiers, equipment, and supplies.

SPANISH INFLUENZA

Although U.S. involvement in the war was relatively short, the country felt repercussions for a long time. One of the most debilitating results of the war was the Spanish influenza. Soldiers returning from European military theaters brought this devastating disease home. Several Irish Sisters of Mercy recalled the loss of families and friends to the flu in Ireland.

This rapidly spreading virus was called the "Three Day Fever" at first. Later, it was recognized as a severe form of Spanish influenza. The flu initially appeared at Camp Dodge in early October 1918, causing an epidemic. During the first week of the illness, more than 3,500 soldiers were under observation and approximately 2,000 of them tested positive. The major complication of pneumonia caused the deaths of 14 soldiers during the first week.

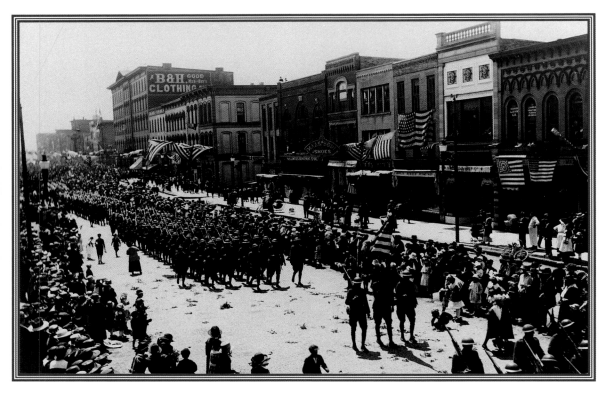

Within two weeks, the epidemic had passed its crisis at the camp, but had taken a firm hold deeper within the city of Des Moines. A special flu committee was formed, and the chairman issued an order to all city hospitals to make room for a percentage of flu patients. The hospital willingly offered 50 of its beds to care for flu victims, saying that as many more beds would be provided by Mercy "to the city as the occasion may demand. Nurses and doctors also will be furnished." [20]

Sister Mary Dorothy Flaherty remembers that Mercy was "full to the brim. We had people in the hallways." [21] Sister Mary DeLourdes Hardiman, who grew up across the street from Mercy, remembered that the nurses used to come down to their house for a break from the strenuous demands placed on them by the flu epidemic:

> *"In 1918, especially when they had that flu, [the nurses] would come down just to get away. I remember down by Harbach's [funeral home] it seemed like all across the street were caskets. They were dying that fast. But thanks be to God, none of [my] family got the flu."* [22]

Sister Dorothy also remembered, while working as a young nurse at Mercy, that none of the sisters died during the flu epidemic. They lost their young chaplain, Father John Galligan, however. [23]

During the war years, Mercy underwent a change in administration. Within four years of becoming Des Moines' first bishop, Austin Dowling separated Mercy Hospital in Des Moines from Mercy Hospital in Davenport.

Soldiers returning from European military theaters brought the Spanish influenza into Des Moines, creating an epidemic that took the lives of 14 soldiers in one week. More than 2,000 servicemen tested positive to this debilitating virus.

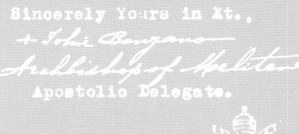
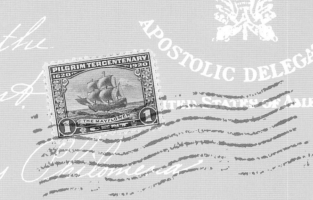

CHANGE IN ADMINISTRATION

For the first 22 years of its history, Mercy Hospital in Des Moines existed as a daughter institution of Mercy Hospital in Davenport. Relations between the two institutions were congenial, and staff moved freely between them on an as needed basis. There was no direct intervention by Mercy Davenport in the daily operations of Mercy Des Moines because of the distance between them. As a result of this goodwill and amiable working relationship, the subject of separating the two organizations rarely surfaced. But when it did come up, there was heated discussion on both sides of the issue.

More than likely, the first request to designate Mercy Des Moines as an independent entity came in 1900 when a prominent Des Moines Catholic men's group wrote a letter to Bishop Cosgrove. It is thought that the request came as a result of the men's dissatisfaction with the removal of Mother Xavier as administrator of Mercy Hospital in Des Moines. Bishop Cosgrove took no action at the time, responding that "for all practical purposes, it was so [independent]; as no projects for its advancement were ever interfered with by Davenport, but on the contrary, cooperation and assistance freely given." [24]

A NEW REQUEST

In September 1913, Bishop Dowling wrote to Bishop Cosgrove's successor in Davenport, Bishop James Davis, saying that the sisters in Des Moines wanted separation from Mercy Davenport. Bishop Dowling decided that the relationship between the two hospitals must be made separate. He acted in response to his own need to exercise executive authority, and more than likely, in response to pressures from prominent Des Moines Catholics. Three new Des Moines hospitals were in the planning stages, and Bishop Dowling feared the competition, especially if it appeared that the Catholic Church in Des Moines was not in control of the Catholic institutions within its jurisdiction.[25]

Bishop Davis and Mother Mary Aloysius, who was superior of Mercy Hospital in Davenport, met to discuss Bishop Dowling's request. Mother Aloysius was not sure it was true that the sisters at Mercy Des Moines wanted the separation. Bishop Davis advised her not to worry. He seemed to think that the move for independence was made only by the two sisters in charge in Des Moines, Mother Xavier and Mother Philomena. Bishop Davis and Mother Aloysius discussed the possibility of changing the operating structure in Des Moines, but due to repercussions following Mother Xavier's removal as administrator a few years earlier, they decided against it. They agreed to wait until Bishop Dowling made his next move. In the meantime, Mother Aloysius counseled the sisters in Des Moines to work quietly and steadily, acting charitably to those in charge.[26]

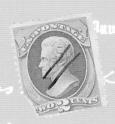

The situation continued to simmer for another year-and-a-half. In March of 1915, Bishop Dowling wrote another letter to Bishop Davis. He asked that Mercy Des Moines be put under "near authority" because of the "condition of spiritual turmoil which prevails at Mercy Hospital." This letter also carried more than a subtle hint that Bishop Dowling actually considered cutting off all Catholic association with Mercy so that it would "cease to be regarded as a Catholic institution." Bishop Dowling said he did not intend to join the hospital to the sisters in Council Bluffs, which was being suggested at that time.[27]

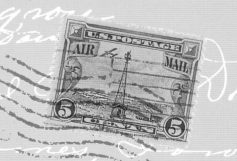

After a series of futile letters between the two clergymen, Bishop Dowling, Bishop Davis, and Mother Aloysius met in Davenport on April 20, 1915, to discuss the separation issue. They came to no decision, and the two in Davenport thought Bishop Dowling had agreed to wait for separation until after the elections of new superiors at Mercy Davenport in one month. With this assumption in mind, Mother Aloysius arranged for several new sisters to go to Des Moines to aid the hospital there. She thought this would smooth things over.[28]

To End The Matter

Bishop Davis and Mother Aloysius were astonished to receive a letter from Bishop Dowling almost immediately after he returned to Des Moines. He wrote that "he had decided to end the matter by making the division effective on Sunday, April 25, 1915." Finances would be arranged later, and he hoped that enough sisters would be left in Des Moines to carry on Mercy's work until those who left could be replaced.[29]

Bishop Dowling later confided several reasons for the separation in a letter to the Apostolic Delegate, Archbishop John Bonzano. Dowling believed that discipline among the sisters was lacking at Mercy Hospital in Des Moines. Evidently, one of the priests who was close to the sisters relayed this to him. The bishop also felt there were lingering ill-feelings toward the late Bishop Cosgrove among Catholics in Des Moines regarding the transfer of land and money from Father Brazill's estate.

One clause in Father Brazill's will had left control of the Des Moines property to Bishop Cosgrove for "the good of the Catholic Church." Some Des Moines Catholics believed the clause was interpreted as the Catholic Church in Des Moines, not Davenport. One rumor suggested Bishop Cosgrove had transferred more than $20,000 from Des Moines to Davenport. Bishop Dowling added that "the lawyer who drew [Father Brazill's] will said he knew Father Brazill...meant the [Catholic] church in Des Moines."[30]

While he wanted to separate the two hospitals, Bishop Dowling feared Mercy would be boycotted by Des Moines physicians if all of the Des Moines sisters returned to Davenport. The threat of a boycott was more real now because three non-Catholic hospitals had opened in Des Moines within the last three years.[31]

After separating the two hospitals, Bishop Dowling immediately established a new foundation of Sisters of Mercy. Mercy Hospital became a motherhouse and Mother Philomena was named superior/administrator. The sisters in residence were told that they could remain in Des Moines with the permission of Mother Philomena. Seven of them felt their allegiance remained with Davenport, and they left Des Moines on April 26. A complete list of these sisters does not exist. Only five sisters remained in Des Moines: Mothers Xavier and Philomena, Sister Anthony, and two unnamed sisters.

A War Of Words

After the division, administrators in Davenport immediately petitioned Archbishop Bonzano to intercede on their behalf. They wanted a nullification of the situation created by Bishop Dowling, or if this was not possible, they would agree to the separation after a fair financial settlement between the two houses.

Mother Mary Mercedes Wellehan, the new superior in Davenport, inherited the long series of negotiations between Des Moines and Davenport. Both sides petitioned to the Apostolic Delegate at one time or another. The Davenport sisters went so far as to send money to ensure that their petition would be considered.

Archbishop Bonzano eventually sided with Bishop Dowling. He felt Bishop Dowling had acted out of good faith because his main concern was the Des Moines community. The Archbishop told the Davenport sisters to ratify the separation according to the constitution of the Sisters of Mercy and to ask a board of arbitrators to arrange a financial settlement.[32]

A war of words began in another exchange of letters between Mother Mercedes and Bishop Dowling. No conclusion was reached. The Davenport sisters still wanted no part of separation and were not willing to decide how much money they needed for financial restitution. The bishop, on the other hand, made it clear that his main plan was a separation so he could bring about "observance of the rule."[33]

During this time, the Davenport sisters asked their attorney, Emmett Sharon, to find out what he could about the "atmosphere" in Des Moines.[34] Mr. Sharon wrote a letter seeking the confidence of an old friend, Des Moines lawyer John Sullivan, who also represented Bishop Dowling. Sullivan replied that although he represented Bishop Dowling, he could provide the benign information Sharon needed.[35] Another letter in which Sullivan changed his mind soon followed this response. He said that it was better that he not have any part in the project, and he recommended that Mr. Sharon consult with Frank Comfort, another Des Moines lawyer.

At the same time, Mr. Sharon requested the clerk of court in Des Moines to send him a valuation of Mercy properties in Des Moines without the Des Moines bishop, sisters, or other Catholics knowing about it.[36] The clerk supplied information provided by a friend who solicited it from Dr. Robert Lynch. The estimated value placed on the hospital was $295,000.[37]

Not long after this, Mother Mercedes wrote another letter to Archbishop Bonzano to ask for his help. She reiterated that the sisters did not want a separation. She also stated that the value of Mercy properties in Des Moines was $500,000.[38]

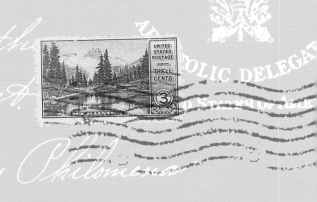

A Settlement

Evidently, the Davenport sisters decided on a more reasonable financial settlement because in February 1916, Bishop Dowling wrote to Mother Mercedes saying that he was glad they had given him the $70,500 figure to present to hospital authorities.[39] He asked for a further itemized statement, and after that was received, he wrote rather pointedly:

> *"I assume that the submission of these figures is a recognition of the division made by me last April and that the informality complained of there has been removed. Lest, however, I may be mistaken, may I ask you as a preliminary to a financial settlement to say whether or not my assumption is exact and also whether there are any other bills or charges not mentioned in this list for which the Motherhouse in Davenport holds Mercy Hospital of Des Moines responsible?"*[40]

As this correspondence passed between Des Moines and Davenport, two additional sisters returned to Davenport, leaving only three in Des Moines: Mothers Xavier and Philomena and Sister Anthony.

Mother Mercedes expressed her concern to Archbishop Bonzano that if Davenport should receive the requested financial settlement, there would not be enough sisters to run the hospital in Des Moines. The Archbishop suggested sending any spare sisters Mother Mercedes had in Davenport to Des Moines. He felt this would be a gesture of goodwill that with the two bishops' permission would show they considered Mercy Des Moines a new foundation.[41]

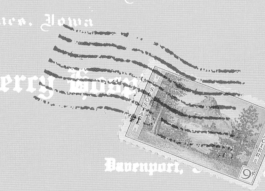

No progress was made during the two months that followed, mostly due to Bishop Dowling's absences from Des Moines.

On May 18, Bishop Dowling forwarded an offer of a $50,000 cash settlement from the sisters in Des Moines. Within a week, Davenport countered with a figure of $60,000. This figure was finally accepted by the Des Moines sisters, and Bishop Dowling informed Davenport of the sisters' acceptance on June 1, 1916.[42] Although the settlement price was agreed upon in June, the deal was not closed until early November. A quit claim deed issued on November 8, 1916, conveyed all of the Des Moines property held by Davenport to Des Moines upon payment of $60,000.[43]

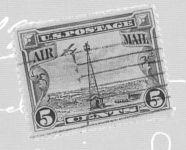

Growth And Separation

Many changes occurred at Mercy Hospital during the prosperous time after 1910. The sisters added three structures to the hospital and new treatments for old diseases were tried. The world's attention focused on Serbia, and those events erupted finally into World War I.

A dispute evolved closer to home as Bishop Dowling separated Mercy Hospital in Des Moines from Mercy Hospital in Davenport. As a result, some Sisters of Mercy who had been in Des Moines for years returned to Davenport. New sisters came from other places, and for a time, the hospital in Des Moines became an independent convent of Mercy.

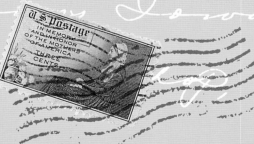

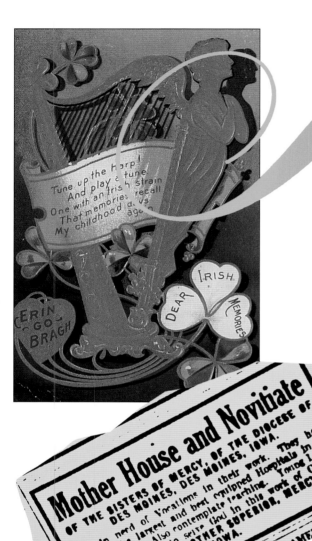

Mother House and Novitiate

OF THE SISTERS OF MERCY, OF THE DIOCESE OF DES MOINES, DES MOINES, IOWA.

Are in need of vocations in their work. They have one of the largest and best equipped Hospitals in the Middle West. Also contemplate teaching. Young Ladies who feel called to serve God in this work of Charity may apply to the MOTHER SUPERIOR, MERCY HOSPITAL, DES MOINES, IOWA.

ROSS CASTLE, KILLARNEY

SAINT PATRICK'S DAY

ERIN, GO BRAGH!
ERIN BE STRONG!
SAINTS BE A WATCH-GUARD
TO SHIELD THEE FROM WRONG!
ERIN, SWEET ISLE,
THO FOES STRIVE TO AWE,
NOW AND FOREVER
ERIN, GO BRAGH!

COPYRIGHT 1911 BY H.M. ROSE

CHAPTER FIVE
A NEW BEGINNING

A new beginning for the Sisters of Mercy shined brightly on the horizon after three additions to the hospital and the acceptance of Mercy Des Moines as an independent community. Their numbers were few, but time was on their side and growth had become a way of life.

A PORT IN THE STORM

Three Sisters of Mercy remained in Des Moines after the separation from Davenport. Sister Anthony, who managed the first floor, was the only diploma nurse with a valid Iowa nursing registration. Mothers Xavier and Philomena were administrators who were not involved in the day-to-day care of patients. As a result, the bulk of the work was being performed by secular employees. Mother Mercedes had complained to the bishops about this fact. She feared the reputation of the hospital and the administration in Davenport was being damaged by inadequate provisions for the care of the sick in Des Moines.

Soon after the separation of Mercy Des Moines from Davenport, Mother Philomena advertised in the Catholic publication, *Our Sunday Visitor*, to attract young women to the new motherhouse. Six Sisters of Mercy from Iowa City saw the ad or heard by word-of-mouth that Mercy Hospital was seeking new members for their community. The sisters at Mercy Hospital in Iowa City had gone through an unsettling period not long before this time as a result of a scandalous lawsuit. A few of them were searching for a "port in the storm," and in October and November 1916, they petitioned Bishops Davis and Dowling to join the Des Moines community. The six sisters who came to Des Moines from Iowa City were: Sisters Mary Baptist and Evangelist L'Estrange, Consilii Finn, Augustine O'Flaherty, Bertha O'Brien, and Josephine Curran.

SISTERS MARY BAPTIST AND EVANGELIST L'ESTRANGE

Sisters Mary Baptist and Evangelist L'Estrange were blood sisters. They were born Caroline Josephine and Susan Louise L'Estrange, respectively, in King's County (now County Offaly), Ireland. There were 10 daughters in the L'Estrange family of 15 children. Five of the girls entered religious orders. Caroline and Susan went to the United States and entered the Mercy Convent in Iowa City in 1907. Their brother, James, settled in the Cummings, Iowa, area, possibly prompting the sisters to join the Des Moines community nearby.

Sister Baptist was about 24 years old when she came to Des Moines, and she was ill with tuberculosis. A trip to Colorado in November to regain her health was unsuccessful. She died at Mercy on April 13, 1917, and is buried in the old St. Ambrose Catholic Church section of Woodland Cemetery. A copy of her obituary reprinted in an Irish newspaper ended:

"As an indication of the respect felt for the deceased it may be mentioned that the motor hearse containing the remains, which were enclosed in a silver-mounted coffin, was followed by over forty motor cars." [1]

The L'Estrange sisters were good nurses, although Sister Baptist was confined to bed during most of her time in Des Moines.[2] Sister Evangelist reportedly was the most valuable member of those who affiliated from Iowa City. This was true especially during the Spanish influenza epidemic of World War I.[3] She remained in Des Moines after her sister's death, until October 1919. Sister Evangelist petitioned to join the Mercy community in Stanton, Texas, a future part of the St. Louis Province of the Sisters of Mercy. She was appointed to the position of mistress of novices and remained in Stanton for many years. She died in St. Louis in 1953.

SISTER MARY CONSILII FINN

Another sister from Iowa City, Sister Mary Consilii Finn, may have immigrated from Ireland at the same time as the L'Estrange sisters. Sketchy convent records say that Margaret Finn was received in 1904 and professed in 1906, in Iowa City. She and Sister Evangelist were friends, and when Sister Evangelist decided to migrate to the Texas community, Sister Consilii petitioned to go there a few months later. In 1929, Sister Consilii was confined to a New Orleans sanatorium. She died at Slaton, Texas, on May 24, 1979, at the age of 99.[4]

SISTER MARY JOSEPHINE CURRAN

The one Iowa City sister about which very little is known is Sister Mary Josephine Curran. Sister Josephine's last name may be incorrect, but if it is Curran as is suspected, she entered the Sisters of Mercy as Emma Curran in Iowa City in 1889.[5] One source says that Sister Josephine was a "floater" or "roamer" who did not enter originally in Iowa City, but came there after profession elsewhere.

It is said that Sister Josephine possessed genteel manners and may have received training as an artist. One of her paintings hung in the choir loft of the convent chapel in Iowa City for many years. She was a fine musician.

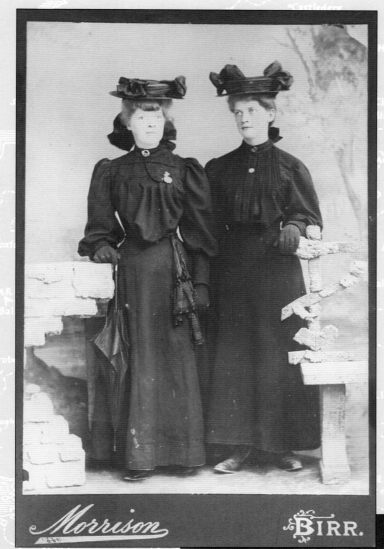

Caroline and Susan L'Estrange, *left*, came from Ireland to become Sisters of Mercy. Their mother sent this photograph to her daughter Delia, saying, "pray for your poor dear sisters who have gone to a Mercy convent in Iowa City, Iowa, USA." Shown *below* with their brother James, the two women became Sister Mary Baptist and Sister Mary Evangelist L'Estrange.

Morrison *BIRR.*

After Des Moines amalgamated with Council Bluffs in 1922, Sister Josephine remained with Mercy Hospital in Des Moines as temporary mistress of novices. She died at Mercy on February 25, 1923, and is buried in Glendale Cemetery.[6]

SISTER MARY BERTHA O'BRIEN

Another sister who migrated from Iowa City was Sister Mary Bertha O'Brien. She was born Elizabeth O'Brien in County Cork, Ireland, in 1880. Sister Bertha was received into the Iowa City community on October 15, 1907. In 1916, she received permission from the bishop to transfer from the Iowa City convent to the Mercy convent in Des Moines. Sister Bertha weathered the changes at Mercy and chose to remain there for 42 years. She was a gentle lady whose special tasks included taking care of the chaplains and interns. She performed her duties until 1939 when she retired to "inactive service." Sister Bertha died on March 27, 1960, just short of her fiftieth jubilee as a Sister of Mercy.[7]

Sister Mary Bertha O'Brien, above, came to Mercy Des Moines from Iowa City. ❧ Mother Mary Philomena Keating and Sister Mary Eugene Dunleavy represented Mercy Des Moines in Milwaukee at the second annual meeting of the Catholic Hospital Association in June 1916, below.

SISTER MARY AUGUSTINE O'FLAHERTY

Of the six sisters who came to Des Moines from Iowa City, five were fully professed Sisters of Mercy who could vote, make hospital policy, and assist with patients and nursing students. The sixth, Sister Mary Augustine O'Flaherty, was a "white-veiled novice." According to Sister Augustine's records, she entered the Mercy order in Iowa City in 1911 and took temporary vows in 1914. She took her final vows in Des Moines on September 10, 1917.

Sister Augustine evidently was a very capable nurse. Bishop Drumm chose her as temporary administrator of Mercy when he amalgamated the Des Moines and Council Bluffs communities. Sister Augustine remained temporary administrator until she was replaced by Sister Mary Evangelist Claherty in June 1922.[8]

SISTERS MARY ALOYSIUS AND JOSEPH BYRNE

At some point during the motherhouse years, two other Sisters of Mercy were allowed to join the small community. These women were blood sisters, Sisters Mary Aloysius and Joseph Byrne. Their community of origin is unknown. However, evidence exists that they may have joined the Sisters of Mercy in 1875 at St. Patrick's convent in East St. Louis, Illinois.

The Byrne sisters were from the same county in Ireland as the L'Estrange sisters. Since they were considered visitors, and they had no place to go, hospitality was extended to them. More than likely, they knew Sisters Evangelist and Baptist

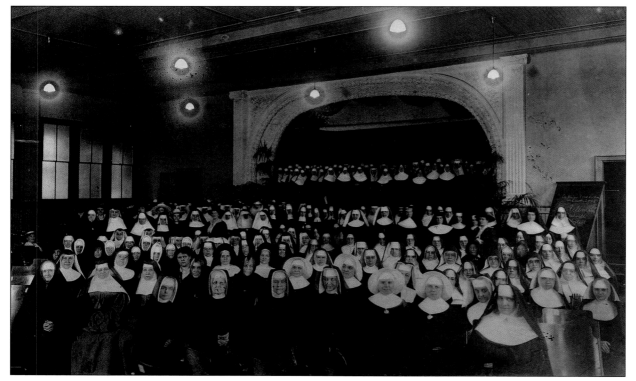

from Ireland. According to tradition, both women traveled extensively in the western United States and may have been part of Mercy communities in Pendleton, Oregon, and Salt Lake City, Utah.

Sister Aloysius Byrne died in Des Moines on May 15, 1918, at the age of 64. Sister Joseph died on August 8, 1921, at the age of 89.[9] The two sisters also are buried in the St. Ambrose Catholic section of Woodland Cemetery. Unfortunately, there are no markers on the graves to show where they rest. Information in an old cemetery log book compiled during the Works Progress Administration (WPA) period lists a "Sr. M. Aloysius" buried in a grave marked with a wooden marker. Time or perhaps vandalism has erased the marks of their burial.[10]

TRYING TIMES

As a motherhouse Mercy was not particularly successful. Only 12 candidates applied to enter the novitiate between 1916 and 1922. With a small number of professed sisters to carry on operations of both the hospital and the convent, there were not enough people to fill the need. Years later, Sister Dorothy Flaherty remembered that she was put into a supervisory position because there was no one else to do it: "I was supervisor for a long time. It felt like a long time. It was only three years, I guess, that I was on the floor. I had no special training in supervising. I just did it." [11]

Stress ran high in those years. World War I created a shortage of supplies and medical staff. Money was a constant worry. At the end of the war, the returning soldiers brought the dreaded influenza, causing as many deaths within the United States as in other countries.

In 1918 when local elections for Mercy's administration were to occur, there were not enough professed sisters to vote, and Bishop Dowling made the appointments. He selected Mother Philomena as superior/administrator of Mercy, and Mother Xavier as mistress of novices.

When Mother Xavier's two great-nieces, Catherine and Evelyn Reed, arrived at Mercy in February 1917, they enrolled in the school of nursing and also in the Mercy novitiate as postulants. Soon, other young women in these same programs grew jealous of the Reeds. Oral interviews in later years hinted that favors shown to the nieces caused considerable friction within the organization.

HEALING ENDEAVORS

Mercy Des Moines struggled as a motherhouse during these days. Those who were part of the effort contributed greatly to the healing endeavors and war-induced shortages at Mercy Hospital. The era ended with Mother Philomena's sudden death on December 28, 1921.

In 1918, Bishop Dowling appointed Mother Mary Philomena Keating administrator of Mercy Hospital. This action was taken because there were not enough professed sisters to properly elect the new superior. Bishop Dowling informed Mother Philomena of her selection in the letter *below*.

MERCY HOSPITAL
DES MOINES, IOWA

Dear Mother Philomena —
May 1st 1918

As your Community lacks a sufficient number of Professed Sisters for a Canonical election of Superior, I hereby appoint you the Superioress for the ensuing three years according to the authority vested in me and recognized by the Guide of your Institute

Austin Dowling
Bishop of Des Moines

CHAPTER SIX
THE END OF AN ERA

In the early morning hours of December 28, 1921, a special bell rang in the Des Moines convent. All sisters, novices, and postulants were awakened. They were told that Mother Philomena was dying.[1] Later, her death was attributed to a lung hemorrhage. She suffered with pleurisy for a long time, but Mother Philomena had given no indication she was ill. Her death threw Mercy into turmoil.

At the time of Mother Philomena's death, Des Moines' Bishop was Thomas W. Drumm. Bishop Drumm replaced Bishop Dowling who became Archbishop of St. Paul in 1919. Bishop Drumm was visiting in Dubuque when Mother Philomena died. Dr. James T. Priestley, as president of the Mercy Medical Staff, telegraphed Bishop Drumm to inform him of Mother Philomena's death. The telegram's text is rather puzzling:

> *"Mother Philomena died this morning. Will you please use your influence to have no change made in the management of Mercy Hospital at the present time—will explain fully upon your return."* [2]

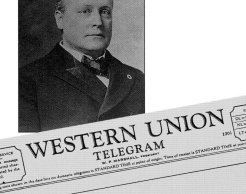

WESTERN UNION TELEGRAM

BISHOP DRUMM =
MOTHER PHILOMENA DIED THIS MORNING. WILL YOU PLEASE USE YOUR INFLUENCE TO HAVE NO CHANGE MADE IN THE MANAGEMENT OF MERCY HOSPITAL AT THE PRESENT TIME – WILL EXPLAIN FULLY UPON YOUR RETURN=
DR. JAMES PRIESTLEY =

Was Dr. Priestley responding to the directives of Mother Xavier because she was afraid of losing control? Or was this telegram prompted by physicians' fear that Mother Xavier might be appointed the new administrator of Mercy?

Several of Bishop Drumm's correspondences hinted there were things happening at Mercy of which he did not approve. In one letter, Bishop Drumm indicated that he almost had gone to Mercy on the day before Mother Philomena died to "clean up the whole mess, but Providence— there is no other explanation—kept me away." [3]

Bishop Drumm decided to act quickly after Mother Philomena's death. Armed with secretly-gathered information, the bishop called for an audit of the hospital. The accounting showed there were severe problems with Mercy's bookkeeping system. It was recommended that the auditors "kindly be allowed to suggest the absolute necessity for an improvement in office management and system, as it is impossible from the records now kept to have any check on the handling or balancing of cash received and disbursed. No proper statements of income and expenditures or financial statement can be made from the records and the information needed for the guidance of the management is not readily obtainable." [4]

Bishop Drumm, acting with the advice of Archbishop John Bonzano, the Apostolic Delegate, took action. He dissolved the motherhouse at Mercy Des Moines and

As president of Mercy's medical staff in 1921, Dr. James T. Priestley, *top,* sent a telegram to Bishop Thomas W. Drumm, *above,* informing him of the death of Mother Mary Philomena.

appointed a temporary administrator for the hospital, Sister Mary Augustine O'Flaherty. The bishop made another sweeping change with the full support of Archbishop Bonzano. [5]

In 1908, a vote had been taken by the resident sisters in Des Moines, indicating that the majority of them favored an amalgamation of all the Sisters of Mercy in the United States.[6] By the end of January 1922, Bishop Drumm had arranged for a less broad, but more real, amalgamation. Mercy Des Moines would be joined with the Sisters of Mercy in Council Bluffs. This move seemed natural because the sisters from Council Bluffs were already operating two Catholic elementary schools and one home for working women in Des Moines.

Earlier that month, Bishop Drumm had written a letter to the "twelve sisters of Mercy Hospital, Des Moines," outlining the outcome of his investigation. He wrote that he found the novitiate "out of harmony with the laws laid down by the Church," resulting in "a very unhappy condition." There were too few professed sisters to hold an election, and he was "handicapped with the meager material for the reconstruction of the government of this community." However, he felt that: "the glory of God, the honor of the church in this community, and the future of this institution depend on the things we are doing now, and I am confident that God is guiding us to make Mercy Hospital worthy of His glorious service, and with this in view I count on the prayerful cooperation of you all." [7] He later outlined his specific plans in this way:

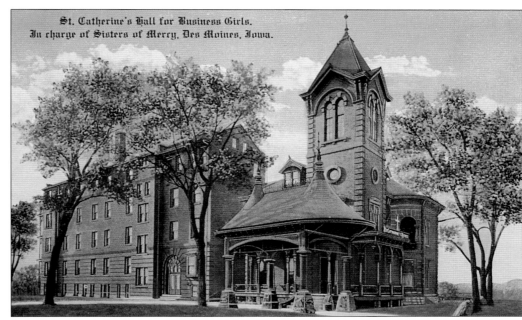

St. Catherine's Hall for Business Girls. In charge of Sisters of Mercy, Des Moines, Iowa.

Bishop Drumm arranged the amalgamation of Mercy Des Moines with Mercy Council Bluffs. The Council Bluffs sisters were already in Des Moines operating St. Catherine's Hall for Business Women shown above and St. Peter's and Holy Trinity Schools.

> *"The present novitiate shall be discontinued within six months. Meantime, the present postulants shall not be received and the present novices shall not be professed. I am not appointing a mother superior, but I hereby appoint Sister M. Augustine, [administrator] of the Mercy Hospital Community with full authority and power under the Bishop to govern and administer the affairs of this community for an indefinite period."* [8]

This directive was delivered by the bishop in Mercy's chapel. Drumm asked Sister Augustine to take her place as the administrator, and for each of the sisters to come forth and make their obedience to her.

THE SWINGING DOOR

In a handwritten plan, Drumm noted that eight sisters promptly came forth to promise obedience. Mother Xavier and her niece, Sister Mercedes, left the chapel without approaching Sister Augustine. The other niece, Sister Genevieve, broke down in tears but did not leave the chapel.[9] Two rather interesting and opposing

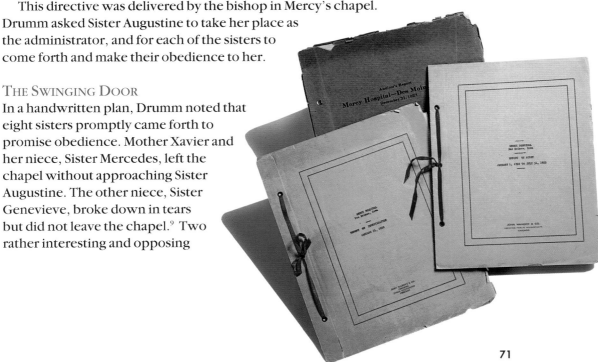

accounts remain of a confrontation which occurred between Sister Mercedes and Bishop Drumm immediately following this meeting. The first was written by Drumm at that time, and the second was related years later by Mrs. Eva Proulx, formerly Sister Mercedes.

Bishop Drumm told the sisters that he would be in the parlor if any of them wished to speak to him. He wrote: "Sister Xavier asked to go to Washington. I granted permission. I even offered to pay her way. I showed Mercedes the swinging doors when she became offensive. [I want you to] submit to [the administrator]. She said she could not." [10] Sixty-six years later, Mrs. Eva Proulx wrote:

> *"[Drumm] asked each one to come and accept Sister Augustine: I did not. He said any one who wants to see me I'll be in the Parlor. I did go to see him: I said I could not save my soul under her: He said do you want me to tell you what to do? Come with me. He walked me down the Hall to the swinging doors and said: That door swings either way. He left me standing there and walked away. I almost died at that moment. But I decided in that moment to leave.[11] I died a dozen deaths I only wanted to become a nun." [12]*

Sister Mercedes left Mercy and Sister Genevieve remained for one month. Sister Genevieve was forbidden to speak to Mother Xavier or the other novices.[13] Her parents and brother arrived on February 17, 1922, and convinced her to return home.[14] It was a sad, confusing time for the sisters at Mercy.

Years later, Mrs. Proulx gave Bishop Drumm credit for inspiring her vocation when she attended his missions in Waterloo as a young girl. She met him at a Catholic nursing conference in Chicago about two years after she left Mercy. He said to her: "Mercedes, even bishops make mistakes." He also confided to her that he became friends with Mother Xavier before she died. Mrs. Proulx and Bishop Drumm exchanged Christmas greetings for several years.[15]

A TIME FOR PATIENCE

Several of the novices were close to making their final vows when all of this occurred, but they were not allowed to do so until after the union with Council Bluffs. As mistress of novices at the time, Sister Josephine was put in charge of these novices until the merger took place.[16] Sister Mary Antoinette Hill, a white-veiled novice, led the School of Nursing. This appointment caused additional problems because Sister Antoinette was not fully-professed and did not have voting rights.

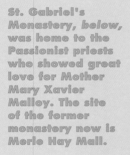

St. Gabriel's Monastery, below, was home to the Passionist priests who showed great love for Mother Mary Xavier Malloy. The site of the former monastery now is Merle Hay Mall.

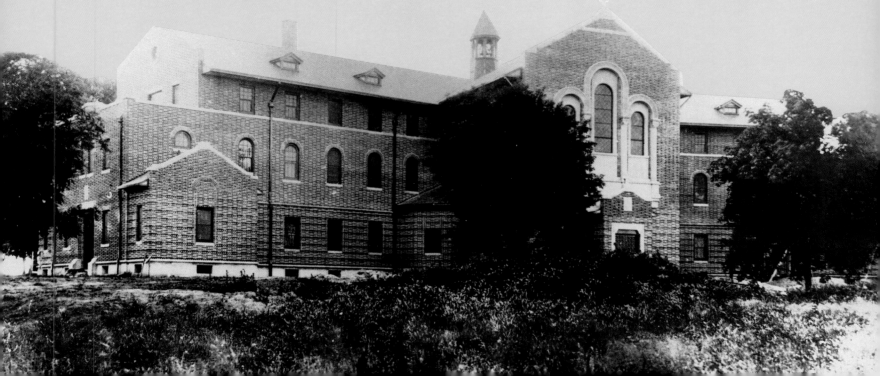

However, Bishop Drumm was in a bind because he had so little professional staff to carry on the hospital work while he was completing the union with Council Bluffs. Sister Antoinette had experience as an American Red Cross nurse during World War I, and she was the logical choice to be in charge of the nursing school. She served in this capacity for a few months until Sister Mary Thomas Wilson was appointed School of Nursing director by Council Bluffs.

Mother Xavier continued to live at Mercy for a little more than two years, trying to gain control by eliciting help from her friends in Des Moines and from Archbishop Dowling in St. Paul, Minnesota. The internal conflict at Mercy ended with the death of Mother Xavier on September 24, 1924. Her final illness lasted only six days. During those last few days, it is said that Sister Mary Theresa Connell of Council Bluffs advised Mother Xavier to make her peace with Bishop Drumm. Sister Theresa Marie McDermott remembers that she did. Bishop Drumm visited Mother Xavier. They talked and "blessed one another." [17]

In his eloquent funeral sermon, Bishop Drumm spoke of the strife and conflict which had existed between him and Mother Xavier. He admitted that he had been the source of additional "burdens to poor Mother Xavier." He added:

"I had no other thought—why should I?—than the welfare of the hospital. And I can also say, and everyone understands it, that Mother Xavier had no other thought—why should she?—than the welfare of the hospital." [18]

Over the years, Mother Xavier had supported the Passionist priests at St. Gabriel's Monastery in Des Moines. The fiftieth jubilee of her profession as a Sister of Mercy would have been celebrated in a few months if she had lived. The Passionists were planning a surprise for this celebration. Instead, as an "act of love toward her who had loved the order so much, the student priests of St. Gabriel sang her requiem Mass." [19] The rector, Father Silvan, was deacon of honor. Remaining in the chronicles of this beautiful monastery (which is now Merle Hay Mall) are the quiet admonitions:

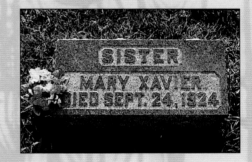

"May the religious of St. Gabriel never fail to pray for Mother Xavier. Let all future generations remember the Sisters of Mercy Hospital. All of us know how our Holy Founder treated benefactors. Oh! Let us never forget these good Sisters. May the soul of Mother Xavier rest in peace." [20]

AMALGAMATION WITH SISTERS OF MERCY, COUNCIL BLUFFS

Thus, the motherhouse chapter of Mercy Des Moines came to an end. The Sisters of Mercy from Council Bluffs quietly took control of the hospital after both houses voted to join together.

After completing details for the union, Bishop Drumm petitioned Rome for the proposed change. The Vatican rescript uniting the two communities arrived in May 1922, and the union took place on June 4. As Mother Mary Bonaventure Carroll wrote so poignantly at that time: "In regard to your letter containing this rescript— Like death, although long enough expected, it came as a shock at last. May God's Holy Will be done." [21]

THE FIBER BECOMES THE THREAD

After 30 years, Mercy Hospital in Des Moines became firmly woven into the fiber of the city. The comforting arms of the Sisters of Mercy ministered to thousands throughout it all, bringing a blessing to the people of Des Moines. Protected by the healing hands of God, the hospital survived the challenges and thrived. In the years that followed, the Council Bluffs sisters continued to provide nurturing care to the suffering poor of the community.

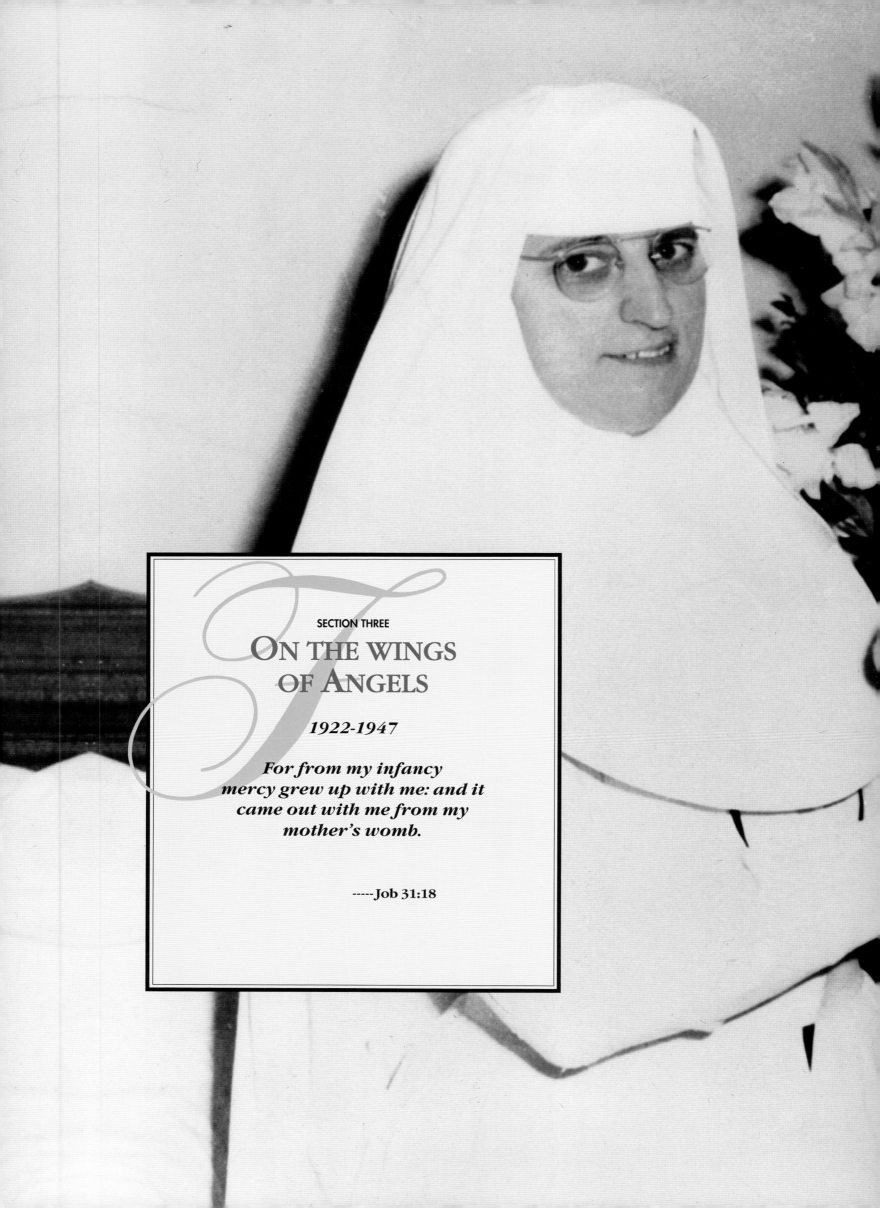

SECTION THREE

ON THE WINGS OF ANGELS

1922-1947

For from my infancy mercy grew up with me: and it came out with me from my mother's womb.

-----**Job 31:18**

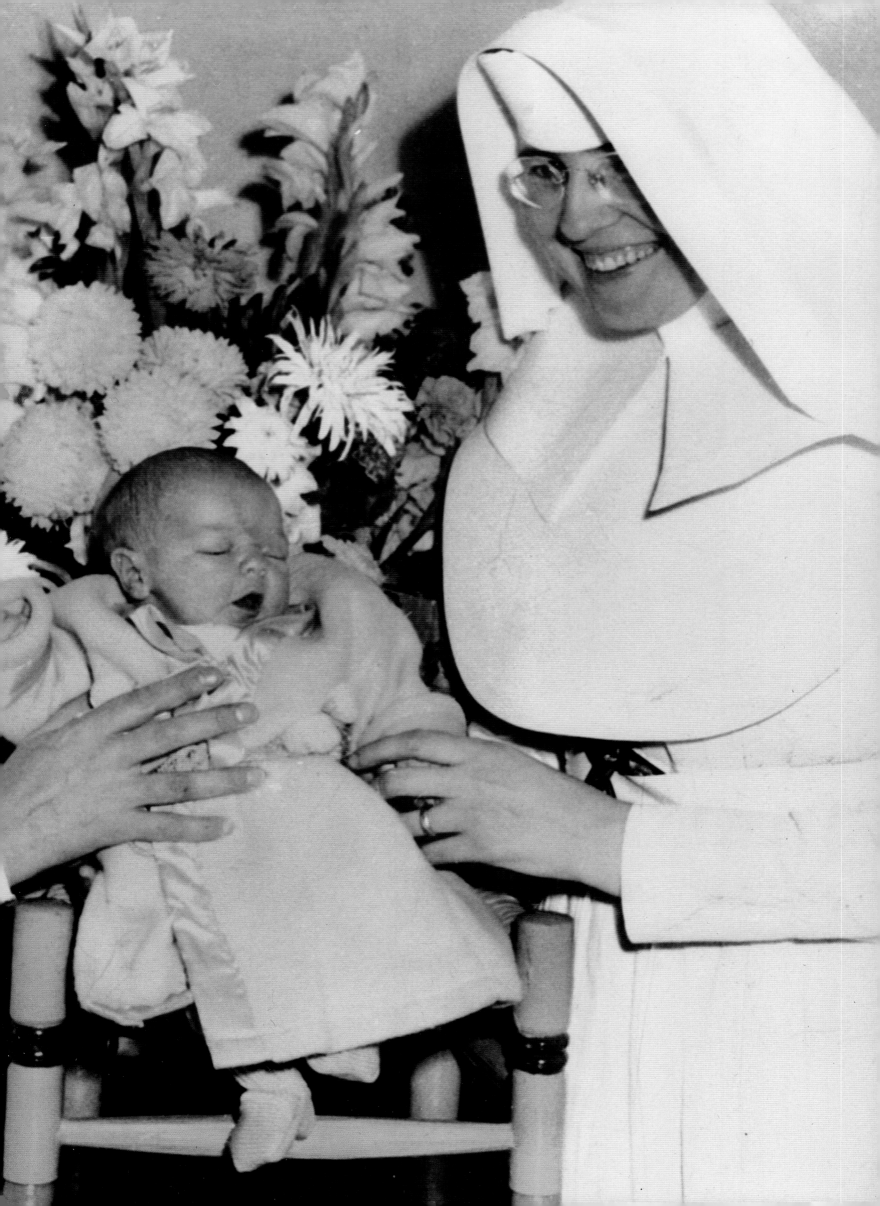

CHAPTER ONE
FURTHER GROWTH: NEW LEADERSHIP

Fresh on the heels of World War I and the problems generated by a weakened farm economy, the Sisters of Mercy from Council Bluffs began managing Mercy Hospital in Des Moines. Council Bluffs' superior, Mother Mary Bonaventure Carroll, prepared a staff to assume leadership roles in Des Moines.

Six Sisters of Mercy came from Council Bluffs to Mercy Des Moines in 1922. They were: Sisters Mary Evangelista Claherty, superior/administrator; Thomas Wilson, superintendent, school of nursing; Winifred Leusen, x-ray technician; Alacoque Lannan, treasurer; Teresa Connell, head housekeeper; and James McDonald, assistant housekeeper.

The sisters approached their new challenge with faith and a bit of trepidation. Along with responsibility for running the hospital came the assumption of Mercy's debts. Mother Bonaventure asked for an immediate accounting of money owed by the hospital. She found the amount to be large and due soon. To help repay this debt, the Mercy Board of Directors, Sister Mary Augustine O'Flaherty, and Monsignor Michael Flavin authorized the sale of all Mercy Des Moines real estate holdings to Mercy Council Bluffs. This included the hospital and surrounding grounds and a 128-acre farm located on the north edge of Des Moines. The new mortgage was $200,000, with a special issue of bonds at five percent interest.[1]

Hard work was in store in order to keep the hospital open. When the first sisters arrived from Council Bluffs in June 1922, they donned long, checkered aprons and scrubbed bathrooms, walls, and toilets on their hands and knees.[2] In the end, their diligence in all efforts produced rewards.

VAST IMPROVEMENTS

Technological improvements such as x-ray and the clinical laboratory, advancements in scientific diagnoses and therapeutics, and discoveries in germ theory that led to aseptic surgery were available in the 1920s.[3]

Improved surgical techniques were being shared by surgeons who had participated in military medical theaters in Europe. These surgeons came home eager to use their new-found knowledge. While their peers learned new procedures, Mercy updated equipment to facilitate changes. They purchased a portable x-ray machine and charged $10 for hospital use; $25 for use outside the hospital. Other equipment improvements during the 1920s came as a result of donations from the medical staff.

Mother Mary Bonaventure Carroll, above, served as superior at Mercy Hospital in Council Bluffs in 1922 when the sisters there began managing Mercy Des Moines. During this time, students cared for rabbits, opposite, and other animals in the hospital laboratory.

The first basal metabolic machine in the laboratory was purchased after Dr. Wilton McCarthy encouraged ten physicians to contribute $100 each toward the $1,005 purchase price. The new machine was installed and put into operation within six months, with a $10 charge for each treatment.[4] It was used to measure activities of glands, particularly the thyroid.

After World War I, the direction of Mercy's laboratory came under the management of Dr. Rodney Fagan, and later, Dr. Julius Weingart. Soon after the arrival of the sisters from Council Bluffs, Sister Mary Joseph Munch became a leader in developing Mercy's laboratory into a first-class clinical setting.

One of the first Mercy laboratory improvements came in the form of a flat fee assessed to all incoming patients. For three-dollars, newly-admitted patients were entitled to all laboratory examinations, excluding x-ray and basal metabolic tests.[5] Upon admission every patient underwent a urinalysis and a complete blood count. Other tests were ordered by the patient's physician.

MERCY'S LABORATORY: FIRST-CLASS

Mercy's laboratory in the 1920s had three rooms. One room was devoted to blood chemistry and other blood examinations. Another was set aside for urinalysis. The third was equipped for tissue and frozen and paraffin section preparations. Sister Joseph recalled early efforts to maintain sterile conditions in the laboratory:

> *"[It was] quite an operation and everything had to be sterile like surgery. Oh, I was very careful. Any infectious materials that I worked with I never let any technicians work with those. I did any cleaning myself...because I didn't want anything bad to happen to any of them."* [6]

Culture media—with the exception of throat cultures—were prepared in the laboratory. Friends at area slaughterhouses provided the hospital with calves' brains used to prepare meat-based cultures. Colloidal gold, hoarded like a million dollars, formed the basis for spinal fluid cultures.

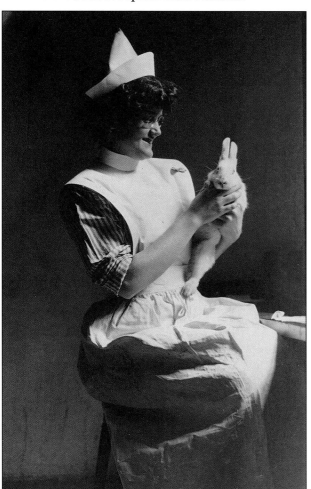

Rabbits and other animals were used for testing in the laboratory. Mice and rats were kept to test for tuberculosis. "The rats were big. You had to be careful that they wouldn't bite you."[7]

WAR AGAINST CONTAGION

The 1920s were marked by many advancements in the containment of contagious diseases. In 1923, Des Moines waged an all-out effort to stamp out diphtheria. Plans were put into effect to use the newly discovered Schick Test for the detection of tuberculosis.[8]

In 1924, cancer and pneumonia became more prevalent and fatal than tuberculosis in Des Moines. Cancer caused 150 deaths; heart disease took 158 lives.

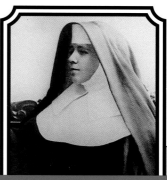

Sister Mary Evangelista

Sister Mary Evangelista Claherty was the first administrator appointed from Council Bluffs. Born in Pennsylvania in 1876, she entered the Sisters of Mercy in 1894 in Council Bluffs, where she also studied nursing.

Sister Evangelista's first administrative position was at Mercy Council Bluffs in 1903. She remained in administration for most of her active life as a religious. Before coming to Des Moines, Sister Evangelista was the first administrator at St. Joseph's Mercy Hospital in Centerville, Iowa, from 1910 to 1913. From 1913 to 1921, she held administrative positions in Council Bluffs.

In Des Moines, Sister Evangelista served as administrator from 1922 until the summer of 1927. Most remember that she was very strict and addressed by the title of Mother. Some young nursing students would go out of their way to avoid her even though she always said, "Good morning."[9]

After the 1929 Amalgamation, Sister Evangelista became assistant provincial in the newly formed Omaha Province. She returned to Des Moines for a short time in the late 1930s to assist the new administrator, Sister Mary Anita Paul.

ADMINISTRATOR 1922-1927

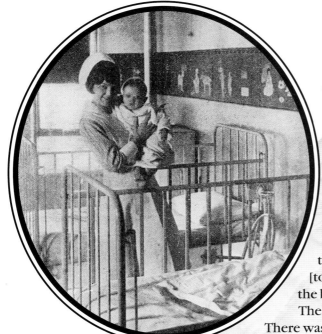

Typhoid was at an all-time low, with one death occurring that year.[10] Treatment of serious disease shifted from the neighborhood doctor's office and the home to the modern hospital.[11]

As these trends continued, Mercy adjusted to meet the changes. In 1925, the hospital opened a children's department. The new facility began service on the first floor of the North Wing. A cheerful wallpaper strip adorned a nursery equipped with painted iron cribs. A ward also contained a play area furnished with pint-sized chairs, rockers, and a desk. This room was used for "light occupational therapy suited to the age and strength of the little patient."[12] Attached to the children's department was a solarium with "helio-glass windows [to] permit passage of ultra-violet rays, [allowing] the little ones to enjoy the benefits of the sun's rays."[13]

The department capacity was 22, with no more than four beds to a room. There was also an isolation room where contagious or infectious cases were treated. Mercy proudly pointed out that the new children's department had "an especially good croup tent and electrically heated inhalation ward."[14] The charge for care was $10 per week.[15]

TENDER CARE

After World War I, more women delivered their babies in hospitals, and Mercy's obstetrical services grew. Accommodations for maternity patients included 19 private rooms and two double-bed wards.

The nursery was located on the second floor West Wing. Baby bassinets were hung in a row along walls. Today, this would not be considered the best way to prevent infection, but at that time, it was standard practice. An abundance of natural light filled the nursery through floor-to-ceiling windows.

The children's department was opened at Mercy in 1925, on the first floor of the North Wing. Equipped with painted iron cribs, the nursery shown *above* was adorned with cheery wallpaper. The ward contained a play area, *below*, furnished with pint-sized chairs, rockers and a desk.

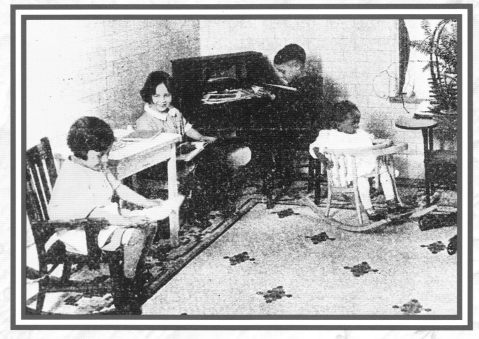

The typical newborn stayed in the nursery during the mother's tenure of confinement, usually about two weeks. A premature baby was kept in an incubator, considered quite primitive today. "It reminded me of an upside down umbrella," recalled Louise Brady, a Mercy nursing graduate. "We had no preemie nipples. The babies were fed with an eye-dropper," she continued. "The only medicines were Coramine and whiskey. And sometimes we saved them. I've often wondered if it was the whiskey or the stick with the needle [that] kept them going."[16]

If a baby developed a rash, the infant was kept in isolation until it was determined if the rash was contagious. Babies were taken to their mothers for feeding four times a day. Bathing and early morning and night feedings were done by the nurse in charge. This nurse usually gave feeding and bathing demonstrations to the mother before she left the hospital with her baby. The baby was weighed each day, and if it was not thriving, feedings were supplemented by baby formula.

Sister Joseph's first assignment was in Mercy's obstetrical department. Sister Mary Clare Clifford became department supervisor in 1924. Sister Clare shared the position with Sisters Mary Aloysius McGuire, Gonzaga McGuire, Winifred Leusen, Austin O'Donohoe, and Eustace Wondrask until 1939 when Sister Mary Zita Brennan was appointed to Mercy Hospital in Des Moines.[17]

By 1927, the average length of stay for obstetrical patients was shortened to 12 days. Standard rate for a two-bed ward at Mercy was $40 for the entire time the new mother was hospitalized. Mercy considered opening a five-bed ward with a lower rate if the "baby business" continued to grow. There were several three-bed wards available.[18] Late in 1927, the sisters changed obstetrical rates, offering the previous prices to those who could not otherwise afford to come to the hospital. For those patients who could afford a private room, a higher rate was assessed.[19]

NEW PROCEDURES

Mercy implemented two new procedures for identifying newborns during the 1920s. In 1924, they became the first Des Moines hospital to give newborns a bead necklace that spelled out the mother's name. In 1925, Mercy introduced the footprint method of baby identification that is still in use today.

As new methods of medical treatment developed worldwide, Mercy moved quickly to add them to their medical skills. In 1924, doctors at Mercy attempted to save a newborn's life by giving the child a transfusion supplied from the blood of her father.[20] Unfortunately, the child did not survive, but Mercy's traditional compassionate innovation continued. Each new procedure was carefully attempted, and the medical staff incorporated the results of these cases into their clinical discussions.

In 1925, Mercy physicians performed a difficult bone transposing operation to set the broken wrist of a 12-year-old patient. The arm had been set six times, but because of the shattered nature of the break and the twisted bone, setting techniques were not successful. In a two-hour operation, Dr. R.A. Weston removed a piece of healthy bone from the arm and used it to support the weak sections until the arm healed.[21]

EXPANDED SERVICES

By the end of 1928, Mercy welcomed a department of urology, a medical library, and an expanded physio-therapy department.

The new urology department was located on the third floor in the West Wing. The rooms included a urologic dressing room with good light and a bathing area that contained the "latest conveniences."[22] Dr. Clifford Losh, Sr. who had received specialized training in urology after World War I helped guide Mercy's efforts to

The nursery, *top*, located on the second floor of the West Wing, had baby bassinets hung along the walls and an artfully-designed Italian tile floor. An abundance of natural light filled the room through floor-to-ceiling windows. In 1924, Mercy became the first hospital in Des Moines to identify newborns with bead necklaces, *above*, that spelled out the mother's name.

establish a strong urological department. One Mercy student remembered with pride: "Our sterilizing record was good. As I remember, we had no urological infections." [23]

The medical library's roots began in 1927 when Mercy became the first hospital in Des Moines to provide a traveling library for patients. The library contained more than 750 books, giving patients respite from the long hours of recovery. Carts filled with books and magazines were wheeled twice a week through each floor, stopping at bedsides long enough for patients to choose something to read. Most books were gifts to Mercy, and the supply was constantly increased. Mercy chaplain, Father Vitus Stoll, and Sister Mary Pauline Hammes regularly donated books to the library's collection.

At the same time, the medical staff opened its own library within the hospital. Physicians were asked to donate subscriptions to augment the professional journal holdings within the hospital. Whenever physicians attended conferences or published papers, they were encouraged to donate copies of materials to the hospital medical library. The intent was to establish a good library, enhancing the education of Mercy's interns. This helped to fulfill a standardization requirement of the American College of Surgeons. It had been a struggle for many years to attract outstanding young interns into service, and it was hoped that this would help.

By the end of the 1920s, Mercy had expanded its physio-therapy department to include more current equipment, such as ultraviolet lamps, deep therapy lamps, infrared surgical and medical diathermy, and auto-condensation equipment. [24] Sister Mary de Paul Collins worked as the physio-therapy technician in this department from 1929 to 1933. Sister Mary Rosaire Keairnes succeeded her.

A TIME FOR CHANGE

By the end of 1926, Mercy's patient capacity was 165. There were 84 private rooms and the rest were two-bed rooms for adults, except for the wards on the children's floor. Admissions for 1926 totaled 2,428. [25]

In July 1927, Sister Mary Benedicta McCarten was appointed superior/administrator of Mercy Des Moines. Sister Benedicta came to Des Moines from a similar position at Mercy Council Bluffs. She remained in administration for 25 years after leaving Des Moines in 1935. [26] Sister Beneditcta had worked with Sister Evangelista on two earlier occasions in nursing at Mercy Hospital in Council Bluffs, and in teaching at St. Patrick's in Imogene, Iowa. [27]

Sister Evangelista possessed many strong leadership qualities and occupied similar positions of authority before coming to Des Moines. The Sisters of Mercy were about

Hospital Has a Perambulatory Library

Helps Patients at Mercy While Away the Long Hours.

Getting behind on your summer reading?

Better take a few weeks in the hospital and catch up.

A traveling library of more than 750 books is one of the means adopted at Mercy hospital for helping the sick while-away the long hours.

The library is in sections, one set of shelves on wheels for each wing of the hospital, two on a floor. Twice a week an attendant wheels it through the wards, stopping at each bedside long enough for those who are well enough to read to make selections.

No particular book enjoys greater circulation than the rest, according to the sisters, but the authors most read and enjoyed seem to be Peter B. Kyne, Harold Bell Wright, Zane Gray, Myrtle Reed, Grace Richmond, Isabel Clark, Kathleen Norris, Francis J. Finn, S. J., Gene Stratton-Porter, Katherine Tynan Hinkson, Eleanor Porter, Martin J. Scott, S. J., Edward F. Garesche, S. J., and Kate Douglas Wiggin.

Several magazines are regularly received and circulated, among them "The Rotarian," the American magazine, Literary Digest, Hygeia, Ave Maria and Messenger of the Sacred Heart.

The books for the most part were ⸱ ⸱ ⸱ to the ⸱ ⸱ ⸱ tion, and

ELIZABETH DAUGHTON, NURSE AT MERCY HOSPITAL, WITH MOVABLE LIBRARY AT THE BEDSIDE OF A PATIENT.

In 1927, Mercy became the first hospital in Des Moines to have a traveling library. Carts were wheeled twice a week through the floors, stopping at each patient's bedside so they could select from more than 750 books.

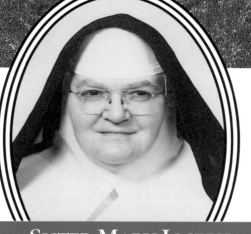

SISTER MARY JOSEPH

As a young girl, Marguerite Munch, migrated with her German family to the United States in 1911. They traveled by ship—*The Lapland*—to New York City and Ellis Island, where they stayed until being relocated to a farm near Chariton, Iowa. Marguerite's first acquaintance with the Sisters of Mercy came when she entered nurses' training at St. Joseph's Mercy Hospital in Centerville, Iowa, at the age of 18. "[The sisters] were very kind. They were an example of generosity and cheerfulness—all beneficial for patient care. One can vision the perfect example the sisters were to me." [28]

She became a postulant of the Sisters of Mercy in 1919 and finished her nurses' training at Mercy in Council Bluffs. Sister Joseph pursued additional education in laboratory, x-ray, and physio-therapy technology at St. Joseph's Creighton Memorial Hospital in Omaha. She took a taxi from Mount Loretto to classes each day. When asked how she came to Des Moines, Sister Joseph replied:

"I came to Des Moines by car. All of a sudden I got word I was to get ready to come to Des Moines. Just like that. And first I was put on floor duty and in [obstetrics]. I loved [obstetrics] and babies, you know, being in charge of the nursery. All of a sudden, I didn't even get orientation, I was told to come down to the [laboratory]. Just like that, I had to pitch right in. Imagine, no orientation. But I took everything as it came along. And the doctors were tickled pink to have me in the laboratory." [29]

Sister Joseph worked in the laboratory without help for a long time. She was finally able to hire a young man, Jimmy Heles, and later on, a young woman, Lillian Schaeffer, to help clean in the laboratory after their school day was finished. Both went on to pursue careers based on their laboratory experience at Mercy.

At one time, Sister Joseph also guided the development of the physio-therapy and x-ray departments. During her career at Mercy, Sister Joseph accomplished many firsts. In 1942, she became the first registered medical technologist in a Des Moines hospital. Mercy was the first hospital in Des Moines to begin the Rh factor test after Sister Joseph learned the procedure at the University of Minnesota. She initiated use of cardiograms and started the blood and plasma banks at Mercy. [30]

"Fame" also came to Sister Joseph for her wonderful jams and jellies. Father Paul Solomia remarked in his sermon at Sister Joseph's funeral in 1987: "Her jelly was delightfully parceled out to those who earned this special reward. I count myself fortunate to have received that particular blessing on a couple of occasions." [31]

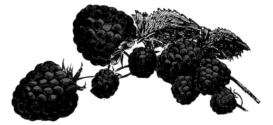

Sister Joseph was an accomplished seamstress who won numerous medals and ribbons at the Iowa State Fair, particularly for her Raggedy Ann and Andy dolls. Many of her works of art were given away. The little she earned by selling her creations paid for material to make more dolls.

After her official retirement, Sister Joseph performed the duties of chapel sacristan, preparing the chapel for daily Mass. On one occasion, she was burning palm branches in preparation for Ash Wednesday services when the flames set off the fire alarm. Her brown eyes twinkled as she later recalled the story of how the fire department came to put out the fire in the palms.

Sister Joseph served Mercy faithfully for more than 64 years. On September 22, 1987, she arranged the chapel for morning Mass, received communion, and two hours later, she was dead. For many of her last years, the strong sister knew she had a potentially fatal condition, but she laughed and said: "Well, I might as well keep going." [32]

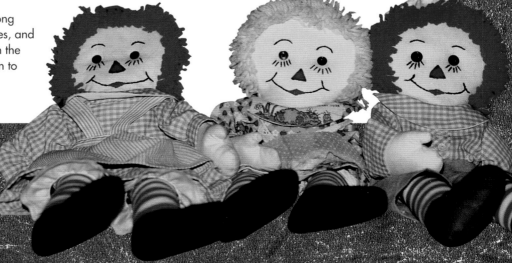

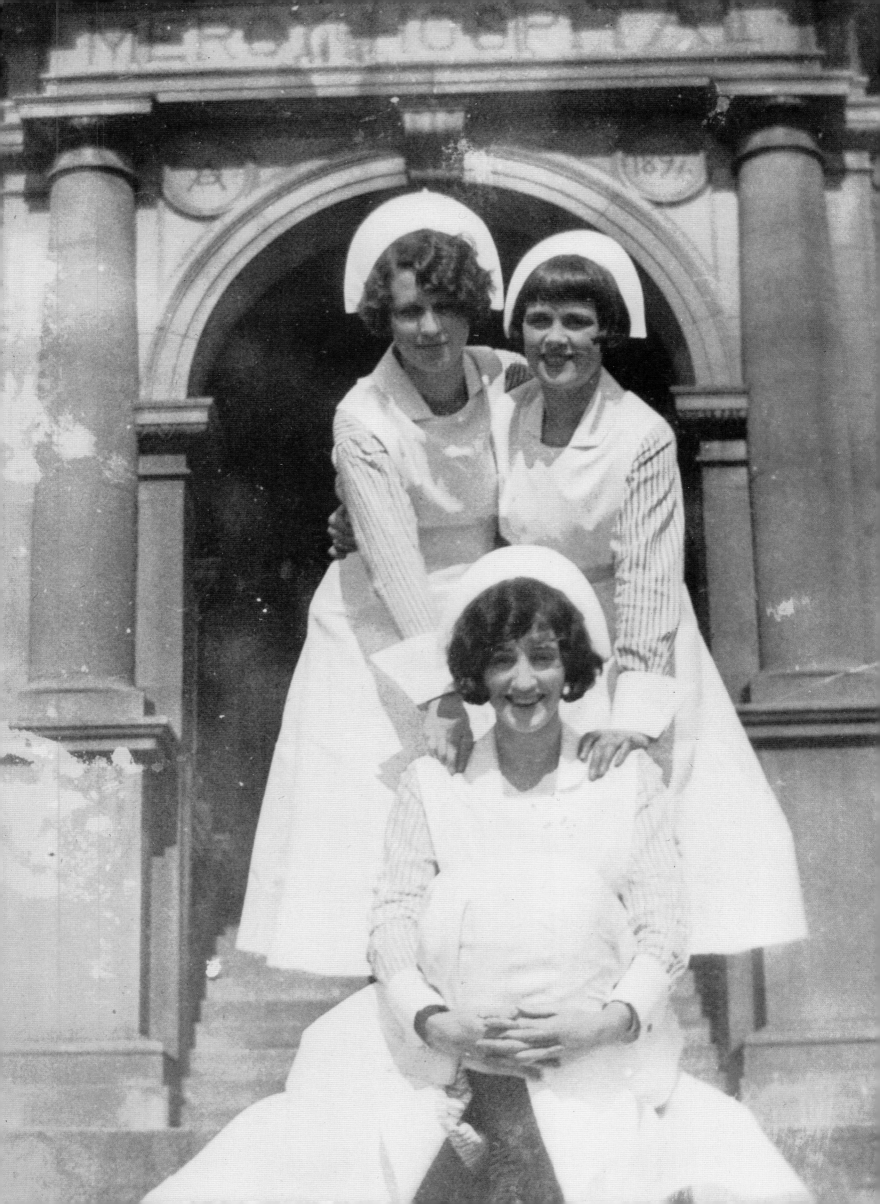

to undergo a major reorganization known as the "Amalgamation." Sister Evangelista played an important part in this revitalization, and her talents were needed in Council Bluffs. This was the fourth administrative change at Mercy Des Moines in 26 years.

COMMITMENT TO EDUCATION

Developments in medical technology and clinical practice were making the education of hospital staff an ongoing and demanding obligation.[33] Mercy became an enthusiastic participant in National Hospital Day activities, the Catholic Hospital Association, and more actively, in the Iowa Catholic Hospital Association.

National Hospital Day: Beginning in the mid-1920s, Des Moines hospitals began participating in National Hospital Day, celebrated on the May birthday of Florence Nightingale. Open houses and nursing school graduation exercises were held in conjunction with this occasion each year. The event became an opportunity for the public to visit hospitals "to focus attention on the many services hospitals render and the important work they are doing, not only in the care of those who are sick or injured, but in maintaining the health of the community, and in safeguarding future citizens through the training of nurses and other health workers."[34]

Mercy participated in this activity with an open house, handing out specially printed brochures and holding graduation exercises the preceding evening. Mercy's participation in National Hospital Day continued for many years. During these observances in 1938, the newly graduated nursing class participated in a tree planting ceremony on Mercy's grounds, with Bishop Gerald Bergan in attendance. More than 600 persons toured the hospital.[35]

Iowa Catholic Hospital Association: Mercy hosted the annual October meeting of the Iowa Catholic Hospital Association in 1926. Fifty sisters from Catholic hospitals in Iowa and Nebraska attended the convention which was held for the first time in Des Moines.[36] The two-day conference began with the celebration of Solemn High Mass by Mercy chaplain, Father Vitus Stoll, in St. Catherine's Hall for Business Women at Seventeenth and Grand. There were eleven educational sessions on topics such as: housekeeping, physician/intern relationships, nursing education, diabetes, public health nursing, hospital care of children, x-ray, basal metabolism, and dietetics. Clinical presentations and tours were held at Mercy and Broadlawns hospitals. The days ended with Benediction of the Blessed Sacrament.[37]

ENDURING THE CHALLENGES

As a result of World War I, Iowa was economically depressed during the 1920s. Many farmers over-extended themselves by purchasing land and equipment in order to increase food production and meet wartime needs. An excess of farm products and the resulting market downturn left many Iowa farmers struggling or unable to pay debts.[38]

The Council Bluffs Sisters of Mercy faced the challenge of returning Mercy Hospital in Des Moines to first-class status. Although plagued by the same kinds of economic problems confronting all Iowans during the 1920s, the sisters succeeded in bringing Mercy to its former glory. Their faith in God and love of people enabled them to endure and prepared them for the arduous tasks they were to meet in the next decade. At the time the Amalgamation took place in 1929, a "Union network" of provinces was established to assist the Sisters of Mercy in their quest to provide the best healthcare in the country.

Trouble lurked around every corner, it seemed, but the healthcare industry felt excited and challenged by the changes in technology and medicine that occurred in the 1920s. In stark contrast, the world economy loomed like a black cloud about to burst and downpour as never before.

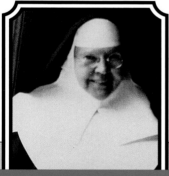

SISTER MARY BENEDICTA

In 1927, Sister Mary Benedicta McCarten became administrator of Mercy.

Born in Michigan as Frances McCarten, Sister Benedicta entered the Sisters of Mercy in 1903. After making her perpetual vows, she studied nursing at Mercy in Council Bluffs. Sister Benedicta taught at St. Patrick's in Imogene, Iowa, and also at the preparatory school at Mount Loretto for several years.

From 1911 to 1927, Sister Benedicta worked at Mercy in Council Bluffs, first in nursing and then as superior. It was from this administrative position that she came to Mercy in Des Moines. Sister Benedicta and Sister Evangelista were very well acquainted because they entered the convent at the same time and had worked together in nursing at Council Bluffs and in teaching at Imogene.

Those who remember Sister Benedicta say she was a very quiet, humble, and kind person, with a cute laugh. She remained administrator until 1935.

ADMINISTRATOR 1927-1935

CHAPTER TWO

A TEST OF STRENGTH: THE GREAT DEPRESSION

No depression in United States history has matched the suffering and long years of poverty spawned by the Great Depression of 1929-1941. "It affected not only the working class, middle class, and poor, but also the many wealthy who became the newly poor."[1]

"For the American hospital system, the Depression was a frightening and dangerous time. Room capacities were overtaxed in typical government hospitals, as the number of those who could not afford to pay swelled, and the sick were forced to find the only care they could afford. On the other hand, not-for-profit hospital admissions dropped, denying these institutions one of their best sources of income. Other income from donations and gifts dwindled significantly. By the end of 1932, the collapse of the voluntary hospital system seemed a real possibility."[2]

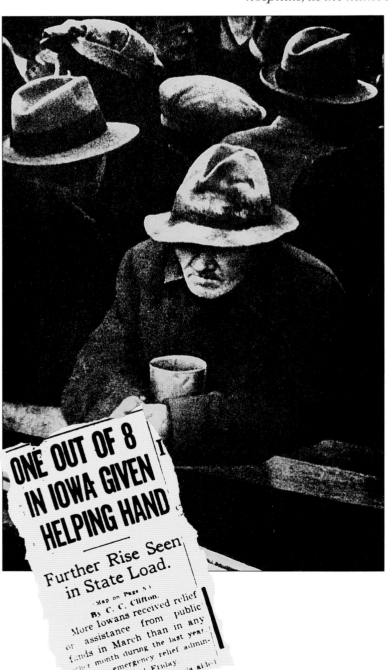

ONE OUT OF 8 IN IOWA GIVEN HELPING HAND

Further Rise Seen in State Load.

Map on Page 51
By C. C. Clifton.
More Iowans received relief or assistance from public funds in March than in any other month during the last year, the Iowa emergency relief administration reported Friday.
The number of individuals aided

One Des Moines healthcare facility became a Depression statistic: Iowa Lutheran Maternity Hospital, located at 1409 Clark Street, closed. This facility was opened in 1914 by the Congregational Church. In 1925, a three-story addition was planned with high hopes, but a year later, the hospital experienced severe financial difficulty.

On January 26, 1926, Iowa Lutheran merged with Iowa Congregational Hospital, expanding Iowa Lutheran's bed capacity to 200 and turning the newly acquired facility into a maternity hospital.[3] This maternity hospital continued to operate until the early 1930s when the financial burden of operating two separate buildings became too great. The maternity service eventually was moved to Iowa Lutheran's main facility on Pennsylvania Avenue. The Clark Street building sat empty for several years. The Sisters of Mercy and the Catholic Women's League rescued the building and turned it into the first Bishop Drumm Home for the Aged in 1939.[4]

THE DARK CLOUD

Words of the generation who lived through the Depression have echoed throughout time: "Anybody that didn't experience the Depression...it's hard to explain to them the situation that really existed then."[5]

The John McIlhon family knew a long association with Mercy. They experienced the Depression when their father lost his job at the Ford Motor Company in Des Moines. Mr. McIlhon had worked at Mercy, but since his first love was automobiles, he secured a job at the automobile factory. When he lost the Ford Motor Company job, Mr. McIlhon returned to his former work at Mercy as a licensed boiler engineer. Not long after returning to work at Mercy, he experienced a 10 percent cut in salary that he never regained.[6] This 10 percent payroll cut at Mercy reflected the climate in many other Midwestern hospitals.[7]

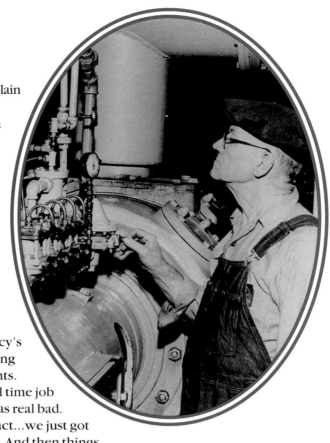

As a young woman, Agnes Hardin worked in Mercy's business office. She remembered that one time during the Depression the staff was asked to pray for patients. "How could I ever forget it," she related. "I had a full time job so another girl and I divided a job between us.[8] It was real bad. You couldn't even pay the bills sometimes, and in fact...we just got enough to rent an apartment. We ate at the hospital. And then things picked up."[9]

As the 1930s dawned, there were several institutions providing health care in Des Moines: Benedict Home, 30 beds; Broadlawns Isolation Hospital, 30 beds; Broadlawns General, 100 beds; Broadlawns Tuberculosis facility, 200 beds; Iowa Lutheran, 150 beds; Iowa Lutheran Maternity, 37 beds; Iowa Methodist, 239 beds; Mercy, 148 beds; Polyclinic, 69 beds; the Retreat, 50 beds; and the Salvation Army Retreat and Maternity Home, 15 beds. Bed counts did not include bassinets.[10]

Five of these institutions were given standardization approval by the American College of Surgeons: Mercy, Iowa Lutheran, Iowa Lutheran Maternity, Iowa Methodist, and Broadlawns Tuberculosis Hospital.[11] Mercy proudly received the stamp of approval from two other accrediting agencies: The American Medical Association and the Iowa State Board of Nurses.

During the spring of 1930, Des Moines hospitals overflowed, and some institutions used the hallways for patient care. In an effort to improve services and to speed the patients' recovery, Mercy, Iowa Lutheran, and Iowa Methodist eliminated morning visiting hours. At the same time, hospitals faced pressures to continue implementing standards. Recognizing the importance of cancer research and tracking, the American College of Surgeons urged hospitals to begin cancer registry programs. Fee-splitting was condemned, and the subject of equal rights for osteopaths and chiropractors as medical physicians became a prominent issue.

A survey at that time showed the startling statistic that the United States ranked highest among civilized countries in infant mortality. There were 6.5 deaths per 1,000 live births. Iowa ranked fairly low on a list of individual states at 4.8 deaths per 1,000 live births.[12]

A SLOWER PACE
The period of the early 1930s at Mercy saw small changes. There were no additions to the existing physical plant. There was little change on the inside in some areas. The staff tried to make do and save money for the sisters. One sister remarked that throughout it all, "the spirit was the best. We tried hard to help each other."[13]

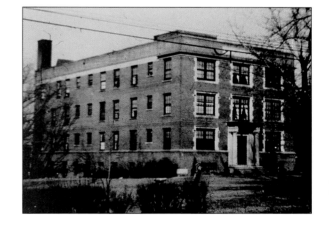

John McIlhon, *top*, came to Mercy during Depression years, after losing his job with Ford Motor Company. One Des Moines healthcare facility, Iowa Lutheran Maternity, *above*, became a statistic of the Depression when it closed in the early 1930s.

In this spirit of cooperation, the Mercy sisters once again turned to their ever-faithful physicians for help. Every surgeon personally purchased instruments worth as much as $5,000 to $10,000. At one medical staff meeting, Mercy's surgeons were asked to donate a few of their surgical instruments to the hospital. It was hoped that as the collection of instruments became adequate, physicians would provide a yearly maintenance fee to keep the necessary instruments on hand.

"[Instruments] were very fragile and [people were] always [taking them] out to be sharpened. A lot of surgeons kept them at home. They kept duffel bags with instruments [inside] wrapped in towels. Regular surgeons [stored them in] lockers; others kept [instruments] in their car.

[The doctors] would bring them to the hospital before a case and turn them over to Sister Mary Pauline who was chief of the surgical section. She would pick out the ones that were going to be used for a particular surgery and have them washed and sterilized and ready to go." [14]

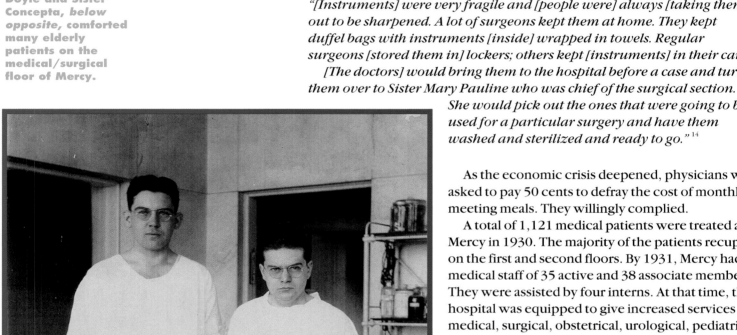

Dr. Jesse McNamee, *below left,* **and Dr. Henry Decker,** *below right,* **were interns at Mercy.** &. Nurse Rachel Doyle and Sister Concepta, *below opposite,* comforted many elderly patients on the medical/surgical floor of Mercy.

As the economic crisis deepened, physicians were asked to pay 50 cents to defray the cost of monthly staff meeting meals. They willingly complied.

A total of 1,121 medical patients were treated at Mercy in 1930. The majority of the patients recuperated on the first and second floors. By 1931, Mercy had a medical staff of 35 active and 38 associate members. They were assisted by four interns. At that time, the hospital was equipped to give increased services in the medical, surgical, obstetrical, urological, pediatric, pathological, radiological, physiotherapeutic, dietetic, and emergency departments.

Mercy's surgical suite consisted of three major operating rooms, as well as a cast room; eye, ear, nose and throat room; sterilizing rooms; and an equivalent doctor's rest room, complete with shower facilities. A total of 1,525 patients came under the care of the surgical staff during 1930. Sister Mary Thomas Wilson supervised the operating room in addition to being in charge of the School of Nursing. She was assisted by Sister Mary Leona Weil.

There were three delivery rooms, a preparation and sterilization room, labor room, an isolation room, and also a doctor's rest room in Mercy's birthing facility. A total of 296 babies first greeted the world at Mercy in 1930. Three-hundred children were cared for in the pediatrics department. Mercy's average daily census for the year was 120. During that same year, more than 17,500 tests were performed in the laboratory.

The x-ray department, supervised by Sister Mary Winifred Leusen, utilized apparatus that would do any type of work desired in this field. A fully equipped splint room stood ready in close proximity to the radiographic room. Sister Mary Jerome Burns became the x-ray technician in 1932 when Sister Winifred left Mercy for a new assignment. Sister Winifred returned to Mercy in 1936 for two years. Sister Jerome became head of the x-ray department in 1939. She went to St. Mary's Hospital in South Bend in 1941 to study for her nursing degree and for additional training as a registered x-ray technician. While Sister Jerome was away from Mercy, her niece, Kay (Tuffield) Hardie worked as chief technician. [15]

SISTER MARY CONCEPTA

Sister Mary Concepta Mullins came to Mercy in 1931 and remained for more than 60 years. Urged not to "give your old bones to God," Margaret Mullins was among the Irish wave of young women who came to the United States around the time of World War I.

Margaret lived with her two aunts and received her nurses' training at Mercy Council Bluffs. She wanted to enter the Sisters of Mercy immediately after graduating, but her aunts asked that she try private duty nursing because they wanted her: "to be prepared to go into the convent, and not expect them to educate you." [16] Margaret practiced private nursing for about two years, learning "the American way, and how the Americans lived. And I found out. No one had nurses then. Only those who could afford private nurses. So that brought me into better homes." [17]

In 1925, Margaret became a permanent member of the Sisters of Mercy as Sister Mary Concepta Mullins. For a few years, she nursed in Centerville, until she was sent to Des Moines in 1931. For the majority of her years at Mercy, Sister Concepta served as supervisor of the second floor in the Central Wing. The patients in her care were mostly medical patients, and those recovering from surgery.

Sister Concepta is remembered as being "always calm and cool and friendly and nice." [18] A graduate nursing student recalls that when her husband lay dying, "Sister Concepta came and stayed with me in the room the whole night until [he] died. She was so sweet to me." [19]

The healthcare profession grew a great deal in the years Sister Concepta was at Mercy: "The changes that came along during those years were enormous, and before beginning any new procedure, I always checked it out." [20]

When asked if many early patients died, Sister Concepta said: "When you look back, it's about the same [as today.] The patients came in. Many got well, and some died. You can't save everyone. [In those days,] we'd get patients that nothing could be done except to keep them comfortable." [21]

Sister Concepta retired from active nursing in 1968. For several years, she worked in the hospital's pastoral care department. In 1973, she joined the public relations department. Sister Concepta retired from active service in 1979. About her life, she said: "Well, I could tell you I've lived three lives." [22]

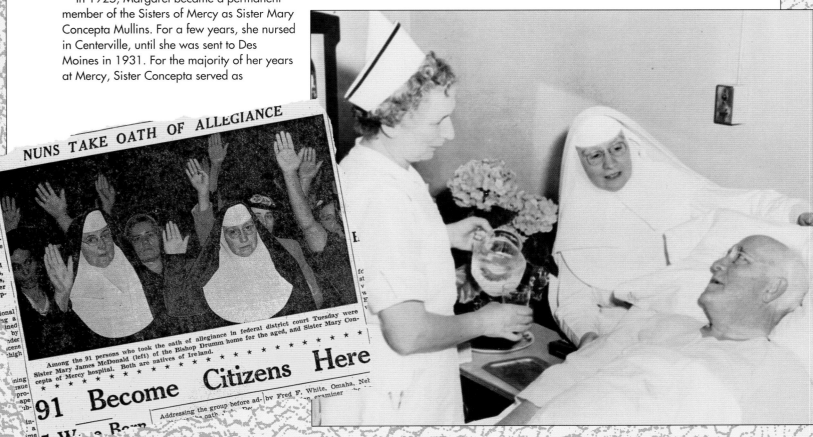

NUNS TAKE OATH OF ALLEGIANCE

Among the 91 persons who took the oath of allegiance in federal district court Tuesday were Sister Mary James McDonald (left) of the Bishop Drumm home for the aged, and Sister Mary Concepta of Mercy hospital. Both are natives of Ireland.

91 Become Citizens Here

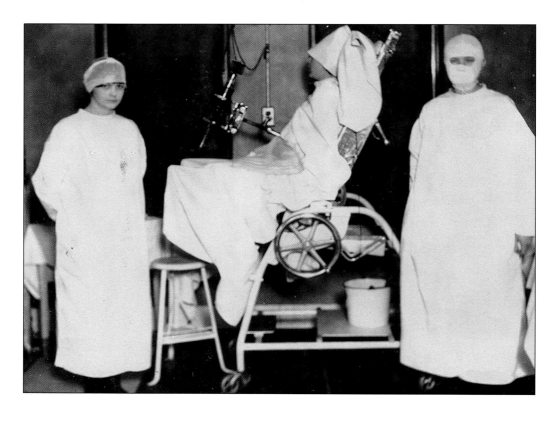

A sidebar note reads:

In 1925, a tonsillectomy cost $11.20. That price included a one-day stay at $4, the operating room cost of $5, medicine at $2, laboratory expenses of $1, and a discount of 80 cents.

A Lower Census

As a result of the Depression, Mercy's census dropped to 99 patients per day by 1931. During the early years, gains were small, and by 1937, the daily census still averaged only 105. The highest per-day census during the Depression years was 150, and the lowest was seventy.[23]

It was an ongoing struggle to keep the hospital operating. Many people could not pay for food, let alone medical care. Their poverty kept them from seeking treatment for illness, and simple cases became critical, forcing longer confinement when the patients finally sought hospitalization. The overflow of poor patients taxed the inadequate facilities at the Polk County hospital to the limit, and the average census of all "church" hospitals in Des Moines was 46 percent capacity.[24] Financial losses to Mercy for the years 1934, 1935, and 1936 totaled more than $100,000.[25] Payment for services came to Mercy in many forms in those days. Some proffered produce or whatever else they could afford, which was very little. One person remembered:

> *"When my mother went [to Mercy] to have my brother, Jim, she had a double room and it cost $2.50 a day....There was no insurance...so for many years...we paid $1.00 a week...to pay it off."* [26]

Another family offered their son's services to pay for his appendectomy. After Jimmy Heles recovered from his surgery, he came to work in the surgery department. He became acquainted with Sister Joseph, and when his bill was paid in full, she hired him to help her in the laboratory after school. Heles pursued a career in science and retired after 33 years as chief metallurgist at the John Deere Company in Ankeny.[27]

Compassionate Service

The idea of hospital insurance was discussed as early as 1933. Staff members were poorly informed on the subject. They had very little to suggest either for or against insurance, and the issue was tabled.[28]

Blue Cross insurance became available in 1939. Among the first to purchase a policy under the new plan were Mr. and Mrs. James D. Brien. Their daughter, Mary Bridget, was born at Mercy on Christmas Day 1940, and her parents received the first maternity benefits from the new plan.

Mercy continued to extend charity to those in need during the Depression. Many "Knights of the Road," as the wandering poor were known, found something to eat in Sister Lucia's kitchen. Sometimes they were offered a chance to do menial jobs in exchange for a meal. Sister Lucia insisted that her guests wash their hands before sitting down to eat.[29]

A NEW BISHOP

Late in October 1933, Mercy lost a great friend when Bishop Drumm passed away. As the second bishop of Des Moines, Thomas W. Drumm had guided the sisters through the turbulent change of administration in 1922. A former Mercy chaplain, Monsignor Raymond Conley, remembered: "Bishop Drumm suffered from intense high blood pressure" during his last few years. He became "unpredictable in his reactions, and his condition became a great distress to all who knew him."[30]

Bishop Drumm was hospitalized several times before he died. Sister Joseph always could tell if he felt well enough to see her when she came to visit him in the hospital:

> "I remember he was a patient in 318 when I went up to see him. We were very good friends....When he called me 'Sister,' that was a sign he wanted to be left alone. When I was 'Joseph,' he wanted me to stay."[31]

Bishop Drumm died at Mercy on October 24, 1933. His final illness lasted approximately one month. Another dynamic man, Bishop Gerald T. Bergan, stepped into Bishop Drumm's shoes.

Bishop Bergan was characterized as one who "gave the distinct feeling that he liked you and was personally interested in your well-being."[32] Bishop Bergan quickly developed friendships throughout the Des Moines Diocese, and his efforts helped Mercy's campaign to acquire community funds for the nurses' dormitory in 1946. He retained close ties to Des Moines even after being appointed archbishop of Omaha in 1948.

ANNUAL SURGICAL CLINICS

Mercy Hospital has been blessed with the talents of gifted and caring surgeons from the time it first opened. By the 1930s, a new generation of surgeons began to influence the direction of Mercy as more surgical specializations emerged.

Under the direction of the president of the Mercy Medical Staff, Dr. Bernard C. Barnes, annual surgical clinics began at Mercy in 1935. Described as a "post-graduate school for physicians," the two-day clinic welcomed more than 250 Iowa physicians in June 1935.

That year for the first time in Iowa surgical history, physicians attempted to restore fertility to a female patient. The woman was given a spinal anesthesia, allowing her to be awake during the entire operation. Other surgeries included eye-straightening for two children, collapsing a tubercular lung, plastic surgeries involving skin grafts,

LUNCH

brain surgery which included the reconstruction of an infant's skull, and a type of blood transfusion involving direct blood flow from donor to patient.

Two new types of anesthesia were introduced at that time: cyclural sodium (Epivol Soluble) which was injected intravenously and tribromethanol (Avertin), introduced into the colon through an enema. These anesthetics were reported to be "hangover" free and particularly beneficial for tonsillectomies or short procedures involving children. During longer operations they were supplemented by gas or ether.

Many notable physicians from across the country gave lectures and case presentations to augment clinical demonstrations. As current president of the American Medical Association, Dr. Walter Bierring from Des Moines, recommended the Mercy clinic as an excellent educational medium. At the closing session, Dr. Barnes announced the decision to make the clinic an annual event. A total of 81 surgeries had been performed during these two days in 1935.

The clinic presented an opportunity for Mercy to announce a restructuring program and the results of its $50,000 modernization. Sister Benedicta outlined the departmental reorganization: The first floor was devoted to pediatrics; the second floor cared for internal medicine patients; the third floor was dedicated to obstetrics and eye, ear, nose and throat; the fourth floor handled surgical patients and orthopedics; the fifth floor—previously a storage area and nursing dormitory—was to be used for the care of urology patients. Forty new beds could be accommodated on the new fifth floor. The nursing students were relocated from the West Wing to the East Wing.[33]

By the time the surgical clinic was offered in 1936, Mercy proudly displayed its remodeled operating facilities. The hospital spent $6,000 to update operating theaters, providing lights that eliminated heat and shadows for $500 each. Sixty-nine surgical procedures, including those done by Drs. H. N. Anderson and D. C. Wirtz, were performed in the new area during the 1936 clinic.[34]

Mercy's annual surgical clinic continued through 1938. During the last two clinics, cataract removal, caesareans, and special orthopedic procedures were highlighted.[35]

EXCEPTIONAL MERCY CARE

Mercy was the only hospital in Des Moines to hold open house for National Hospital Day in May 1937. More than 400 interested citizens toured the hospital that day. Special exhibits had been set up in the diet area, pharmacy, laboratory, nursery, x-ray, and operating rooms. The star of the day was a premature baby thriving in an incubator located in Mercy's nursery.[36]

Two interesting cases were treated at Mercy during this time. One involved a young lady who was injured while performing in a flying show over Des Moines. Her parachute failed to open on her fifth jump from a hot air balloon at an altitude of 150 feet. Miraculously, she survived with no broken bones although she did have severe tissue damage. Recovering at Mercy, she said:

"I suppose I'll have to return to the old crowd and the old tiresome way of doing things. I would rather be up there in the air, where things are clean and fresh. If that's what they call 'living dangerously,' then that's what I want."[37]

Another case involved the waiter who kept forgetting the soup, at a club where Dr. Walter D. Abbott frequently ate. Instead of firing the man, the club arranged for him to see Dr. Abbott for an evaluation. As it turned out, the patient had a very large cyst at the base of the brain, presumably caused by a fall as a child. Dr. Abbott removed the cyst and the prognosis for recovery was good. The club's patrons looked forward to getting what they ordered.[38]

Mercy participated in National Hospital Day and yearly Iowa Catholic Hospital Association conventions. From 1935 to 1938, the hospital also held annual surgical clinics that became known as post-graduate education for physicians.

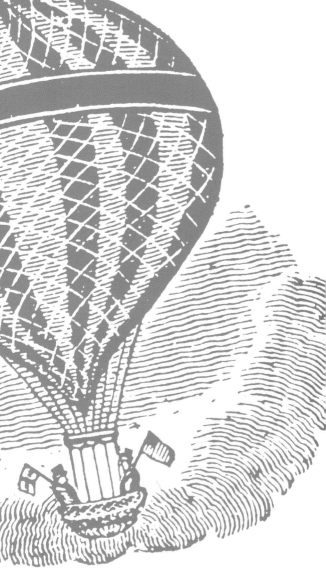

THE IRON LUNG

As the desire for sophistication in patient care evolved, so did the need for specialized equipment to treat patients. A cure for polio eluded researchers for many years. In 1910 and 1916, there had been severe outbreaks of this crippling disease in Iowa. The death toll stood at 37 children and adults for the first ten months of 1937. The disease brought about a new type of patient care management in 1937 when the iron lung was first introduced in Iowa. Three patients who would not have survived polio in earlier outbreaks, were alive because of the introduction of the iron lung.

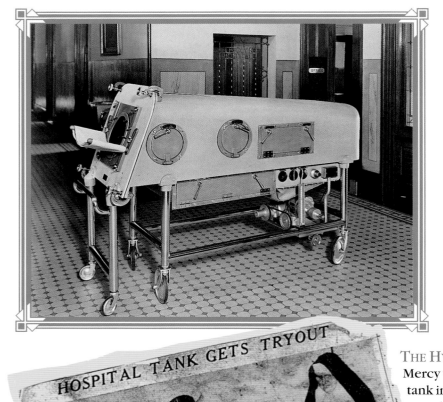

The first piece of this specialized respirator in Des Moines was used at Iowa Methodist in September of 1937.[39] Mercy first began using the iron lung after the Des Moines Police Department Auxiliary donated $1,500 to purchase the equipment in the fall of 1939. The donors requested that services be provided for free. The special feature of the iron lung was the ease with which it could be moved from room to room in the hospital, and, if necessary, outside the hospital.[40]

THE HYDROTHERAPY TANK

Mercy was the first Iowa hospital to use a hydrotherapy tank in their physical therapy department. The purchase price of $3,000, astronomical during this time, was partially funded with dollars left over from the purchase of the iron lung.

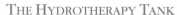

The huge tank, shaped like a figure eight was nearly 10 feet long. Powerful turbines agitated water around the patient. The device helped to relax nerves, strengthen muscles, and improve circulation. The temperature and the force of the water added a buoyancy which helped patients learn to move their limbs, while taking the stiffness out of joints.

The hydrotherapy tank promised to aid victims of polio and similar diseases.[41] The first Mercy patient to use this equipment was the father of one of Mercy's School of Nursing students, Margaret (Niles) Albertson.[42]

OTHER INNOVATIONS

A new portable x-ray camera became a useful tool during many hip-pinning operations performed at Mercy at the end of the 1930s. When the surgeon had placed the pin, a technician would take an x-ray with the portable unit. The technician would run down the stairs from surgery to the ground floor of the West Wing. The surgeon would wait five to seven minutes until the x-ray showed whether or not the pin placement was correct.[43]

Mercy began using the iron lung, top, to treat polio victims, after the Des Moines Police Department Auxiliary donated $1,500 to purchase the equipment in 1939. ❧ Mercy was the first hospital to use a hydrotherapy tank, above, in their physical therapy department.

Another innovation began at Mercy in the late 1930s: the electrocardiograph machine. Dr. Harold Anderson reported on the use of this new piece of equipment during a 1937 medical staff meeting. He stated that between 80 and 90 electrocardiograms had been performed at Mercy during the previous year. Mercy offered the option of giving an official interpretation to the attending physician. Or, if the physician desired, the actual tracings would be sent to him. The total charge for the test was five dollars.[44]

Another medical advancement during the late 1930s was the widespread use of sulfa drugs. These drugs came into worldwide use and quickly earned a reputation as "wonder drugs." Sulfa drugs did not have the best effect on certain types of bacteria.[45] Shortly after their appearance, a new drug—penicillin—began to make waves in medical circles, replacing sulfa as the "one to watch."

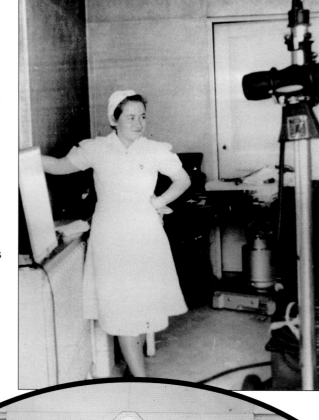

LOSS OF ACCREDITATION

Many stories which made news when they happened have another side rarely mentioned. Such was the case late in 1939 when Mercy, Iowa Methodist, and Iowa Lutheran lost their accreditation with the American College of Surgeons.

Historically, the suspension lasted two years, until the examining body could visit again. This time, another problem added fuel to the fire. Des Moines' physicians were accused of practicing fee-splitting, which was not allowed by the American College of Surgeons. There was another side to the story, however.

According to Dr. James Chambers, a new intern at Mercy in 1939, Des Moines surgeons were in great demand throughout the rural areas. Many of these surgeons kept an extra set of instruments in the trunks of their automobiles. A rural physician would call upon a surgeon-specialist for help with a specific type of surgery. The surgeon would travel to the requesting physician's town, and perform the surgery.

"They would go up to Boone, [or] to Stuart and operate on a patient. Then, the family doctor would do the postoperative work. The surgeon would come back to Des Moines, and they would converse on the telephone and he would go back out there in three or four days to see how they were. That was popular with most of the Des Moines surgeons I knew who were reputable and trained surgeons....[They went] out of town three days a week. It was a lucrative practice for them.

Fee-splitting was a dirty word, but it was customary. The surgeon would pay the doctor that would scrub for him a portion of the fee, whether he did anything or not. He might just stand there, but he was paid a portion of the fee and that was considered ethical. Later, it

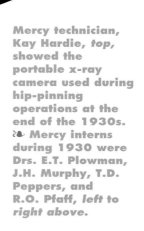

Mercy technician, Kay Hardie, *top*, showed the portable x-ray camera used during hip-pinning operations at the end of the 1930s. Mercy interns during 1930 were Drs. E.T. Plowman, J.H. Murphy, T.D. Peppers, and R.O. Pfaff, *left* to *right above.*

Miss Leah C. Cameron, *below*, worked as Mercy's pharmacist from 1916 to 1938. Children found Miss Cameron to be a loving, caring person. ఊ Peter Markunas, *middle opposite*, began working as a janitor at Mercy in 1916. In the 1930s, he cooked in the kitchen, *top opposite*, where he also provided moments of glee to employees' children. Dan, John, Mary, and Pat McIlhon, *bottom opposite*, watched in awe many times as Pete jumped over the kitchen table at their whimsical beckoning.

became unethical and finally was dropped, but it was an accepted thing. I don't know whether it was good or bad but one way or another that was what was happening." [46]

Administrators of the three suspended hospitals met and found they shared common inconsistencies in record keeping, irregular staff meetings, and rumors of fee-splitting. Each of the hospitals prepared a pledge against fee-splitting, for all of their physicians to sign . A copy was presented to the American College of Surgeons, and in 1940 after just one year without certification, the accrediting agency was satisfied that the hospitals met requirements for accreditation, and they all were reinstated. [47]

WORKERS' UNIONS ARRIVE

The late 1930s brought unions to workers, and the threat of strikes plagued hospitals. Mercy experienced two strikes during this time. Student nurses staged a two-hour strike in 1936 because they did not like the new roommate schedule. This resolved itself when the students served a suspension lasting for several days, and the desired roommates were reassigned.

Eleven janitors and maids lost their jobs at Mercy in 1937 for "disloyalty to the hospital." According to a hospital spokesman: "The employees held secret meetings and we were informed that they planned to call a strike for higher wages." [48] The Building Service Employees Union claimed the incident was just a misunderstanding. They said no strike was planned for the hospital, but several of Mercy's janitors had recently joined their union. One young wife and mother at that time remembers: "The union wanted to get into Mercy. My husband, Jimmy McLaughlin, and several others joined the union. They were fired by Mercy. My husband was not a strong man, and so, one of the sisters got his job at Mercy back for him." [49]

HARD TIMES, GOOD MEMORIES

In spite of the hard times experienced during the 1930s, good memories remain. Two young men—Dr. Daniel F. Crowley, Jr. and Monsignor John McIlhon—have vivid childhood memories about their fathers who worked at Mercy during that time. Dr. Crowley's father, Dr. Daniel F. Crowley, Sr., was an intern who came to Mercy from Creighton in 1906. The senior Dr. Crowley continued his long association as a general practitioner/surgeon with Mercy until his death in 1959. Dan, Jr. remembers accompanying his father to Mercy for rounds after Sunday Mass. However, he and his brother and sister frequently were left in the care of Miss Leah C. Cameron, Mercy's pharmacist. Most adults found her intimidating, but the Crowley children thought she was a loving, caring person:

> *"She always had candy for us, and she always had a mark on the wall somewhere. She would see how tall we were and how we were growing. So it was an entirely different picture of Miss Cameron than the one [other] people had. We were crazy about her."* [50]

Monsignor McIlhon also had fond memories of Miss Cameron. He recalls: "My dad liked Cameron....You would see them together and pretty soon they would be roaring and laughing. I suppose they were telling stories." [51] Miss Cameron left Mercy in the fall of 1938 and joined the pharmacy staff of St. Mary's Hospital in Rochester, Minnesota. She is remembered there for her good heart and for teaching pharmacy interns two things: "Put things in the WANT Book and date everything." [52]

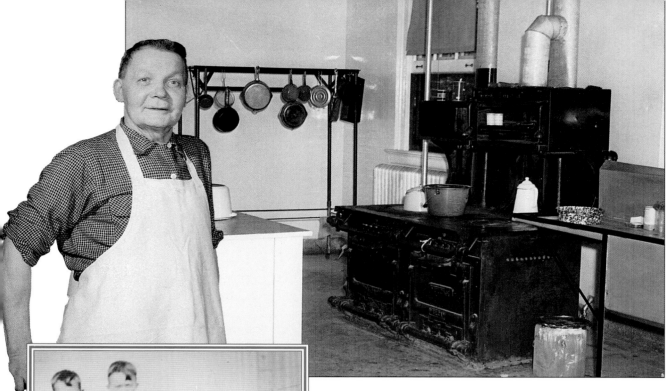

Other Mercy employees were memorable as well. Young boys at that time were said to have "hollow legs," and they managed to get invited with great frequency to the Mercy kitchen. There, they were fed by Sister Lucia or one of her helpers, Stacia McLaughlin or Pete Markunas.

The McIlhon children anxiously awaited these invitations. The greatest time of all was on certain Sundays when Sister Lucia made ice cream. This treat was virtually unheard of during the Depression.

"Now it wasn't every Sunday, but apparently they made their own ice cream. She would serve us great, big balls of ice cream and cookies. I would just sit there as if [this] was the final ultimate goal of my life's purpose, sitting in the kitchen with Sister Lucia, eating ice cream." [53]

And there was entertainment as well. Peter Markunas was the cook. At the children's bidding, he would place one hand on the table and jump over it. "I would just stand there amazed, and always wondered if I got as big as he, could I jump over the table like that. But I wouldn't dare try it in front of Sister Lucia." [54]

CHANGES IN THE ECONOMY

The economy was showing gains as the 1930s drew to a close, and the interns thought this would be a good time to approach Mercy's administration for an advance in salary. After reviewing the request, the executive committee decided that the salary should remain at $25 per month.[55] However, to one of Mercy's interns, the monthly fee was a godsend. "We were magnificently paid here. In addition to the $25, we received board and room. When I came here I thought, 'I'm going to be rich.'" [56]

As if the monetary challenge to keep hospitals open was not enough during the 1930s, it was a challenge for administrators to keep up with the deluge of newly implemented federal legislation. The Catholic Hospital Association allied itself with the American Hospital Association and the Protestant Hospital Association in a committee to strengthen the voluntary system. By the mid-1930s, although eleven percent of church-sponsored hospitals closed, those that stayed open soon returned to financial stability.[57]

PREPARING FOR THE 1940s

As one hurdle after another was met and cleared during the 1930s, another presented itself. The final challenge of the decade turned all eyes to the other side of the world. Barely 21 years had passed since the "War to End All Wars," and it appeared there was to be another.

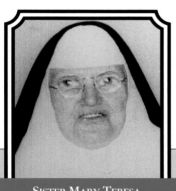

SISTER MARY TERESA

Mercy's administrator from 1935 to 1941 was Sister Mary Teresa Connell. Caroline Connell was born in Providence, Rhode Island, in 1875. She became a Mercy sister in 1900.

Sister Teresa worked primarily in office and domestic work before coming to Mercy Des Moines in 1922 as head houskeeper. Sister Teresa remained in Des Moines for the rest of her life.

In 1927, she was appointed superior of St. Catherine's Hall for Business Women. In 1935, Sister Teresa became administrator of Mercy. She left Mercy in 1941 to return to St. Catherine's. In 1948, she became superior of Des Moines' Bishop Drumm Home.

Sister Teresa returned to Mercy in the early 1950s and died in the hospital on February 6, 1953. One person remembers Sister Teresa as "the fairest person." [58]

ADMINISTRATOR 1935-1941

CHAPTER THREE
UNITING FOR FREEDOM

As war clouds loomed on the eastern horizon, those who believed in freedom united to fight the enemy. This endeavor proved to be the impetus that kept the thin margin of economic recovery, which had occurred during the late 1930s, growing within the United States.

An immediate need developed for medical personnel to administer physical examinations for draftees as soon as the Selective Service was inaugurated in 1941. More than 740 Iowa physicians served in this capacity, rendering their services free of charge. When it was apparent that many physicians would be needed for overseas duty, the sisters feared Mercy would not have enough physicians to care for their patients. Through voluntary enlistment, the quota of physicians was met.[1] At one time during World War II, twenty-nine of Mercy's medical staff physicians were in active duty.[2]

When the conflict ended 12 Iowa physicians had lost their lives, including Dr. Richard Morden and Dr. Ralph Snodgrass from Des Moines.[3]

A SHORTAGE OF INTERNS

In the summer of 1941, there were no interns at Mercy. One young man found work as Mercy's "house officer" through a Chicago employment agency. In this position, Dr. Frederick Katzmann, performed the same duties as a rotating intern. He had completed two internships, and Mercy's position did not qualify as a residency because he did not receive training in a specialty.

Dr. Katzmann prepared histories and physicals for the patients, and assisted in surgery or obstetrics—anything he was assigned to do. His pay of $100 per month was somewhat better than the regular rate. However, as the only Mercy intern for six months in 1941, Dr. Katzmann performed the work formerly done by four men who were each paid $25 per month.

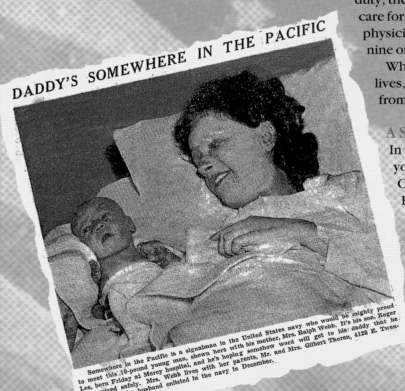

DADDY'S SOMEWHERE IN THE PACIFIC

Somewhere in the Pacific is a signalman in the United States navy who would be mighty proud to meet this 10-pound young man, shown here with his mother, Mrs. Ralph Webb. It's his son, Roger Lee, born Friday at Mercy hospital, and he's hoping somehow word will get to his daddy that he has arrived safely. Mrs. Webb lives with her parents, Mr. and Mrs. Gilbert Thoren, 4128 E. Twenty-ninth st. Her husband enlisted in the navy in December.

"I walked up to Mercy for the first time in July 1941. Sister Pauline was the one who received me. The first thing she said to me was: 'We want you to work very hard.' I was the only one and I had to take care of the emergency room. I hardly left the hospital. When I did, I could be reached on a beeper that I carried already then."[4]

World War II separated families, and many children were born while Daddy was fighting overseas. Often, the first word soldiers received about births came from newspapers.

Eventually other interns came to join him. During 1942, help came to Dr. Katzmann when Dr. Erich Hollander arrived from Germany. Dr. Emmett Mathaison from Council Bluffs was "a very nice chap, red hair. And he and I and some nurses had pretty good times together."[5] There also was a Japanese lady doctor. "She was very efficient and

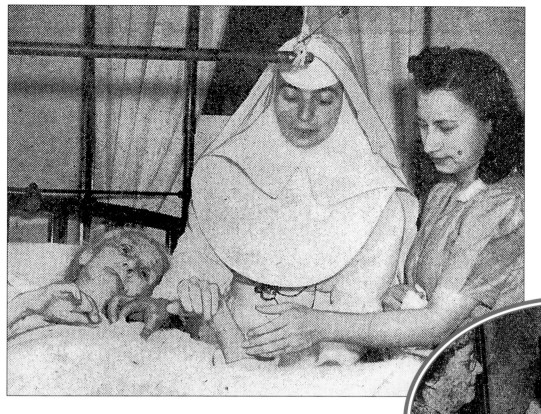

very competent." [6] This was Dr. Tsutayo N. Ichioka. Dr. Ichioka was born in Hawaii, although her ancestory was Japanese. The climate in the United States at that time made things difficult for the Japanese. However, Mercy welcomed Dr. Ichioka as resident house physician.

AN ACT OF CHARITY

The early 1940s were characterized by a massive volunteer effort by all citizens. Contributing to the World War II cause was on the mind of everyone. Hospitals faced staff shortages and asked for volunteers, encouraging them by offering special training classes through programs sponsored by the American Red Cross. Training was given in first aid, nurses' aid, hospital supplies, home service, hospital corps, home nursing, disaster corps, and Braille. Mercy participated in many training areas. Classes were held at Mercy to train the "Gray Ladies, hospital men volunteers, and nurses' aides." [7]

Sister Mary Sebastian Geneser remembered teaching some of these Red Cross-sponsored courses:

> *"Sister Mary Kevin [O'Sullivan] and I went out to the Presbyterian Church on Grand Ave. I think we had one class at St. Augustin's. It was home nursing. After that they wanted us to teach classes in nurses' aid. Then of course, they would come and work [at Mercy] on Saturdays and Sundays....They were doing it for nothing."* [8]

Many hours of service were given to Mercy by its dedicated corps of volunteers. One volunteer said:

> *"I worked full-time at the insurance company. Then I worked Saturday and Sunday where my heart was [at Mercy]...for the best part of a year. I did not get paid—I didn't expect to. No, that was my act of charity."* [9]

97

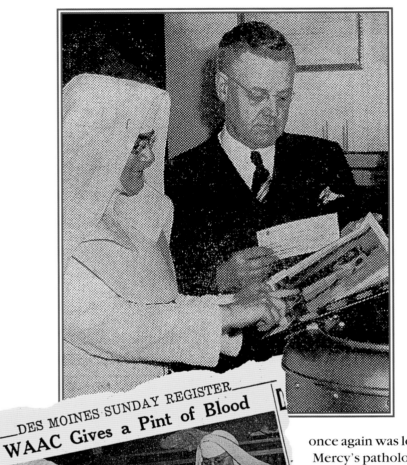

DES MOINES SUNDAY REGISTER

WAAC Gives a Pint of Blood

WAAC Auxiliary Frances Evans of Malone, N. Y., dropped into Mercy hospital Saturday to give a pint of her blood, for a blood-bank. After giving the blood to Sister Mary Joseph (left) and Sister Gonzaga, Miss Evans drank a pint of milk and was on her way.

Sister Mary Joseph Munch, *top,* **accepted the Des Moines Lions' Club's contribution to Mercy for a special refrigerated cabinet that stored donated blood.** *&* **Sisters Joseph and Gonzaga drew blood from an auxiliary member volunteer,** *above.*

THE MERCY LABORATORY

As part of the early World War II effort, Mercy established a blood plasma bank in its laboratory. Funds from the Des Moines Lions' Club made possible the purchase of a special refrigerated cabinet in which to store and process the donated blood.[10]

In 1943, Mercy received an award for its voluntary work in establishing this plasma bank. In a special KRNT radio broadcast sponsored by Banker's Trust Company, the laboratory staff accepted a citation of merit. Recognition was given to several groups and individuals who helped finance the blood-plasma equipment. More than 200 Des Moines citizens had already responded to the call for plasma donors, and the radio program encouraged donors to phone Sister Joseph to set up future plasma appointments.[11]

The 1940s marked many other changes for Mercy's laboratory. Dr. Franz Lengh was hired as resident pathologist in October 1940. Within six months of his arrival, Dr. Lengh had improved many photographic capabilities within the laboratory and encouraged the purchase of equipment to perform agglutination tests within 48 hours.[12] Dr. Lengh served as Mercy's pathologist until 1943, when Dr. William Hardesty replaced him. By December 1944, however, Mercy once again was looking for a pathologist.[13] Dr. Frank Coleman became Mercy's pathologist in 1946.

IN SPITE OF THE WAR

Mercy's staff kept quite busy during the war years. Events on Iowa soil followed the tides of time and nature. On New Year's Eve in 1941, a snowstorm created a bit of memorable history when it dropped 12 inches of snow on Des Moines. This, added to a previous accumulation of 10 inches, completely paralyzed the city.

"Nothing whatsoever moved. No car moved. No street car moved. A couple of doctors were caught in the hospital, among them Dr. Peasley. I remember it distinctly. Between [sic] two or three staff men, we took care of all of the 180 patients for maybe half a week before the traffic moved again and people could get in and out of the hospital. The snow caused total paralysis." [14]

One of the nurses finally managed to make it home, only to find the telephone ringing when she opened the door. It was the hospital asking if she had taken home the keys used on the floor where she worked. She found the missing keys in her pocket. "The staff said they could wait until I could get out to bring them by. The sister in charge had been able to patch together a set of keys they could use." [15]

New Deal legislation and the need for additional hospital beds provided funds to expand or develop community facilities for the defense program, commonly called the Lanham Act. In September 1941, Sister Mary Anita Paul, Mercy's new administrator who replaced Sister Mary Teresa Connell, applied for funds to expand the hospital.

Mercy planned to construct a new nurses' home and move the nursing students out of their dorm rooms in the main hospital and into the new building. This would allow Mercy to increase the number of patient beds to meet anticipated wartime needs. In early April 1942, however, Mercy's application was denied in favor of Broadlawns Hospital. Undaunted, Sister Anita applied for assistance from the Kansas City Public Health Service. This also was denied, but after applying a third time, monies were secured for Mercy based upon new legislation under the Bolton Act.

The 1943 Bolton Act established the Cadet Nursing Program, a federally subsidized program to encourage young women to pursue nursing. After finishing their training, graduate nurses pledged to serve in a civilian or military capacity until World War II ended. Mercy applied for the Cadet Nursing Program, and in return, qualified to apply for federal funding to expand its facilities to accommodate the expected influx of nursing students.

The Public Health Service and the Federal Works Agency informed Mercy that they would favor a construction project to house an additional 50 nurses. When the monies finally were allocated, Mercy received two grants: $72,000 given in September 1943, and $60,000 awarded in April 1945. The first grant came as a result of Mercy's participation in the Cadet Nursing Program. The second grant was given by the Federal Works Agency. The additional funds allowed Mercy to make the planned nurses' home longer and add a fourth floor, more than doubling the space of earlier plans.

A GOLDEN ANNIVERSARY

The year 1943 marked an important Mercy milestone: the golden anniversary of the opening of Mercy Hospital in Des Moines. Unusually—perhaps because of the war— the year passed without any notable celebration. It is more likely, however, that the sisters decided to celebrate Mercy's anniversary in 1944, fifty years after the East Wing first opened. On December 12, 1944, they did just that.

A Solemn Pontifical Mass of Thanks-giving was celebrated by Bishop Bergan and held at St. Ambrose Cathedral. Monsignor Stoll, former Mercy chaplain gave the homily.

In keeping with tradition, the Sisters of Mercy held open house, giving visitors a complete tour of Mercy with stops in the chapel, pediatrics department, and the obstetrics observation window. One of the guides stated that the census was down because "no one wants to be in a hospital on Christmas." This line was reported in the local newspaper the next morning, which caused the superintendent of Iowa Methodist to ask Mercy to take its patient overflow the next day. Sister Anita quickly answered: "Unoccupied rooms! We haven't even an empty crib."

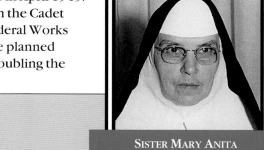

SISTER MARY ANITA

Sister Mary Anita Paul came to Mercy as administrator in 1941 and served in this capacity until 1947. She also held a second term from 1953 to 1959.

Catherine Paul was born in Kalo, Iowa, a small coal-mining town south of Fort Dodge. She knew prejudice at a young age when she and her family were referred to as "Catholickers" because they were the only Catholics in the small country school she attended.[16]

Eventually, Catherine and her family moved to the Des Moines area, and she began working in Mercy's business office. Miss Paul, as she was known then, admitted patients, escorted them to their rooms, and discharged them when it was time.

Influenced by the exceptional ladies for whom she worked, Catherine traveled to Council Bluffs in 1929 to become a novice with the Sisters of Mercy. In 1932, she returned to Mercy Des Moines as Sister Anita. This was to be a temporary assignment. She was told: "You needn't take your trunk along because you're not going to stay very long."[17] As it turned out, she did not leave Mercy again until after her first term as administrator ended 15 years later in 1947. Sometime during her tenure at Mercy, Sister Anita's trunk did arrive from Council Bluffs.

Sister Anita's business skills grew with her responsibilities. It was not long before she became Mercy's office manager, supervising four positions. In 1941, she was appointed as Mercy's superior/administrator. This promotion brought with it awesome responsibilities, as she later described:

"I began to 'administrate' as well as become Superior to 18 other nuns. Besides the affairs of the religious community and the overall responsibility of the hospital, I was also in charge of coordinating the functions of the Medical Staff, being ultimately responsible for the Doctors."[18]

Sister Anita guided Mercy Hospital through the difficult years of World War II. She was characterized by her quiet, reserved manner. Those who really knew her, however, knew that she had a great sense of humor, trademarked by a sly smile.[19]

After leaving Mercy in 1947, Sister Anita became administrator of St. Catherine's Hall for Business Women in Des Moines. Six years later, she once again assumed the leadership reins at Mercy Hospital, becoming the only Sister of Mercy from Council Bluffs to serve two non-consecutive terms as the hospital's administrator.

ADMINISTRATOR 1941-1947 and 1953-1959

The Sisters of Mercy request the honor of your presence at the Pontifical High Mass in commemoration of the Fiftieth Anniversary of Mercy Hospital Tuesday, the Twelfth of December at ten thirty o'clock Saint Ambrose Cathedral Des Moines, Iowa

Open House Two to Five Seven to Nine

1944

50

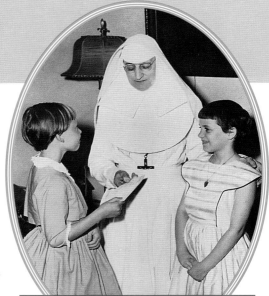

SISTER MARY ZITA

ister Mary Zita Brennan, known as Mercy's "baby sister," was born to a poor Kilkenny family on a cold, damp St. Patrick's Day. A premature baby, Sister Zita recalls being told that she was so frail her "parents put her basket in front of the open hearth for extra warmth." A goat provided the extra milk she needed to survive. Sister Zita's parents felt education was important and instilled this belief and a deep and fervent Catholic faith in their seven children.

It was this strong, faith-filled spirit that sustained Ellen Patricia Brennan as she made her way alone at the age of 15 from her beloved Ireland to the strange shores of America. In 1922, she left her Uncle Richard's farm in Colo, Iowa, and traveled to Mercy Des Moines to begin nurses' training. She was a typical, shy, yet wide-eyed girl, who loved to learn. She loved American History classes taken at North High.

During a late winter snow storm in 1926, Ellen traveled to Council Bluffs to enter the Mount Loretto novitiate of the Sisters of Mercy where she became Sister Mary Zita. Sister Zita finished nurses' training during her novitiate years, and then worked at Mercy Hospital in Council Bluffs until she was reassigned to Des Moines in 1939. She returned to the obstetrical department at Mercy and found it physically unchanged from her student years in the 1920s. There were war-induced shortages, crowded conditions, and other inconveniences.

Sister Zita started the milk laboratory located at the opposite end of a "block-long" hallway from the nursery. Mothers' rooms were situated in the West Wing, a great distance from the delivery rooms positioned on the east end of the Central Wing.

Sister Zita and the staff suffered from chronically chapped hands because they used lye rinses to help prevent the spread of infection. She spent long days making sure every comfort possible was given to the new babies and their families. Little touches added by her became well-known in Des Moines. Perhaps the best known of these was the hand-written birth certificate which accompanied each birth. Sister Zita's famous

calligraphy graced these announcements, as well as thousands of comforting letters and special prayers addressed to "Mommy and Daddy."

Sister Zita also inaugurated a "care package" which the new families took home. The package included a six-pack of formula with specific instructions on the care and feeding of the new Mercy nursery graduate.

For more than 34 years, Sister Zita applied her comforting ministry to families who came to Mercy to participate in the miracle of new life. Her greatest pleasure came from "getting to do for people—the mothers and the babies. And the fathers, God bless them. Don't forget the fathers." [20]

hrough the years, Sister Zita rejoiced with each move of the maternity department. In 1959, a new obstetrical department opened in the South Wing. When Sister Zita retired in the 1970s, she continued in an advisory capacity in the newly completed obstetrical unit in the Mercy tower complex.

Sister Zita taught maternity nursing, gynecological nursing, and newborn care in the hospital. She also taught courses targeted for licensing practical nurses through the adult education program of the Des Moines Public School system.

In 1968, Sister Zita was named Nurse of the Year by the Seventh District Iowa Nurses' Association. In 1979, Sister Zita accepted the Des Moines Citizens Community Betterment Award. In 1988, she was given the Distinguished Achievement Award in the Fields of Human Relations and Community Service from the National Conference of Christians and Jews.

Sister Zita thanked God for her life: "It is through being a Sister of Mercy that I have been able to do those things I feel I was sent to America to do. I love Des Moines...it is through this community that I have been able to be challenged and rewarded time and time again." [21]

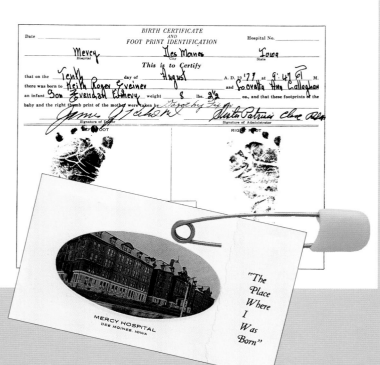

Mercy cared for 193 patients per day, but squeezed in 202 patients, with four beds set up in a parlor. The hospital's administration was eagerly awaiting the completion of the nurses' home so the students could move out of the main hospital and free up that space for patient care.[22]

In conjunction with this anniversary, Mercy sent a letter of solicitation to friends, requesting assistance to raise money in order to finish the new nurses' home. A stipulation for receiving the federal monies was that 40 percent of the total dollars must be provided by Mercy.[23]

G. Ralph Branton, a leading Des Moines businessman, responded to Sister Anita's letter. He outlined a plan arrived at during an earlier meeting he attended with other Catholic businessmen, Mercy physicians, and Bishop Bergan.

The men promised to solicit $50,000 from the Des Moines community for the purpose of building the nurses' home. They shared the concern that federal monies might not come through. The committee had written another "very confidential" letter to Washington, D.C., urging the federal funding. They pledged their support, however, and if the federal money should not fall into place, they promised to return any monies to the donors.[24]

By the time the fund raising effort was over, the businessmen—spearheaded by Bishop Bergan—had raised more than $100,000 for the new dormitory. This amount more than doubled their original projection. Mercy's Medical Staff donated $15,000. Combined funding reached the $300,000 level by the time the home was completed. The money allocated from the federal government totaled $132,000. With the added funds, the new home now could accommodate 120 nurses instead of the originally planned 50 students.[25]

THE NURSES' HOME

Construction on the new nurses' home, facing Fifth Street just off the northwest corner of the North Wing, began on January 1, 1945. The winter weather cooperated so that the walls of the brick structure were at second floor level by April. Bishop Bergan laid the cornerstone on July 1, 1945. The terrible destruction of World War II laid heavily on everyone's mind, and Bishop Bergan's words echoed the concerns of all. The final dedication of the nurses' home came on June 30, 1946.

After the student nurses were relocated in the new facility, Mercy's bed capacity increased by 65. Remodeling for the new beds—targeted to care for increased medical and surgical cases—centered in the East Wing. Other plans called for enlargement of the laboratory, a chemistry laboratory, and two classrooms in the main wing. Dr. Coleman upgraded Mercy's professional laboratory staff shortly after he arrived in 1946, doubling the staff and increasing the number of tests and diagnostic services the laboratory provided.[26]

During the construction of the nurses' home, the Sisters of Mercy made several improvements in the physical plant. A new boiler and stoker were added to the heating plant, increasing the number of boilers to three. Tuck-pointing secured the

We are proud to lay the cornerstone of a building devoted not to the production of arms, but to construction, progress, and salvation. Had the world's building been on the cornerstone of Christ, the heartbreak and suffering of the last few years never would have occurred. If we make Him the foundation of our national, family, and individual lives, such disaster will not occur again. With God's blessing, we dedicate to suffering humanity this nurses' home.

Bishop Gerald Bergan
Cornerstone Ceremony
for the Nurses' Home
July 1, 1945

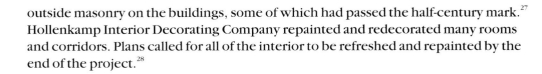

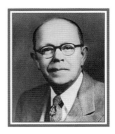

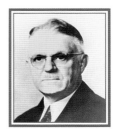

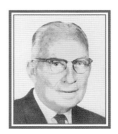

outside masonry on the buildings, some of which had passed the half-century mark.[27] Hollenkamp Interior Decorating Company repainted and redecorated many rooms and corridors. Plans called for all of the interior to be refreshed and repainted by the end of the project.[28]

MEDICAL ADVANCEMENTS

Penicillin passed its initial research period in the early 1940s. Its lifesaving reputation grew and production swung into high gear with the outbreak of World War II. Thousands of casualties were averted because penicillin was available in medical military theaters. During the Mercy Medical Staff meeting in June 1944, a special Penicillin Committee was appointed to work toward acquiring penicillin for use at Mercy. Dr. Harold Anderson, Dr. Clifford Losh, Sr., and Dr. Harry Collins were on this committee.[29]

Open-chest surgery was not that common in Iowa in the late 1930s and early 1940s. The chest was not invaded unless a bullet wound or some kind of accident forced the procedure. Pleural effusions were the main chest procedure, until the late 1930s when thoracotomies for tuberculosis became a common method of treatment. Another procedure, incredulous by today's standards, was the insertion of ping pong balls into the chest cavity to collapse the diseased part of the lung. As one physician commented: "It would scare the heck out of you when you took an x-ray of a chest and you saw all these big round things in there...if you didn't know that they were there purposely."[30] Anesthesia was a major problem with more difficult surgeries:

> *"They couldn't keep the patient alive and still put him to sleep. They didn't have a way to keep his breathing going. When they got a little more sophisticated with that [procedure], they started to...do thoracotomies and take out tuberculous lungs."*[31]

It was not until the late 1940s that Mercy began to perform major chest surgeries. Dr. Daniel Crowley, Jr. was trained not only in general surgery, but also in chest surgery. Dr. Crowley observed: "I had a very difficult time getting a nurse on private duty to accept a chest case because they never had any [experience]."[32]

THE LAY ADVISORY BOARD

Throughout its history, Mercy benefited from the aid of many in the form of prayer, physical assistance, advice, and money. During the campaign to secure funds for the construction of the new nurses' home, Mercy received immeasurable assistance from key people in Des Moines. Times were changing and the sisters realized that these same people could help guide Mercy in its continually expanding mission to the Des Moines community. Sister Anita invited several members of the former Nurses' Home Committee to join the hospital as an advisory board.

The first Mercy Lay Advisory Board meeting was held on November 6, 1946. Those present were: Bishop Bergan, Mrs. James J. (Genevieve) Kelly, Mrs. Maurice L. (Mary) Northup, Mrs. John (Florence) Normile, Mr. Ralph Branton, Mr. J. Woolson Brooks, Mr. E. F. Buckley, Mr. Harold Klein, Mr. E. H. Mulock, and Mr. Morey Sostrin. At this first meeting, Sister Anita explained some of the problems facing Mercy. She indicated that the most pressing was the shortage of nurses, and she asked for advice about recruiting nurses to fill the nursing school.

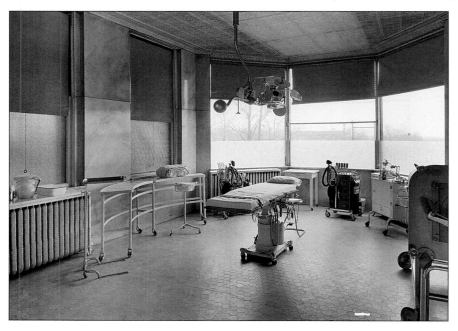

Members of the 1944 Penicillin Committee included from *top to bottom above,* Drs. Harold Anderson, Clifford Losh, Sr., and Harry Collins. ?? Funding came to Mercy from the 1940s Des Moines Variety club. *Front row, left to right opposite:* G. Ralph Branton, Nate Sandler, Sister Helen, Bishop Bergan, Sister Zita, Milton Feinberg, and William Toney. *Back row:* Max Rosenblatt, A.G. Stolte, Lou Levy, and Harold E. McKinney.

Within a few months, Father Raymond Conley, C. W. Gifford, and Arthur T. Gormley joined the board and were included on the first roster. The board considered several topics during 1946 and 1947: the bad condition of the parking lot located to the south of Mercy across Ascension Street, hospital advertising and promotion, an in-house publication on a regular basis, adequate telephone service, and remodeling within the hospital which would require soliciting federal aid, as well as aid from the Des Moines area.

Ten years after the creation of Mercy's Lay Advisory Board, Sister Anita was asked to give her advice to another Catholic hospital contemplating the establishment of such a board. She wholeheartedly supported the idea and added:

> *"In its initial organization...the Constitution and By-laws...established, in effect, that the Board shall act in an advisory capacity. However, in connection with our recently completed capital funds campaign and our current planning for an expansion program, their efforts have gone far beyond mere advice. Without their vigorous leadership and untiring efforts, our campaign might not have been the tremendous success that it was....An Advisory Board is an excellent means of accomplishing better hospital care for the patients in a Catholic Hospital."* [33]

Mercy's Lay Advisory Board took on long-term projects such as the Mercy Hospital Guild and the first regular hospital publication, *Mercy News*, created in 1947. They continued to provide advice to Mercy's administrators for more than 35 years.

A Sigh Of Relief

The 1940s drew to a close as World War II ended, and the world breathed a sigh of relief. Filled with excitement, Mercy's professional staff returned from war theaters, anxious to share new training and knowledge. Medical technology and knowledge grew at a phenomenal rate and brought new challenges to provide even better healthcare.

As the decade passed, Mercy entered a time when bed capacity would be taxed beyond limits as technology changed almost overnight. The cost of health care began to increase, and the methods of payment presented ongoing problems of balancing compassionate care with fair compensation. After 54 years of service to the Des Moines community, Mercy prepared to extend its comforting aid to an ever-widening circle of people.

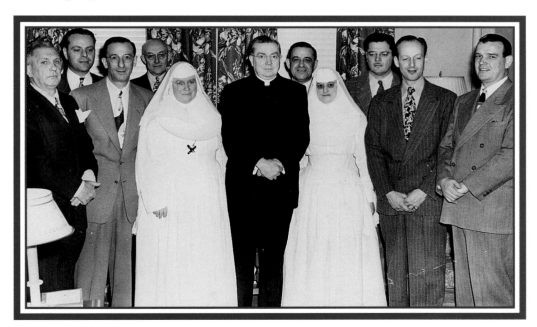

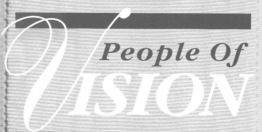

People Of VISION
1922-1947

LAY ADVISORY BOARD, 1946

J. Woolson Brooks
· *Brooks-Borg Architects*

G. Ralph Branton
· *First Lay Advisory Board President*

E.F. Buckley
· *Central National Bank & Trust*

C.W. Gifford
· *Des Moines Railway Company President & General Manager*

Arthur T. Gormley
· *Des Moines Register & Tribune Vice President & Business Manager*

Mrs. J.J. (Genevieve) Kelly
· *Mercy Guild President, 1951 & 1952*

Harold Klein
· *Iowa-Des Moines National Bank*

E.H. Mulock
· *Central Life Assurance Company*

Mrs. J. (Florence) Normile
· *First Lay Advisory Board Secretary*

Mrs. M.L. (Mary) Northup
· *First Mercy Guild President*

Morey Sostrin
· *Younker Bros.*

CHAPTER FOUR
SCHOOL OF NURSING: 1922-1947

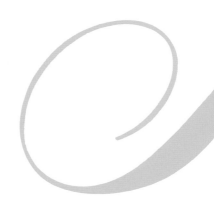

Mercy Hospital and its School of Nursing accomplished an almost unbelievable task of reorganization in the 1920s. The steady and tireless efforts of sisters and supervising nurses made these results possible.

When the Council Bluffs sisters began managing Mercy Hospital in Des Moines, there were 30 students in the School of Nursing. In 1922, Sister Mary Thomas Wilson assumed the position of superintendent of nurses in addition to being in charge of the operating rooms.

SISTER MARY THOMAS WILSON

Sister Mary Thomas Wilson was born Gertrude Wilson in Council Bluffs in 1880. At the age of 17, Gertrude converted to the Catholic religion, and entered nurses' training at St. Bernard's Hospital. Influenced by the merciful sisters who trained her, Gertrude entered the Mercy order in 1903, and upon profession, became Sister Mary Thomas. She supervised in nursing, anesthesia, and surgery until 1922, when she came to Mercy Des Moines as director of the school of nursing. Sister Thomas served as director until September 1, 1930. She remained at Mercy as operating room supervisor until the following April.

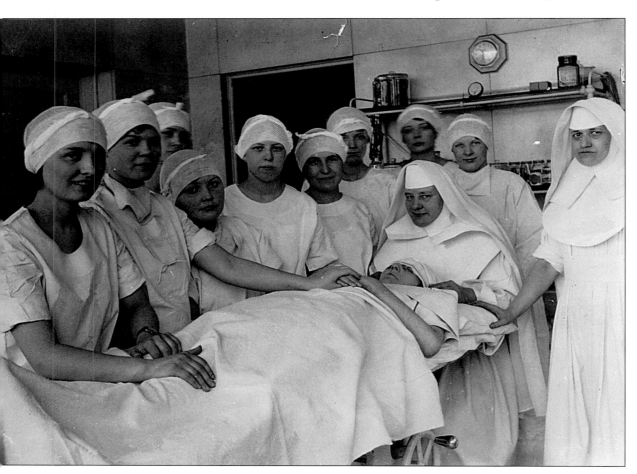

Sister Thomas was described as "kindness personified" by Sister Mary Josephine Collins. One nursing student echoed these sentiments when she said that Sister Thomas was "very kind when I came back to training [after an extended leave of absence]. Sister was very likeable."[1]

Sister Thomas was very particular about her habit. She liked the way Mrs. Esser laundered it. "Well...one time, I did the habit," recalls Angela Biondi. "Sister Thomas came in and asked who laundered her habit. I told her I did, and she said: 'Well, you shrunk it. You can see my ankles!'" After Sister Thomas left Mercy, she nursed in Council Bluffs, until her death on May 7, 1940.

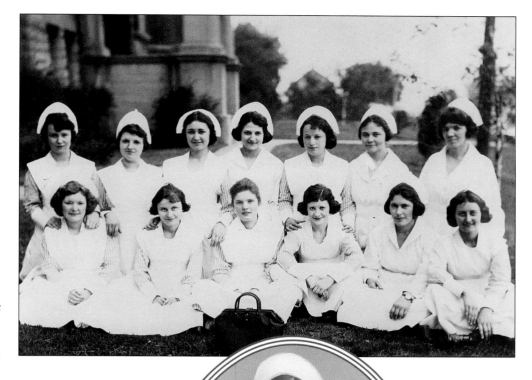

CURRICULUM

During Sister Thomas' time as director, she gradually upgraded the school's curriculum. She successfully acquired the first full-time instructor, Sister Mary Aloysius McGuire, in 1925 and another, Sister Mary Clare Clifford, in 1926.

Two hours of nursing technique were taught each day. A great teaching aid was added in 1926 when a separate room was set aside in the northwest wing of the first floor, fully equipped with the same apparatus as that used in the wards. Another change to the curriculum occurred when only two classes of students were accepted each year, in the fall and in January. Before that time girls were brought into the program throughout the year, and their time was marked from their starting date. All applicants were required to be high school graduates by 1929, and the probationary term was extended to four months.

Miss Lee Aldera remembers how they decided that she had sufficiently finished her training:

> *"One Sunday, it was March 17th, St. Patrick's Day, Sister Mary Thomas called me into her office. She said: 'Are you ready to go to work?' I said that I guessed that would be okay. Sister said she thought that since I was 'the only Irishman' that today would be a good day to mark the end of my student days and get out of training two weeks early." [Miss Aldera was Italian by nationality.].*[2]

DORMITORY FACILITY

During this era, students' quarters were in the East Wing. A report made by the Iowa Division of Nursing Education observed that:

> *"No thought was given in the early construction of the hospital to make adequate provision for student nurses. The best arrangement that could be made, later, seemed to be to take over the east wing of the hospital which is kept entirely separate from the patients' quarters. It is not an ideal situation, but much thought has been given and time spent to make the available space as habitable as possible. The majority of rooms are for two people with single beds for each, a dresser, table, two or three chairs, and a rather small closet. There is excellent provision for light and air. Bathing and toilet facilities are inadequate, but those available are in good condition. Quiet rooms are provided for night nurses on the first floor of the hospital."*[3]

THE PRIMARY FORCE

The student nurse was the primary labor force for the hospital during the 1920s. They worked long days, 12-hour shifts from 7:00 A.M. until 7:00 P.M. One student related that "you were supposed to get three hours off each day," but were "lucky if you got an hour and a half."[4]

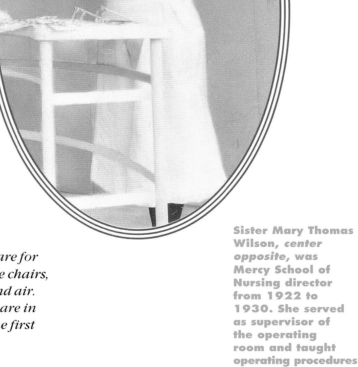

Sister Mary Thomas Wilson, *center opposite,* **was Mercy School of Nursing director from 1922 to 1930. She served as supervisor of the operating room and taught operating procedures to student nurses. ❧ Mercy's class of 1922 is shown** *top.* **❧ Miss Lee Aldera graduated from the school of nursing in 1928.**

Mercy Hospital
Des Moines, Iowa

LATE PERMIT

Miss .... *Young*

Date .... *7/4* .... Time ....

Time returned *5MC*

Signed ....

Director, School

Students were learning nursing, and they were learning basic dietetics by preparing patient trays. They also rolled bandages and cut sponges by hand for use in surgery.[5] They learned how to operate sterilizers and autoclaves. Bedmaking then was an art, especially under the watchful eye of Sister Mary Alacoque, with her ever-present tape measure. She would follow behind the young nurses and measure the distance between the draw sheet and the top of the bed. If it was not correct, the student remade the bed.[6] Sometimes the students were called on for the most unusual duties. All items for each patient room were numbered with red paint. After repeated cleaning, the paint wore off. One of the sisters used to have the students on her floor paint new numbers on each item.[7]

Whenever Sister Geraldine found a missing item from a patient's room, work on the floor would cease, and the girls were dispersed to all points to locate the missing object. One student remembered that Sister Joseph taught a "class in sewing. She was most meticulous."[8]

Many women who took their nurses' training at Mercy during this time have fond memories. One remembers how hot it was the first weeks of the probationary period: "We folded bandages out on the lawn that first week."[9] With long working hours and little money, entertainment pleasures were simple. "We used to go up to Sixth and Laurel to Reed's ice cream and for 15 cents, buy a big dish, bring it back, [and] sit on the lawn out front to eat it."[10] One of the girls was a good piano player: "She would play ragtime, and we would dance."[11]

Two students asked to be changed to a new room. The change was okayed and a new room assigned near the fire escape with the added stipulation that for the new room, the occupants "were to report anyone who came in the back stairs after hours. So, I told everyone that I would turn them in....That's not to say that some didn't come in that way when I wasn't there."[12]

If the girls had dates they had to get late permission signed by the director. Coming in late meant explaining to Miss Clark, the night supervisor, and later to Sisters Thomas or Clare. If the offense was severe enough the student was grounded, meaning she could not go anywhere off campus.

Sister Mary Clare Clifford

Sister Mary Clare Clifford replaced Sister Thomas as director in 1930. Sister Clare was born in County Cork, Ireland. She entered the Sisters of Mercy in Council Bluffs in 1906 and received nurse's training at St. Bernard's Hospital and St. Joseph's Mercy Hospital in Centerville. Sister Clare came to Mercy in Des Moines in 1924 and supervised the obstetrical area for two years. She became an instructor in the school of nursing in 1926.

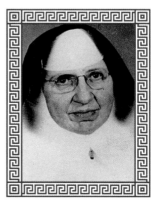

In 1928, Sister Clare accompanied Sister Mary Xavier Clinton to Ireland. They recruited Irish women to enter the Sisters of Mercy. Fifteen young women returned with them to the United States. Several became professed Sisters of Mercy who served in Des Moines.[13]

Sister Clare was a firm believer in professional associations as a means for further education for nurses. She insisted that her nurses belong to the Mercy Alumni

Mercy's student nurses worked long hours. Free-time was spent with friends and family, and strict curfews could be broken only if one had a late permit issued by the school director.

Association and the Seventh District Iowa Nurses' Association.[14] Sister Clare was described as "a very fair supervisor with an Irish temper. But she had such a twinkle in her eye all the time you were talking to her, you couldn't help but feel she was in sympathy with you. However, she had to deal out whatever had to be dealt with."[15] When one prospective graduate came to Mercy for admission, she mentioned that she had been rejected for admission to another nursing school because she was small. Sister Clare replied: "Oh, you poor thing. Some of our best nurses are little people."[16]

CHANGES WITH THE NEW DECADE

The 1930s brought more changes to Mercy's school. In 1930, the blue striped, apron-covered student uniforms were replaced by white uniforms, shoes and hose. The length of the uniforms was very important. Through this period, it varied from 10-14 inches from the floor. Many of the graduates remembered "how beautiful we looked. We would all line up...caps to a point, and all the hems in a row."[17]

Special aprons were used during operating or obstetrical procedures, and in the diet kitchens. The students also were required to subscribe to the *American Journal of Nursing*. The monthly five-dollar stipend students relied upon to buy hose, treats, and toiletries was discontinued in September 1931. More than likely, this came as a result of the Depression.

By January 1932, there were 85 nursing students enrolled in the school of nursing. The fee for entering students was $75; $50 upon admission with the remaining $25 paid at the end of the probationary period. Uniforms and books were purchased by the students. Mercy bought the uniforms and sold them to students for $2.50.[18] The library subscribed to the *American Journal of Nursing, Trained Nurse,* and *Hospital Progress* to supplement the nurses' reading.

Beginning in 1933, Mercy's nursing program became affiliated with Dowling Junior College. Credit was given for courses taught at Mercy. In 1939, nursing students began a three-month rotation at St. Bernard's Hospital in Council Bluffs for classes in psychiatry and psychiatric nursing, hydrotherapy, social service, and occupational therapy. Ward and practical nursing experience were additional courses taught at St. Bernard's. Earlier classes in psychiatry were taught at Iowa Lutheran Hospital.

One student remembers that they all had to walk up to Lutheran after lunch each day.

"We would get off for lunch, and grab a bite, if we had time. Then we would walk to Lutheran. Well, we didn't have money for a bus. The classes were held in a warm room...and everybody would get so sleepy."[19]

Some classes were taught at the old Broadlawns location on Center Street. The girls walked there as well.[20]

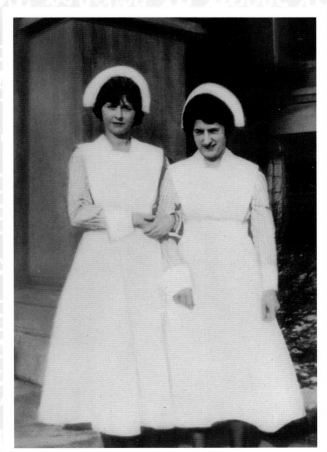

Student nurses, Ellen Patricia Brennan (later Sister Mary Zita), *below right,* and Norah Ryan, *below left,* were chums during their training in the 1920s. Ellen spent many holidays and days off with the Ryan family.

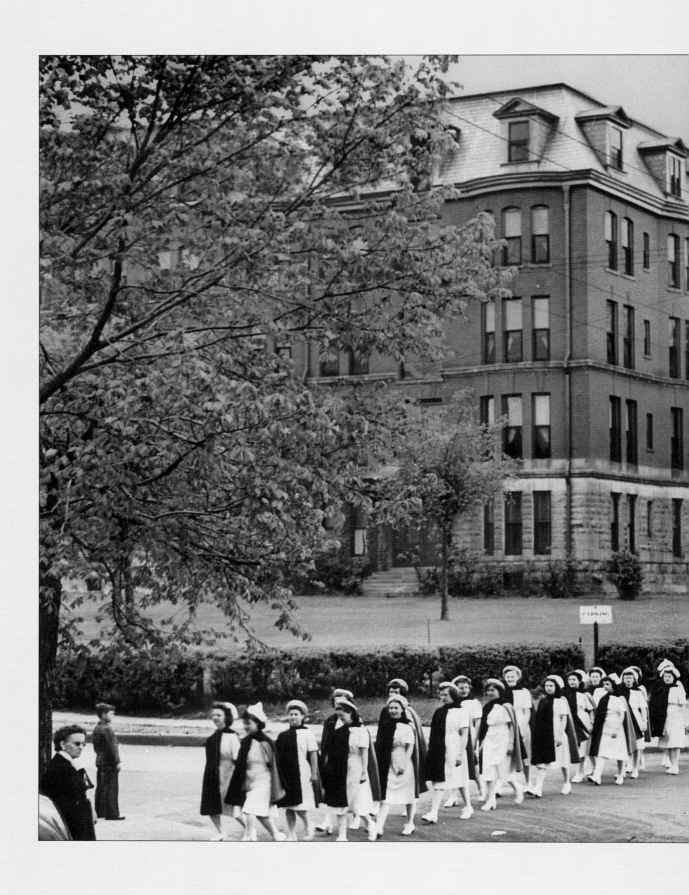

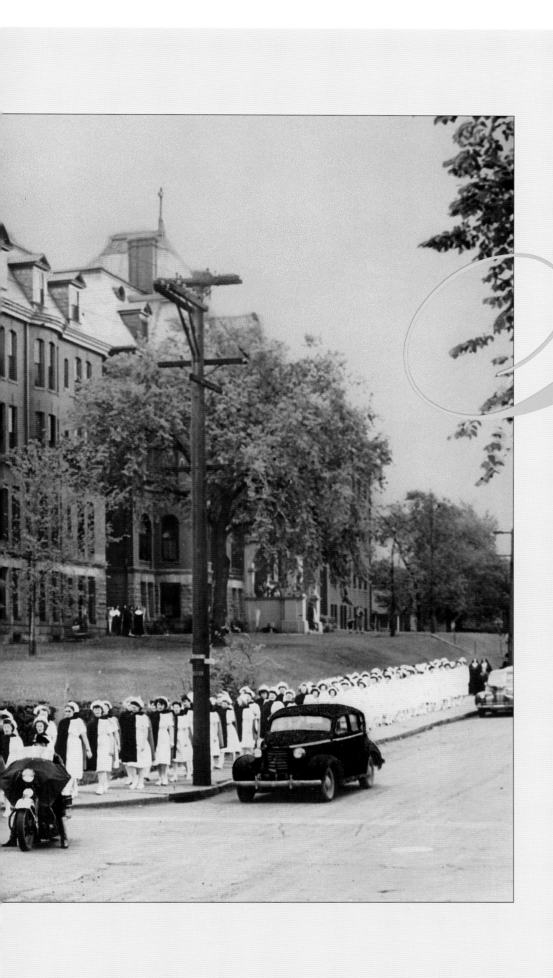

*I*t was graduation Sunday for Mercy Hospital student nurses in 1946. The graduates, along with other students, faculty, and sisters, walked from the hospital to St. Ambrose Cathedral for ceremonies. The march up Ascension Street and down Sixth Avenue was a tradition that began in the 1930s and ended in the 1960s. Mercy re-established the ritual early in the 1990s.

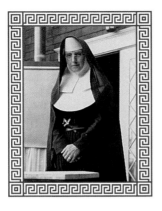

SISTER MARY IMMACULATA STRIEGEL

Sister Mary Immaculata Striegel followed Sister Clare as nursing school director in 1935 and served in this position for about two years.

Sister Immaculata was born in Germany. She entered the Council Bluffs Sisters of Mercy in 1913 and studied nursing. The majority of Sister Immaculata's career was spent in nursing education, and in 1931, she was elected as secretary of the Iowa State League of Nursing Education. She spent 19 years between Council Bluffs and Centerville, with her last assignment before coming to Des Moines as superintendent of nurses in Centerville.

It was Sister Immaculata who arranged for four Mercy graduates to take an additional six-week course at Creighton University in Omaha during the summer of 1936. The course covered hospital administration for nurses, and the women were sent with the encouragement that they would live to see the day when nurses would need a degree.[21]

FOND MEMORIES: NURSING IN THE 1930S

The School of Nursing at St. Joseph's Mercy Hospital in Centerville closed in 1935. Eighteen students who were enrolled in the nursing program there transferred to Mercy Des Moines. One student remembered: "I came in the summer of 1935. We had no trouble fitting in. We were able to continue right on with our class work."[22] A total of 14 students who had begun their training in Centerville graduated from Mercy Des Moines.[23]

As always, there were rules. In the dining room, the students were expected to appear in complete uniform "or in respectable civilian clothes." They were assigned to specific places at table and were

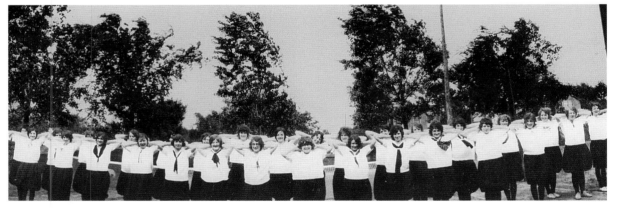

Nursing student activities included exercising bodies as well as minds. Fresh air and physical activity were emphasized.

expected to sit at those places at all times. Silence was to be observed until "Grace" was said. After meals, prayers were a private matter but were expected to be practiced. There was to be absolutely no gum chewing on the way to or in the dining room. The only electric iron could be used any day except Wednesday and the lone electric presser could be used on Mondays until 10:00 P.M. and on Friday and Saturday afternoons.

During this period, student dormitories were located in the East Wing. Freshmen were housed on the third floor; juniors on the second floor; and seniors on the first floor. Late curfew was 11:30 P.M. For the most part the girls obeyed the rules, but they always tried to bend them a bit. An intern remembered being rudely awakened in the wee hours of the morning by a foot in his face, as one late-returning student removed the screen from his ground floor room, trying to sneak in past curfew.[24]

One student's best-remembered prank involved a pilfered chicken from Sister Lucia's walk-in cooler. She and another student tried to cook the chicken in the surgery autoclave. The project backfired because the chicken did not get cooked, and the autoclave was a mess to clean. The whole episode came to a halt when Sister Aloysius caught them trying to clean up.[25]

One incident of student unruliness resulted in a dismissal of several nurses in 1936. Dissatisfied with the way roommates were assigned, six of the student nurses decided not to show up for duty. This strike resulted in instant dismissal. The suspension was short-lived. Administrators decided the girls could come back after seven days. The outcome: "We had to make up the lost time, but we got the roommates we wanted." [26]

SISTER MARY HELEN MACKENZIE

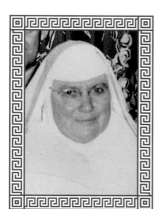

A new nursing school director was named in 1937, Sister Mary Helen Mackenzie. Sister Helen came from a non-Catholic background. She completed her nursing education at Mercy in Council Bluffs in 1906. Inspired by the sisters from whom she received her education, Sister Helen not only became a Catholic, she also entered the novitiate with the Sisters of Mercy in Council Bluffs.

After becoming a Sister of Mercy, Sister Helen taught for 28 years in southern and central Iowa. In 1936, she was appointed superintendent of nurses in Council Bluffs. From there, she came to Mercy Des Moines in the same position. Sister Helen served as school director until 1947 when she became Mercy's administrator.

One young nurse thought Sister Helen had it in for her because she was the first in her class to be assigned night duty.

"She was always picking on me...she didn't like the fact that I would go out to Fort Des Moines to the dances. I was engaged to a soldier, and we won all the dance contests....But when my father was sick and dying some of the nuns came down and presented me with my pin and diploma, so he knew I would graduate. Sister Helen let me go home and care for him until he died. She turned the tide, and she was my friend." [27]

Shortly after Sister Helen arrived, Mercy began to hire nurses who were graduates of the school of nursing on a regular basis. Prior to that time, Mercy's graduate nurses mainly did private duty nursing, either within the hospital or outside through the nurse registry, at the request of a physician. One of the first women hired after graduation was Marie (Jones) Bloomquist. She was unable to find a job in Des Moines other than private duty. After working in that capacity for a short time, Mrs. Bloomquist was thrilled when Sister Helen asked her to work at Mercy. She received room and board, plus $40 per month in salary. She jumped at the chance. "I was so grateful...I just stayed...I never looked for work anywhere else." [28] Mrs. Bloomquist nursed at Mercy until her retirement in 1975.

Kathryn Byrnie, *below,* **was a student nurse who loved to have fun.** ❧ **Sister Gonzaga posed with four members of the school of nursing graduating class of 1931,** *bottom.*

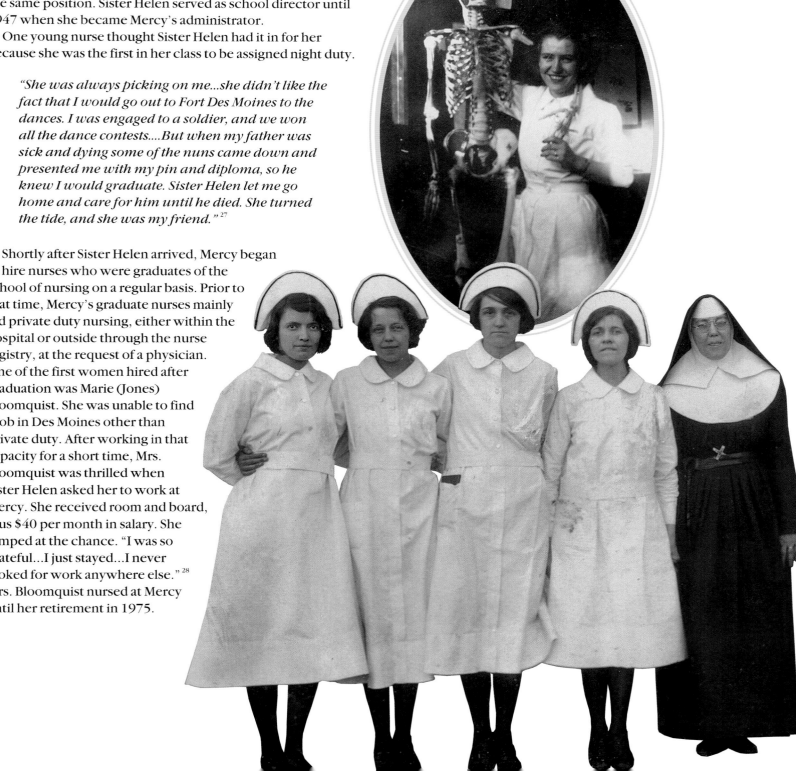

As A Result Of War

Under Sister Helen's leadership, Mercy's School of Nursing met the challenges of World War II, which impacted the hospital in several ways. A serious shortage of nurses developed nationwide when graduate nurses left their civilian jobs to enlist in the military services. Two bills introduced by Mrs. Frances Bolton were aimed at increasing the number of trained nurses to fill the immediate need caused by this event. The first Bolton Bill enacted on July 1, 1941, provided federal funds or further preparation and refresher courses for graduates. The second Bolton Bill enacted in July 1942, and put into effect one year later, was more popularly known as the Cadet Nursing Program. This bill aided Mercy in two ways: increasing the potential for training more nurses and easing the way for application of federal monies under the earlier Lanham Act, which had been denied Mercy on its first requests. Mercy became the third hospital in Des Moines to receive funding under the Cadet Nursing Program.[29]

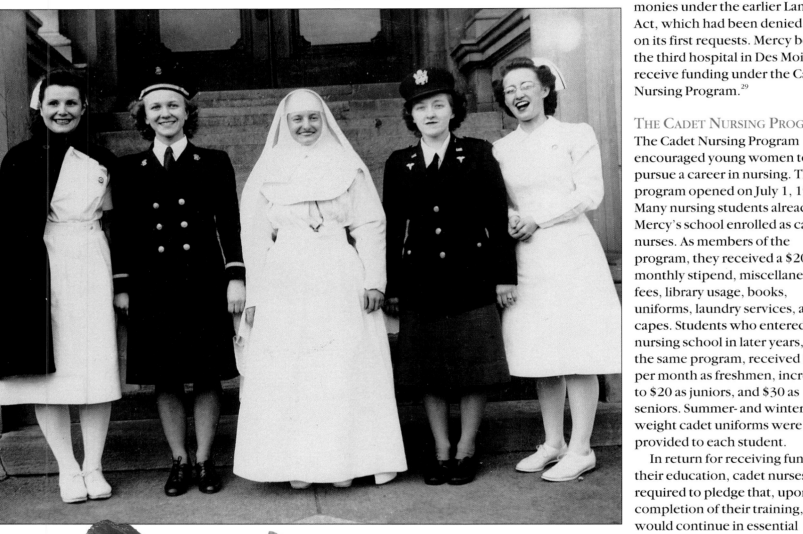

The Cadet Nursing Program

The Cadet Nursing Program encouraged young women to pursue a career in nursing. The program opened on July 1, 1943. Many nursing students already in Mercy's school enrolled as cadet nurses. As members of the program, they received a $20 monthly stipend, miscellaneous fees, library usage, books, uniforms, laundry services, and capes. Students who entered nursing school in later years, under the same program, received $15 per month as freshmen, increased to $20 as juniors, and $30 as seniors. Summer- and winter-weight cadet uniforms were provided to each student.

In return for receiving funds for their education, cadet nurses were required to pledge that, upon completion of their training, they would continue in essential nursing—civilian or military—for the duration of the war. In return, the program ensured graduates of their eligibility as registered nurses.

Nearly 90 percent of 1943 nursing school graduates entered a military branch, and more than 50 percent of the 1944 class were commissioned for the nurses' corps. Approximately 240 of Mercy's nurses participated in the program until it ended in 1948. Nurses who served in the war sometimes found friendly faces in the crowds when they landed on alien shores. One nurse remembered meeting a familiar Mercy surgeon during her tour on Guam. He asked what her assignment was and she told him she was working in linen supply, a duty she found to be quite tedious. He replied: "Oh, Queenie of the Sheet House, huh!" The nickname stayed with her and continued when she and the physician met again at Mercy after the end of the war.[30]

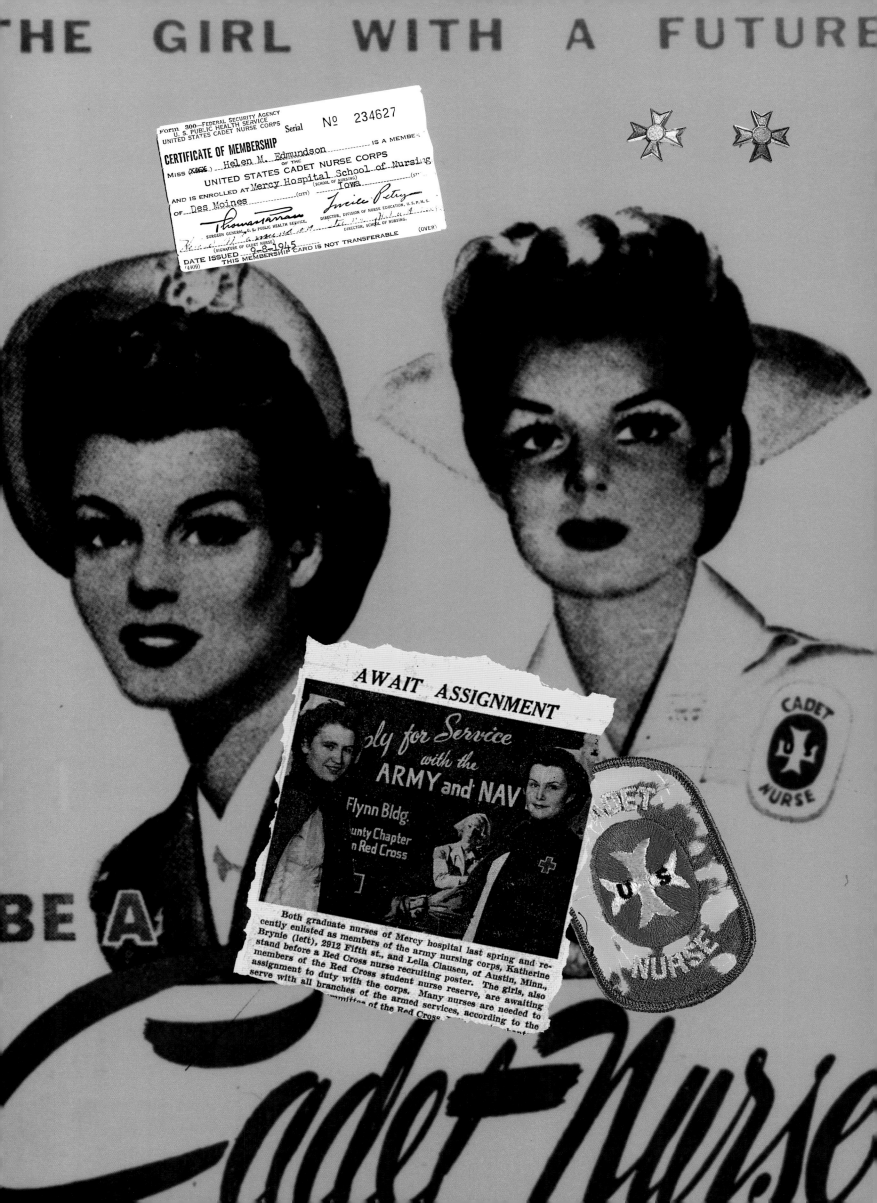

A NEW HOME

Mercy's school had operated under cramped and crowded conditions for many years. In 1942, an additional December class was enrolled, increasing the usual enrollment from 90 to 150 students. An immediate need arose for housing the extra students. Mercy purchased a house and leased another on Fourth Street to provide dormitory space. Two house-mothers were employed to staff the annexes: Mrs. Ella Foster and Mrs. Isabel Meiggs.[31]

Mercy applied for funding to build a dormitory but they were turned down several times. After Mercy's School of Nursing was accepted under the Cadet Nursing Program, however, it was given the approval for funding to construct a nurses' home.

Construction on the new dormitory was completed at the end of June 1946. On the last Sunday of June, Bishop Bergan dedicated the new building. After the program, which consisted of songs by the nurses' glee club and Benediction of the Blessed Sacrament, tours were given by the sisters and nurses.

The home accommodated 110 students. Each bedroom was attractively furnished and coordinated in shades of canary yellow, pale blue, salmon, and sea green. Two students were comfortably housed in each room.

A new nurses' dormitory was added to Mercy's campus in 1946. The dedication, *right,* took place on the last Sunday in June. Rooms were attractively furnished and coordinated in shades of salmon, canary yellow, pale blue and sea green as shown *bottom opposite.* The Mercy nursing class of 1946 posed in front of their new home, *above opposite.*

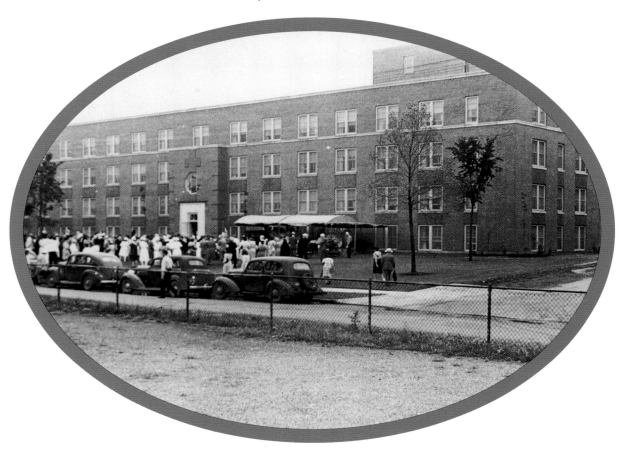

In addition to housing the students, the new facility contained a library, two lecture rooms, a nursing arts demonstration room, science and dietetics laboratories, and a laundry. Offices, a reception room, and a lounge were located on the second floor. After the opening of the new home, three house mothers were employed: Mrs. Margaret Bennett, Mrs. Foster, and Mrs. Meiggs. Eventually, the sisters included a chapel in the nurses home. It was dedicated on November 19, 1947.

Within a few months, another wing—the recreational wing—was connected to the east side of the dormitory. It contained a 275-seat auditorium with a special motion picture booth and a stage for capping ceremonies, lectures, musicals, and plays. The basement under this wing contained a small kitchen, game room, storage space, and a laundry for the nurses. During the opening ceremony for the new auditorium, Bishop Bergan sang and danced a jig on stage with the nurses' glee club.[32]

A YEAR OF CHANGES

The largest graduating class in Mercy's history completed the program in 1946. Fifty-three women received their diplomas in St. Ambrose Cathedral on May 6. With this graduation, 789 young nurses had passed through Mercy's doors into the proud nursing profession.[33]

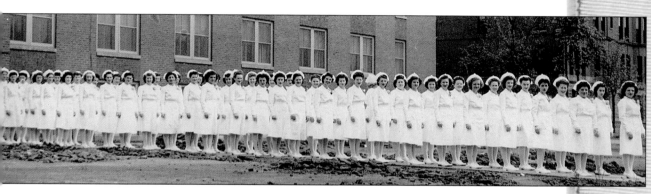

By the end of the 1946 school year, Mercy had six full-time assistants aiding Sister Helen. Sister Mary Catherine Carroll was in charge of the records and clerical department. Sister Mary Jerome Burns taught biological sciences and also supervised Mercy's x-ray and physical therapy departments. Sister Mary Sebastian Geneser taught nursing arts and assisted with the general supervision of the nurses' home. Sister Mary John O'Leary was the school librarian. Miss Beatrice Bender acted as coordinator for the school curriculum and taught clinical case studies. Miss Leona Sweeney was an assistant instructor in nursing arts. Other instructors were hired on a part-time basis to present special lectures.[34] Physician-specialists presented lectures and nurse clinicians trained the students in nursing technique.[35]

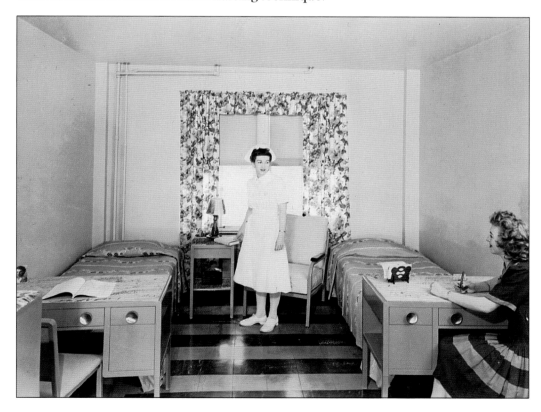

People Of VISION

1922-1947

MERCY SCHOOL OF NURSING DIRECTORS

Sister Mary Thomas Wilson, *1922-1930*

Sister Mary Clare Clifford, *1930-1935*

Sister Mary Immaculata Striegel, *1935-1937*

Sister Mary Helen Mackenzie, *1937-1947*

CHIEFS OF STAFF
F. E. V. Shore, 1922
R. A. Weston, 1923-24
J. C. Rockafellow, 1925
Howard D. Gray, 1926
D. F. Crowley, Sr., 1927
J. R. Condon, 1928
R. J. Lynch, 1929
L. M. Nourse, 1930
C. W. Losh, Sr., 1931
H. C. Schmitz, 1932
J. E. Kessell, 1933
Harold Peasley, 1934
B. C. Barnes, 1935
Earl D. McClean, 1936, '44
Walter D. Abbott, 1937, '48
Harold N. Anderson, 1938, '45
Harry Collins, 1939-40
E. J. Kelley, 1941
Herbert A. Sohm, 1942, '47
Frank E. Foulk, 1943
John M. Griffin, 1946

For the first four months of their schooling, students went through a "pre-clinical period." This time was spent primarily in classroom and laboratory work. After two months, two hours each day were spent in ward practice. Caps were awarded at the end of the pre-clinical period. The remaining 32 months of the three-year nursing program were called the "clinical period." Students spent most of their time in the classroom, acquiring ward experience on the medical, surgical, pediatric and obstetric floors.

The senior year provided students the opportunity to study psychiatry in a three-month rotation at St. Bernard's Hospital in Council Bluffs. Additional child-care experience was

Recruiting brochures of the 1930s and 1940s highlighted training, birthdays, May crownings, and other social activities.

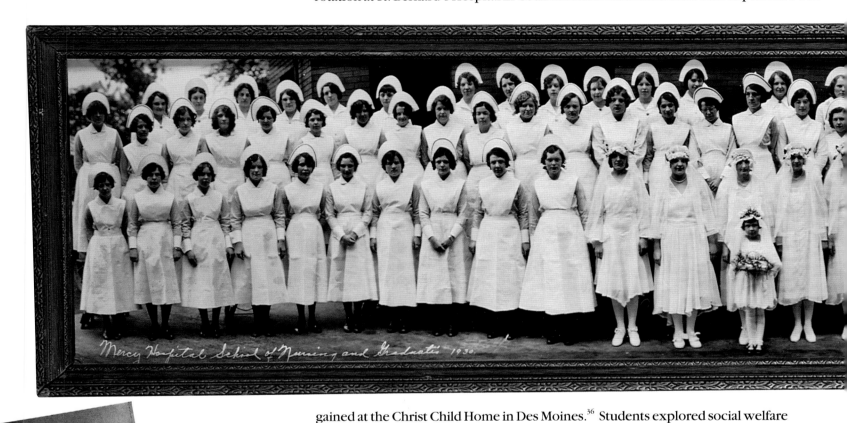

Mercy Hospital School of Nursing and Graduates 1930.

gained at the Christ Child Home in Des Moines.[36] Students explored social welfare problems through work with field case workers at the office of Catholic Charities.[37]

Although busy with class work and floor duties, students managed to find time for extra-curricular activities. Classes in swimming and basketball were held at the Jewish Community Center. A choir and glee club were made up of volunteers from the nursing classes. The choir performed for many hospital events and sang for special church feast days. Many of the Catholic nurses joined the Sodality of the Blessed Virgin. May Crowning, held in the spring of each year, was a time-honored tradition in Mercy's School of Nursing during this era.[38]

A TIME FOR FUN
Like those who preceded them, students of the 1940s managed to have fun whenever they could. "We worked like dogs, but we had such fun...good clean fun. And we never hurt

Who me?

Would I Be Proud of My Chosen Profession?

To feel 'needed is emotionally important to a woman. That's why girls who make a career of nursing can't imagine doing any other kind of work. As one student nurse smoothly stated it, "When you see anyone who is ill, you naturally want them to get well. And when your encouragement and knowledge has helped them do that—it's a *wonderful* feeling." There is a stimulating challenge about the profession, too. A nurse must have the ability to meet daily emergencies, to assume responsibilities. There's pride in the fact that people respect a nurse's ability and knowledge and her advice is always unquestionably accepted as the gospel truth. Her professional rating earns her a solid social standing in any community and that's no small potatoes, either!

ow Would My Wages ompare with Those in Other Fields?

you ever dreamed of NOT willfully by the really lush clothes found in the plushier f stores and once . . . *just once* that which you sigh for? Not corners all the time is just things about the nursing profession. Of course, earnings depend in part on your experience, ability, specialized training, on the cost of existence in different parts of the country, and on other factors . . . but here in Iowa, you *even start out* at $175 to $200 a month. And there are rainbow-end opportunities to work yourself into responsible positions which will pay from $325 a month to $450 a month. Besides that, salaries are on the upswing, locally and nationally.

Would the Profession of Nursing Give Me Security?

A nursing education would be your personal Tiffany property all thru life and no one could take it from you. It'd insure you of a position in any community, state or country, with air and steamship lines or the armed services. Not only is nursing excellent preparation for the responsibilities of homemaking and child-care, but it is also a reliable source of income when the family budget shows signs of collapse. Many women have returned to nursing after years in the home; others have made it a fruitful, lifetime career. Increased use of hospital facilities; new developments in medicine and treatments; veteran care; health insurance plans; and the growing consciousness in schools, industry and the home of the value and need of good health practices create an ever-growing demand for a nurse's professional service.

anybody. I think the sisters instilled a lot of that in us. Of course I don't know how much of that they really knew."[39]

Two months were very important in Mercy's yearly cycle: August and July. In August, the sisters were moved into new assignments. July held an even greater significance for the young nursing students. That was the month the new interns arrived.

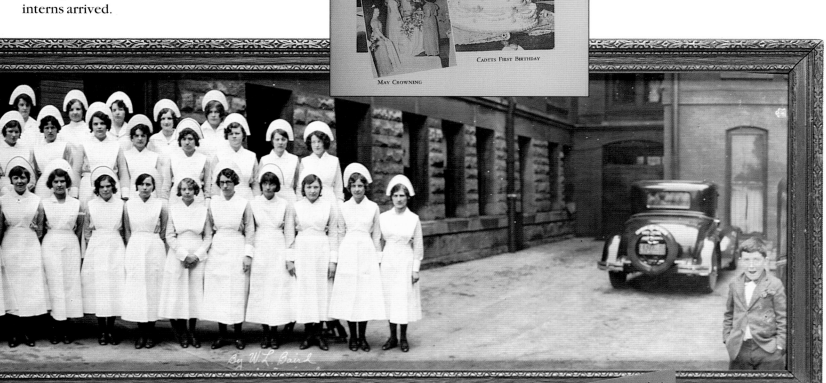

"Then the fun started—they were a ball. Did we have fun in those days. Those two came from Cuba, Echemendia and Pocuruell, and the first day that it snowed...the other interns got them out making snowballs. They got them boxes and had them pack the snowballs in boxes to mail to Cuba. That's the kind of stuff....They were such good doctors. They would have the switchboard page 'Dr. Frank Breech', or 'Dr. R. H. Factor.' You had to keep alert because you never knew who would be the next victim. We all had fierce loyalty."[40]

APPROACHING A BENCHMARK

Slowly through the 25 years from 1922 to 1947, Mercy's School of Nursing grew within the changing framework of health care. Tested by severe economic depression and wartime challenges, the school survived and grew stronger. By 1947, Mercy's School of Nursing was nearly a half-century old. Everyone was looking forward to celebrating that benchmark in history.

CHAPTER FIVE

MERCIFUL ANGELS: THE COUNCIL BLUFFS SISTERS

Mercy Hospital has been blessed with the talents of strong and comforting "angels of Mercy" since its beginning. These dedicated ladies spent months, and at times, their entire lives promoting and developing Mercy Hospital as a place of healing.

When the Council Bluffs sisters began managing Mercy Hospital in Des Moines, there was only a handful of professionally trained or professed religious to administer the hospital. Sister Mary Bonaventure Carroll, superior of the Council Bluffs sisters, established a strong administrative structure, and during the years 1922-1947, more than 50 Sisters of Mercy gave their unselfish service to the Des Moines community. Complete records for each of the sisters who served at Mercy in the 1920s and 1930s are not available. At the time of the 1929 Amalgamation, an effort was made to create a record for the active Sisters in each province. Beginning in 1937, yearly lists were compiled for all convents in each province.

Several Sisters of Mercy who came to Des Moines during 1922 to 1947 spent the majority of their lives giving comfort at Mercy Hospital. They were: Sisters Mary Geraldine Gleeson, Louise Owens, Lucia Endes, Pauline Hammes, Salome Grimes, and Aloysius and Gonzaga McGuire.

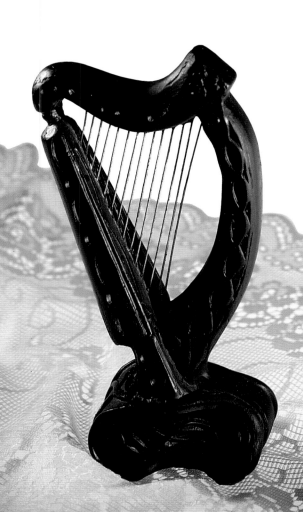

SISTER MARY GERALDINE GLEESON

Sister Mary Geraldine Gleeson was born in Monroe, Nebraska, as Kathryn Gleeson. She entered the Sisters of Mercy in Council Bluffs after finishing her nurses' training at Clarkson Memorial Hospital in Omaha and at Mercy in Council Bluffs. Her first assignment after profession came in 1923 when Sister Geraldine was sent to Des Moines. She spent the rest of her life in nursing at Mercy.

In her later years, Sister Geraldine was known as a "martinet" due to her reputation as a supervisor who ran a "tight ship." Sister Geraldine's influence keenly marked the lives of young nursing students who trained on her floor. They thought she ruled her floor with an iron hand, and they witnessed her rampages whenever she found something out of place. Sister Geraldine instilled in the students that attention to detail must be foremost in patient care. She kept close watch on her patients and a Mercy chaplain remembered that when called to administer the last rites

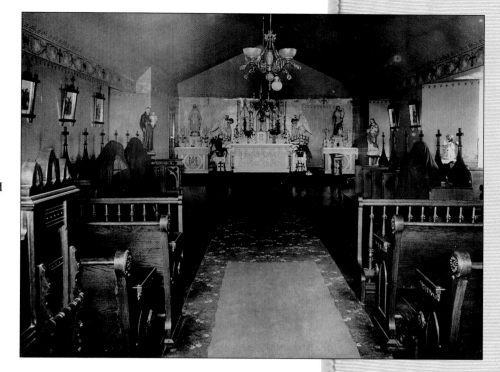

on Sister Geraldine's floor, "you didn't know whether to anoint the patient or Geraldine."[1]

One family whose son was admitted to Mercy found a gentle and compassionate Sister Geraldine:

> *"She had charge of the third floor surgery when our son who was only ten-years-old had a ruptured appendix. Of course, you were supposed to go to pediatrics, but I don't know why he didn't want to go to pediatrics, so I said to sister: 'Could you take him on your floor?' She did, and you know Sister Geraldine was so good to him."[2]*

Sister Geraldine supervised surgical nursing at Mercy for over 40 years. She continued to visit patients until her death in December 1976.

SISTER MARY LOUISE OWENS

Sister Mary Louise Owens was born in England in 1873. She immigrated to the Rhode Island area and became a Sister of Mercy in Council Bluffs, Iowa, around the age of 40. Sister Louise served in Centerville where she was one of the "kind" sisters who influenced Sister Joseph. She transferred to Mercy Des Moines in 1923 and worked as records librarian there until she died.

Sister Louise was known for her quiet, unassuming manner and her pleasing personality. She was a ready conversationalist and equally entertaining to young and old. She was deeply spiritual. Sister Louise died on May 6, 1954, in Des Moines, five days after her annual retreat.

SISTER MARY LUCIA ENDRES

Several postulants were transferred from Des Moines to Mount Loretto to complete their novitiate when the Council Bluffs sisters took the reins at Mercy Hospital in Des Moines. One who returned to Des Moines endeared herself to all for 45 years.

When she left Des Moines for Council Bluffs to complete her novitiate, Sister Mary Lucia Endres' temporary religious name was Sister Mary Agatha. There was, however, another sister named Agatha, so, Sister Mary Agatha Endres became Sister Mary Lucia.

After completing her novitiate, Sister Lucia worked at Mercy Council Bluffs in the dietary department until 1924 when she received her assignment to Des Moines. She remained at Mercy Hospital for the rest of her life.

Sister Lucia endeared herself to everyone who came to Mercy's kitchen. She extended her comforting and nourishing aid as she supervised all of the dietary preparation within the hospital. Sister Lucia was famous for her works of charity. Memories of a "somewhat retiring, very modest, hardworking sister" are forever etched in the minds of those who grew up within Mercy's shadow.[3]

People Of VISION
1922-1947

SISTERS OF MERCY

Alacoque Lannan
Aloysius McGuire
Ambrose Schaub
Anita Paul
Austin O'Donohoe
Basil (Agnes Marie) Smith
Benedicta McCarten
Carmelita Manning
Catherine Carroll
Clare Clifford
Concepta Mullins
Consolata Wagner
Damian Novak
DePaul Collins
Evangelista Claherty
Gabriel Bruce
Geraldine Gleeson
Gonzaga McGuire
Helen Mackenzie
Immaculata Striegel
James McDonald
Jerome Burns
Joachim Dutton

(Continued on page 121.)

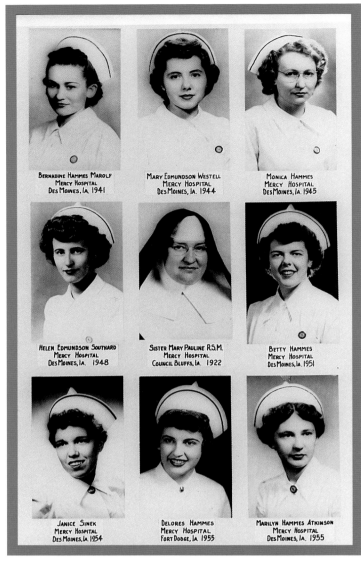

Bernadine Hammes Marolf
Mercy Hospital
Des Moines, Ia. 1941

Mary Edmundson Westell
Mercy Hospital
Des Moines, Ia. 1944

Monica Hammes
Mercy Hospital
Des Moines, Ia. 1945

Helen Edmundson Southard
Mercy Hospital
Des Moines, Ia. 1948

Sister Mary Pauline R.S.M.
Mercy Hospital
Council Bluffs, Ia. 1922

Betty Hammes
Mercy Hospital
Des Moines, Ia. 1951

Janice Sinek
Mercy Hospital
Des Moines, Ia. 1954

Delores Hammes
Mercy Hospital
Fort Dodge, Ia. 1955

Marilyn Hammes Atkinson
Mercy Hospital
Des Moines, Ia. 1955

Sister Mary Pauline Hammes, right, kept close ties to members of her family, above. One of her sisters and seven nieces graduated from Mercy's School of Nursing. One nephew, John, fulfilled his pharmacy internship at Mercy. Another niece, Molly, graduated from Mercy's School of Radiology. ❧ Sister Mary Salome Grimes, above opposite. Sisters Mary Aloysius and Gonzaga McGuire, middle opposite, left to right.

"She made the best chicken and noodles. My brother used to bring chickens to Des Moines from the farm near Atlantic...to her."[4]

Nursing students loved to be scrub nurse for Dr. Losh because his catheters had to be kept cool and the only cool place was the big walk-in cooler in Sister Lucia's kitchen. The scrub nurse would go down to the cooler and bring the catheters back to the surgery area. Many used the opportunity to "stuff up the sleeves, like oranges...fresh fruit. We didn't have much opportunity to have things like that. I remember one time I came out of there...I was just loaded down...and Sister Lucia met me and said: 'Are you hungry, dear?' She had a dish of doughnuts. I could hardly reach out to get them. I was never so humiliated in my life."[5]

Sister Lucia gradually and gracefully retired from active duty at Mercy after having served faithfully for more than 65 years. She died in April 1969, and is buried in Glendale Cemetery.

SISTER MARY PAULINE HAMMES

Sister Mary Pauline Hammes wore many hats during her 35 years of service to Mercy. She supervised the surgery areas, administered anesthetics, and at one time, supervised central supply and the stockrooms.

Emma Hammes was born in Portsmouth, Iowa, near Harlan in 1898. Her family relocated to the Pocahontas area where they built a thriving shoe store business. Emma received her nurse's training at Mercy Hospital in Council Bluffs, and entered the Sisters of Mercy in 1924, becoming Sister Mary Pauline.

Sister Pauline spent several years between Council Bluffs and Centerville as a floor supervisor in the x-ray and laboratory areas. She came to Des Moines in 1933 in surgery and delivery. Two of Sister Pauline's nieces remember making the trip from Pocahontas to Mercy for tonsillectomies because "aunt" Sister Pauline was in charge of surgery.[6] Another remembers she really did not like to sit on Sister Pauline's lap "because she always smelled like ether."[7]

Sister Pauline was well known for her frugality. While she was in charge of central supply, Mercy's staff had to "almost sign their life away" when getting supplies. If she found a light on in an unoccupied area she was heard to comment: "Well, who's paying the light bill this month."[8] Sister Pauline kept close ties to her family. One of her sisters and seven nieces graduated from Mercy's School of Nursing.

One long-time Mercy employee credits Sister Pauline with saving her life. Frieda Steele was helping to move a patient from the bed to a gurney when the sheet ripped. The force threw Frieda backwards toward one of the long, Central Wing windows. Sister Pauline grabbed her just as Frieda was about to go through the glass. "I can still feel the sensation."[9]

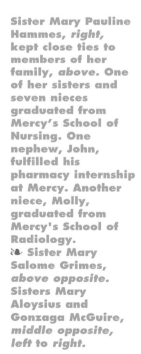

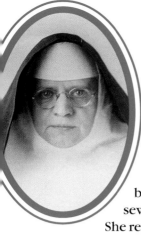

SISTER MARY SALOME GRIMES

Sister Mary Salome Grimes was another of Mercy's "Irish-born" ladies who became a Sister of Mercy in 1906. She served at St. Bernard's novitiate and St. Catherine's Hall for Business Women before coming to Mercy in 1925. Sister Salome plied her skills in sewing from her own little nook on the Fourth Floor for many years. She remained at Mercy until her death in 1961.

SISTERS MARY ALOYSIUS AND GONZAGA MCGUIRE

There have been several blood sisters who came to Des Moines from Council Bluffs and served as religious Sisters of Mercy. The earliest set of these "sister Sisters" was Sisters Mary Aloysius and Gonzaga McGuire.

They were born in Illinois and their family of 12 children migrated to Iowa and settled in the Audubon area. Sister Aloysius entered the Council Bluffs novitiate in 1905, eight years before Sister Gonzaga. Her first assignment was at St. Bernard's in nursing. Sister Aloysius was the first of the McGuire sisters to be assigned to Des Moines. She became supervisor of Mercy's obstetrical floor from 1925 to 1927. She was replaced by Sister Gonzaga, who was in charge of obstetrics from 1927 until 1931. Sister Gonzaga left Des Moines for one year in 1931 to go to Denver. She returned in 1932 and remained in Des Moines until 1954.

Sister Gonzaga dominated the first floor "Gold Coast," following its earlier supervision by Sister Anthony:

> "She admitted her own patients for the most part. If you came to the hospital and Sister liked the looks of you, you got to go on her ward. She managed that whole area like it was her own property. She set the prices, she picked the nurses, she had the rooms painted and decorated whenever she felt like it. This was common knowledge and everybody knew it and laughed and enjoyed it because she ran a tight ship." [10]
>
> "She had her own friends...Babe [Bisignano] loved her and she loved Babe. Sister and Babe were close and when she wanted to get a room decorated she would call up Babe and say 'Babe, I need some money', and he would send her a check. But when Babe got sick, he got a room." [11]

Sister Gonzaga spent more than 27 years in service at Mercy. She worked with surgical and eye, ear, nose and throat patients. Sister Aloysius served 18 years in administration at St. Joseph's in Centerville. It is said that both sisters developed cancer, but did not tell each other. Sister Aloysius returned to Mercy to be with her sister. She died there on September 19, 1950. She is buried in Glendale Cemetery.

By the time of her sister's death, Sister Gonzaga walked with a cane. "I learned later that she had multiple metastases to bone and was actually in the process of gradually dying." [12] Sister Gonzaga retired from active duty in 1953. She returned to St. Bernard's Hospital in Council Bluffs where she died in 1962. [13]

AN INDELIBLE PRESENCE

During the 25 years from 1922 to 1947, more than 50 remarkable "angels of Mercy" ministered their caring arts on the people of central Iowa. These self-sacrificing, strong women created an indelible presence as they guided the direction of Mercy Hospital to its permanent place in the healing history of Iowa.

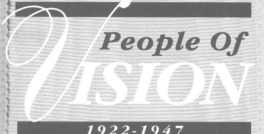

People Of VISION

1922-1947

SISTERS OF MERCY
(Continued from page 119.)

John O'Leary
Joseph Munch
Kevin O'Sullivan
Leona Weil
Loretta Laughlin
Lorraine Daniels
Louise Owens
Loyola Kelleher
Michael Huban
Natalie Senecal
Pauline Hammes
Pierre Brennan
Rosaire Keairnes
Rosalita Culjat
Salome Grimes
Sebastian Geneser
Thomas Wilson
Teresa Connell
Veronica Ryan
Winifred Leusen
Xavier Clinton
Zita Brennan

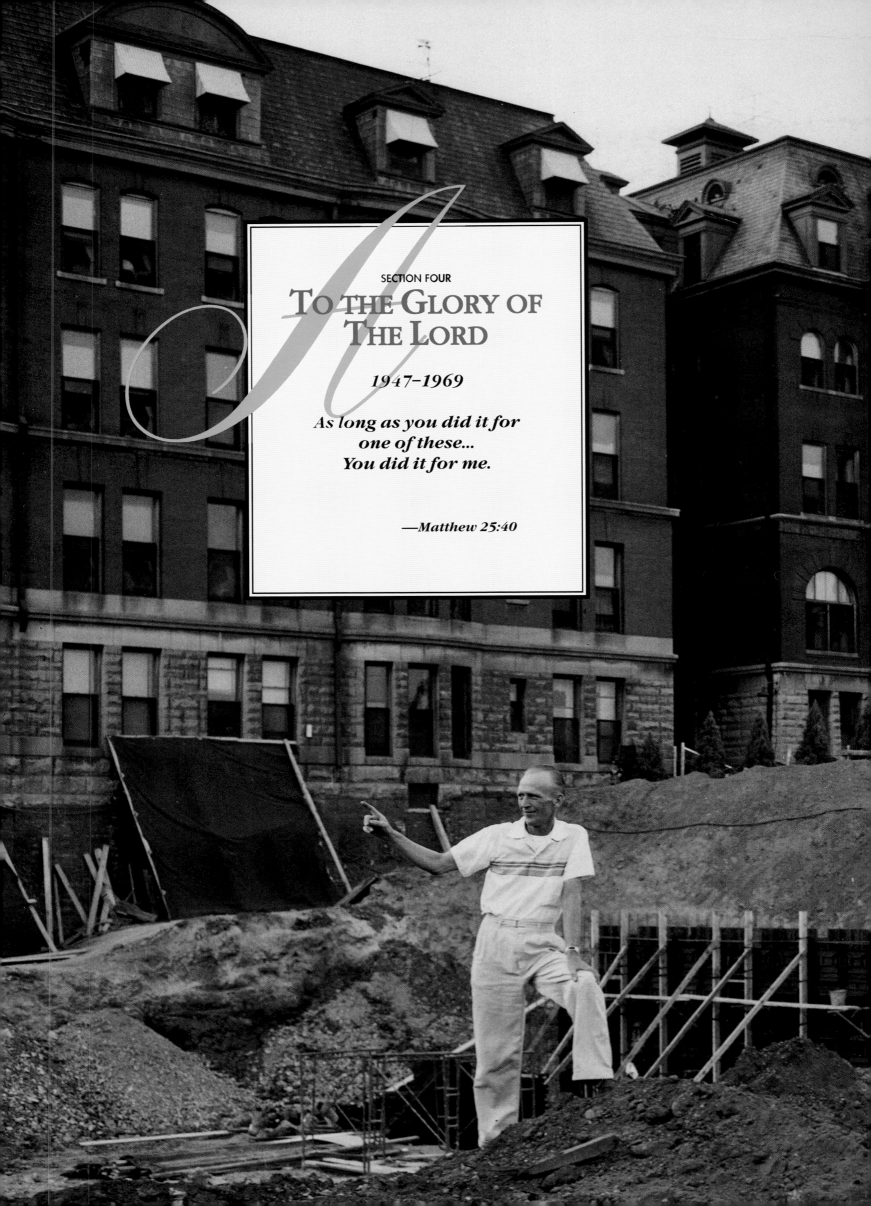

SECTION FOUR

TO THE GLORY OF THE LORD

1947–1969

*As long as you did it for
one of these...
You did it for me.*

—*Matthew 25:40*

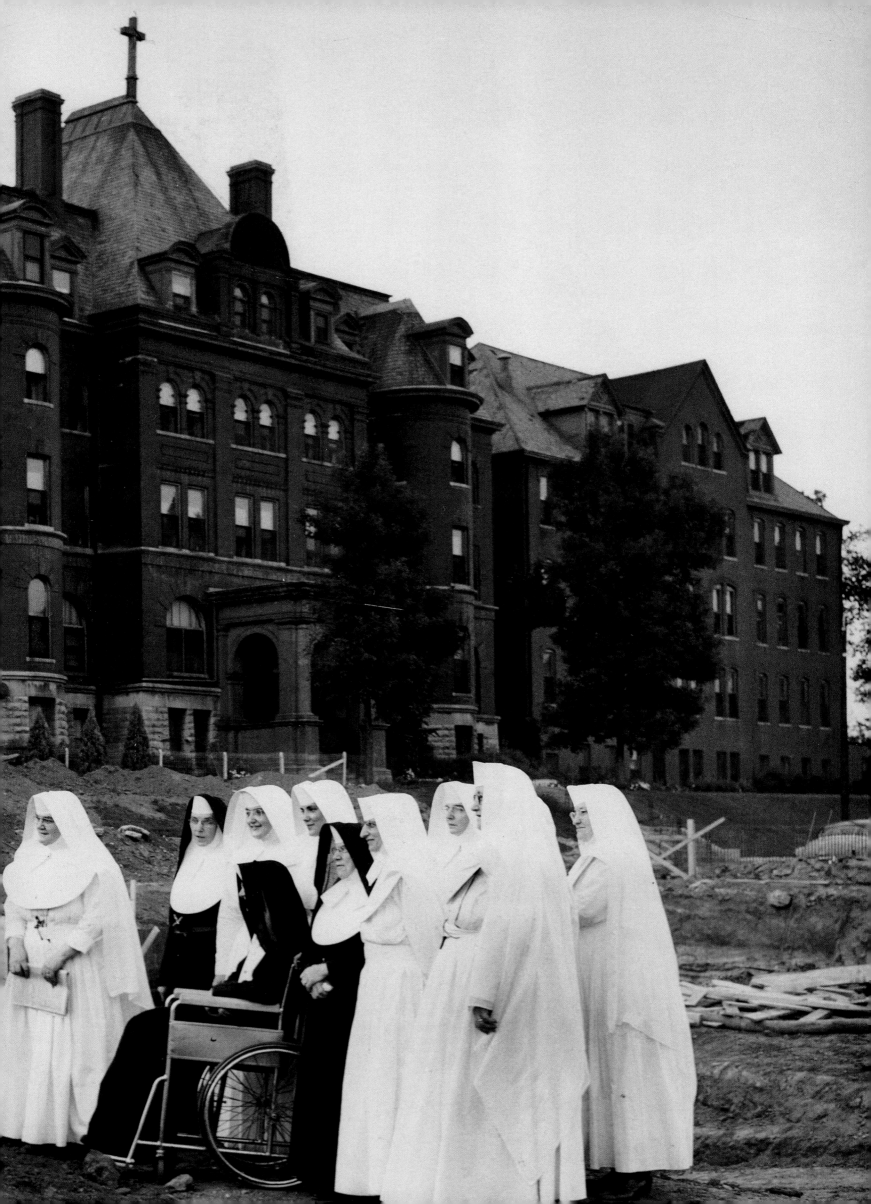

CHAPTER ONE
PATHS NOT YET TAKEN: A NEW DIRECTION

As World War II ended, Mercy eagerly looked forward to a time filled with the promise of change and redirection. Mercy and the Des Moines community had experienced the stifling effects of the Depression and the fears of war. Now it was time to leave behind the memories of those years and move confidently into the future.

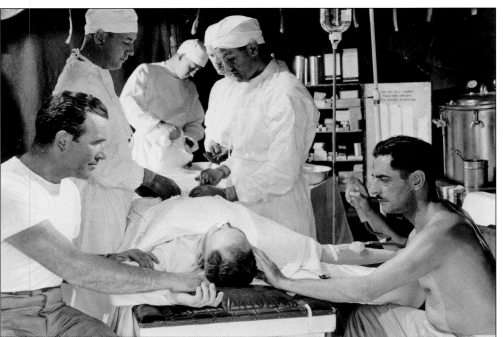

THE MEDICAL STAFF

When Mercy's physicians left for service in World War II, Sister Pauline carefully wrapped their surgical instruments and put them in storage. After their safe return, the physician-heroes were joyfully welcomed home. Their surgical instruments were unwrapped and returned to service. Military clinical experiences were then shared with fellow physicians at medical staff meetings.

Mercy entered the post-war years with a medical staff of 136 members, 38 active and 98 associate. There were three residents: John Dooley, chief resident; R.C. Schropp, resident in pathology; and W.W. Sawtelle, resident in urology. This staff was supplemented by three interns from Creighton: Patricia Phelan, Lawrence Hickner, and James Maynard. The residents and interns comprised Mercy's "house staff."[1]

Dr. Walter Abbott served as president of the medical staff in 1948. Dr. Bernard Barnes was vice president and president-elect. Dr. J.H. McNamee served as secretary, succeeding Dr. James Chambers. Two standing committees, appointed by the sisters, were the Records and Laboratory Committees. Regular staff meetings were held in the hospital on the Tuesday following the first Monday of the month. Annual dues were $4, and attendance at monthly staff meetings usually averaged 40 members.

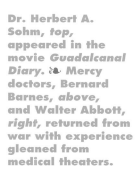

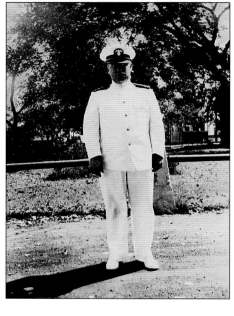

Dr. Herbert A. Sohm, *top,* appeared in the movie *Guadalcanal Diary.* ❧ Mercy doctors, Bernard Barnes, *above,* and Walter Abbott, *right,* returned from war with experience gleaned from medical theaters.

A New Medical Library

The Library Committee of the medical staff was created in 1948 to organize a new medical library. Physician-members of this committee were: Chambers, Foulk, Losh, and Hayne. Within a year, a new medical library was established. For a few years, there was no librarian, and visitors helped themselves. At other times, people were guided by a medical staff secretary. Mercy celebrated the library's tenth anniversary in 1959. Under the direction of a full-time librarian, the library housed more than 1,000 volumes and received 22 periodicals. Smaller libraries were kept in the radiology and pathology departments.[2]

Laboratory Growth

Dr. Frank Coleman became Mercy's pathologist in 1946. Educated at Tulane Medical School, with post-graduate work in New Orleans, Dr. Coleman brought extensive public health experience to Mercy. Under his leadership, Mercy's laboratory doubled in physical size within two years, and the professional staff grew to 12. Three distinct divisions evolved in this new laboratory: pathology, chemistry, and bacteriology. During this period, Dr. Coleman initiated the practice of using commercial plasma at Mercy to minimize the possibility of jaundice. Dr. Coleman held the chair positions on several medical staff committees and supervised the house staff of six residents and interns. When Dr. Coleman's many achievements were presented to Mercy's Advisory Board, he remarked : "This was really a Mercy appointment."[3]

Mercy's Laboratory experienced other professional growth during the mid-1950s. The first chemist in Iowa to be certified by the Registry of Medical Technologists as a biochemist was Mercy's Joe Zaletel. He was sixth in the nation to receive this honor.

Surgical Advancements

Surgical advances as a result of war experiences were enthusiastically embraced by Mercy's operating staff. A young Mercy orderly, who later became a medical staff member, Dr. Roy Overton II, remembers some of the innovations vividly:

> "[Surgical closures moved] from catgut to cotton, then, to wire right after World War II. Of all the improvements I saw [the best] was in anesthesia. John Connell had a great big old gas machine—ethylene. The changes in anesthesia were rapid and progressive."[4]

Clinical presentations during medical staff meetings were filled with news of modern surgical techniques learned in World War II. Two lucky pediatrics patients—one with a severed finger—benefited from the new procedures:

> "The family brought the child in, and the finger, and it was successfully re-attached....There was the 12-year-old with gas bacillus infection and a compound fracture as a result of a fall from a tree in a pasture. The surgeon made longitudinal incisions above and below the injury and laid oxygen catheters on the surface of each incision. That was one technique we hadn't covered in orthopedic nursing! But, the child went home with the arm intact."[5]

Walter Abbott, Des Moines' only neurosurgeon for a time, pioneered many uncharted areas of neurosurgery during his long association with Mercy. A special eight-bed area on the third floor of the Central Wing became known as "Abbott's

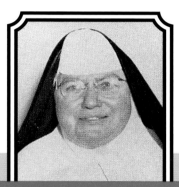

Sister Mary Helen

Sister Mary Helen Mackenzie was the first administrator during the period of Mercy revitalization that began in 1947. Sister Helen was no stranger to the hospital. She arrived in 1937 and served in various positions within the school of nursing, eventually as its director.

Jessie Mackenzie was born in Omaha, Nebraska. She did not become a Catholic until she finished her nurses' training. Jessie then entered the novitiate at Mount Loretto and became a Sister of Mercy in 1907.

Sister Helen spent more than 18 years at Mercy, working closely with Sister Mary Anita Paul. During this time, the advisory board was organized. As a result, when she became administrator late in 1947, Sister Helen was well-acquainted with the goals of Mercy. She served as administrator until 1953 when she was reassigned to Mercy Hospital in Council Bluffs. Sister Helen returned to Mercy Des Moines in 1954 and worked in assigned duties until 1956. She died at Mercy Council Bluffs in September 1963.

ADMINISTRATOR 1947-1953

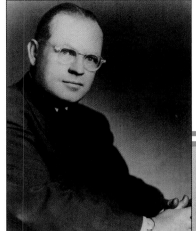

Alley" for recovering neurosurgery patients. Some of Dr. Abbott's young patients recuperated in the pediatric wing: "As they recovered to the point of walking around, you could encounter every variation of haircut long before the age of punk! Some of them were long-term patients who broke our hearts when they couldn't recover, or who caused full-scale celebrations when they went home."[6]

One young patient became so smitten with a white-robed Sister of Mercy that he gave her his most-cherished possession, a Hopalong Cassidy pocket knife. He asked her to "wait 'til he was old enough to get married."[7]

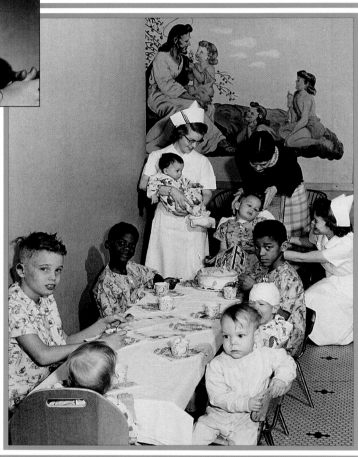

Mercy made news early in 1956 with the daring treatment of one of its youngest patients. For the first time on record, a lobectomy was performed in Des Moines on a 4-day-old baby. In a successful operation, a tumor the size of a baseball was removed from the young man's lung, and the future looked promising for a full recovery.[8]

Mercy continued pioneering in successful chest surgery on very young infants. One newborn was operated on for congenital cystic disease of the lung. Quick detection on the part of Mercy's diagnostic team was credited with saving the child's life.[9]

At this time, Mercy's children's department was located on the fifth floor of the West Wing. At least 30 patients between the ages of one day and 13 years could be cared for at any given time. Sister Mary Kieran Harney supervised this department from 1949 until 1954. Sister Mary Timothea Sullivan (now Sister Patricia Clare Sullivan) became supervisor in August 1955. Special comforting care, given out freely in large doses by the staff and by Mercy Guild members through their Child Health Program, not only helped young patients but eased the worried minds of their parents.[10] Sister Patricia Clare, remembering her time spent on Mercy's pediatrics floor says:

> *"Medicine wasn't so hectic then. I used to take some of the kids out in the backyard of the school of nursing, and have a ball game. Sometimes we would bake bread up in pediatrics....We formed life-long relationships with the families and the sick children."*[11]

THE RADIOLOGY DEPARTMENT

Drs. Thomas Burcham, Harry Dahl, and Floyd Springer served consecutively as Mercy's radiologist through the Depression and for a short time after World War II. One person remembered Drs. Burcham and Dahl suffering from burned fingertips as a result of early radiology treatments.[12]

In 1951, Dr. Noble Irving joined Dr. Springer as Mercy's associate radiologist. Dr. Irving was familiar with Mercy because he had practiced as a general practitioner, beginning in 1942. He left in 1948 to take a residency in radiology at the Kansas

In 1956, Mercy located pediatrics on the fifth floor of the West Wing. An eight-bed ward on the third floor of the Central Wing was named "Abbott's Alley" after Dr. Abbott, *top*. Children in both areas were often treated to parties. The birthday celebrated *above* featured ice cream and cake.

University Medical Center, returning to Mercy in 1951. Drs. Irving and Springer served at Mercy as radiologists for about six months, until Dr. Springer left to pursue other interests.

> *"Dr. Ralph Hines joined us in 1952, serving...until he retired in 1979. Sister Mary Nolasco was administrative head of the x-ray department until she left for Coos Bay, Oregon, in 1960. Dr. Irving was appointed director sometime later."* [13]

A forerunner in Iowa, Mercy was the second hospital, after the University of Iowa Hospital, to use radioactive isotopes as a diagnostic tool. In November 1953, a small closet in the x-ray department was designated for the use of isotopes.

The Atomic Energy Commission, as the regulatory agency, issued Mercy's license for radioactive substance use. In order to pass the stringent regulations for licensing, Mercy hired Dr. Adolf Voigt, a nuclear physicist working for the AEC at Iowa State University, to help prepare the facility for nuclear imaging. The measuring device used in those years—a Geiger counter—was primitive and inefficient by today's standards. Dr. Voigt served as Mercy's physicist for several years. He was replaced later by Milo Voss, who helped design the new isotope laboratories in the South Wing and tower additions.

NURSING SHORTAGE

At the end of the 1940s, Mercy once again faced a nursing shortage, this time as a result of the "baby boom." Patient admissions increased as the population grew like never before. Year-end Mercy statistics for 1947 heralded a record 1,675 births and inpatient admissions of 9,600—the highest in Mercy's 54-year history.

Nationwide, hospitals found themselves in the position of competing for nurses with the military services and other professions. Many nurses were able to find better paying employment as typists or seamstresses after the war. Typical salaries for staff nurses averaged $36 for a 48-hour work week.[14]

VOLUNTEER EFFORTS FORM AND GROW

Effects of the tremendous volunteer effort that took place during World War II continued to be felt throughout the city for many years after the war ended. There was a "good-neighbor" feeling in the community, and Mercy benefited from the good works of several volunteer groups.

The spirit of cooperation among Mercy leaders forged a new direction that generated a key internal support group—the Mercy Guild. This organization began at the urging of Ralph Branton, Mercy's Advisory Board chairman.

Another volunteer group that aided Mercy was the St. Camillus Guild. This branch of the Des Moines Diocesan Council of Catholic Nurses provided registered nursing care to the sick-poor, without compensation or remuneration and without regard for race or creed. Mercy's volunteers also included teenagers who served as Candystripers under the direction of the Guild. Many men gave their spare time to Mercy as members of the Holy Name Society from their home parishes.

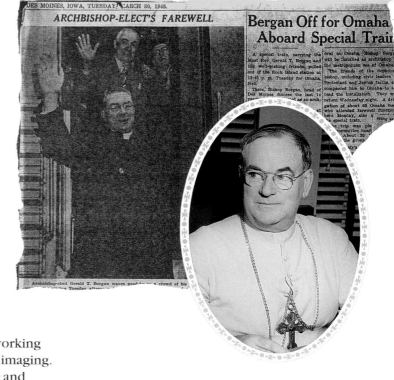

Bishop Gerald Bergan was named Archbishop of Omaha in 1948. Edward C. Daly, *above,* **replaced Bergan as bishop of the Des Moines Diocese. Bishop Daly proved to be a staunch supporter of Mercy Hospital.** ❧ *Below:* **Patricia Connolly, a Mercy Guild member, delivered mail to a patient.**

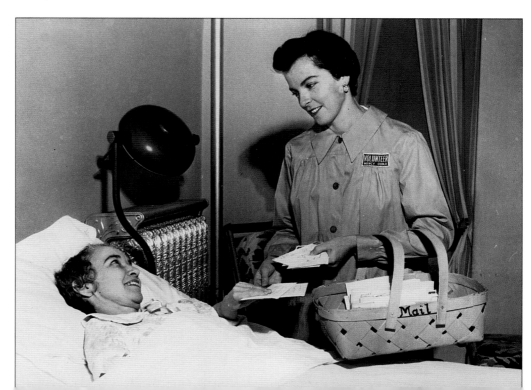

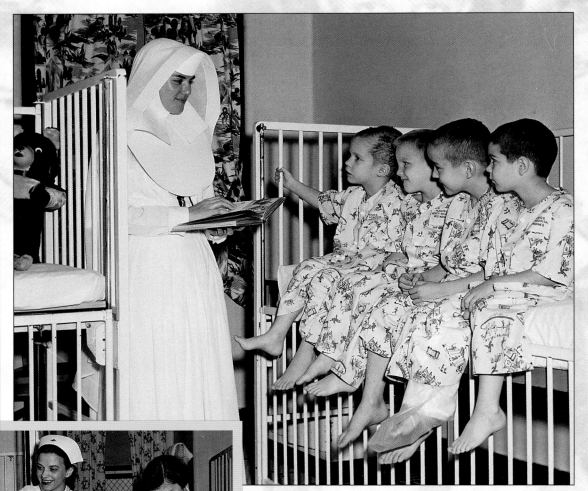

The beginning of the 1950s found Des Moines in the fear-stricken grip of a major polio epidemic. During 1952, Mercy converted 14 beds to the care of convalescent polio patients in order to relieve other hospitals who were overloaded with acutely ill and contagious polio patients. The smell of wet wool forever brings memories of those days to one Sister of Mercy who considers Dr. Jonas Salk a hero:

"I returned from summer school...to find that three of our pediatric nurses were on loan to Blank [Raymond Blank Memorial Hospital] to help meet the emergency. Blank had also borrowed most of the polio equipment. Mercy was asked if we could take a few patients as they came out of isolation since Blank was overloaded. [Mercy] agreed and [we] immediately found ourselves trying to cope with 20 to 25 polio patients. Each of them required six to eight hot packs a day—and all of our equipment was at Blank! Maintenance rigged up a Maytag washing machine with a heating coil in the bottom. In this machine we boiled woolen packs from 6:00 A.M. to 4:00 P.M. These packs were applied to the affected part of each patient. For most of them, we were doing full-body packs [which consisted of] a layer of hot damp wool, a layer of plastic, a layer of dry wool to hold the heat, and a light blanket over all. And this in Des Moines in August! Packs were changed hourly to renew the heat. Salt tablets were given and fluids were offered as frequently as children would accept them to prevent dehydration." [15]

Mercy's Guild members extended aid to patients afflicted with this painful and frightening disease. Countless hours were donated by the Guild as they fed, positioned, read books to, and changed hot packs for recovering children. Special parties were arranged by the Guild to celebrate birthdays or going home.

One of Mercy's student nurses, who was incapacitated by polio during training in 1939, was able to come back to work at Mercy in the late 1940s, thanks in part, to a lot of support from the Mercy laboratory director and staff. After a long recuperation, Florence Stumbo returned to Mercy as a laboratory technician. The hospital provided Miss Stumbo with a microscope equipped with special left-handed controls, a special chair, and several other pieces of modified equipment. Miss Stumbo worked at Mercy until her retirement in 1983.

Spirits were kept as high as possible in Mercy's pediatrics department by Sister Timothea (Patricia Clare) Sullivan, *top*, as well as nurses and members of the volunteer Mercy Guild, *above*. Times were not always jovial, but games and bedtime stories eased the pain.

TWO NEW DEPARTMENTS

As patient census began to grow, Mercy inaugurated two new departments devoted to short-term care in 1951: the tonsil ward and the outpatient department.

The tonsil ward made its debut on the east end of Mercy's third floor. Fifteen beds staffed by Sister Mary Herbert Kaufmann and three full-time employees gave care to patients who came for a tonsillectomy and adenoidectomy.

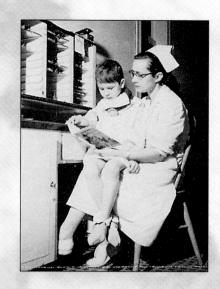

The tonsil ward was open from October to June each year. More than 1,000 tonsillectomies and numerous dental surgeries were performed each year. The patients ranged in age from eight months to 69 years and usually stayed no longer than 24 hours. A trend toward tonsil removal occurred during this time because they were blamed for many illnesses. It became the norm to remove tonsils and adenoids during certain times of the year, and many times, all children in one family were operated on during the same day. The record number of children from a single family to have their tonsils removed at one time was seven.[16] "We just didn't have the antibiotics that we have now. You took out the tonsils, and the kids just seemed to get better." [17]

Another much-performed surgery was done in the tonsil ward before the regular addition of fluoride to Des Moines' drinking water.

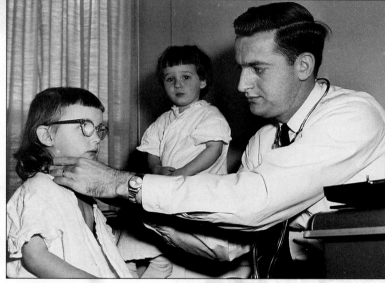

"One of our major surgeries here was taking kids to surgery and putting caps on their teeth. Drill them, clean, and put these little caps on their teeth to try to keep the infection from going into their adult teeth." [18]

Outpatient care had been provided by Mercy as early as the 1930s. Emergency and outpatient care were located in the same area. Mercy treated numerous mining accidents, burn victims, and indigents in this single room.

Expanded outpatient services developed when Mercy Hospital recognized the need to care for emergency patients and to provide service for those requiring treatment while recovering at home. As many as 2,530 persons were treated in this newly specialized department in 1951. The typical charge for this treatment area was two dollars.[19] One of Mercy's young interns said:

"This was in the days when we called it the emergency 'room,' rather than emergency department. The doctors would come and see their patients. Many times they would call us to check on their patients. [We had] lots of responsibility, especially at night after 10:00. Emergency work is either feast or famine...looking for patients or you've got too many. We were working with more than one patient at one time...everything from heart attack to a baby with a cold." [20]

A long-time Mercy employee recalled that one of her duties on the evening shift in the accounting department was to answer a special buzzer connected to the emergency room door. One evening, she answered the door to find a woman in the final stages of labor:

"I was only 19 and didn't know what to do. I ran across the hall and yelled in the interns' quarters for help. The intern came, and delivered the baby right in the room. Afterwards, he said: 'Well, Miss Savage, have you ever seen a birth before?' I said, 'No.' And he said; 'Well, no wonder you look a little green.' " [21]

The tonsil ward made its debut in 1951 when tonsillectomies were as frequent as the common cold. Mercy's young patients recovering from this surgery were treated with the comforting hands of nurses, such as Veronica Abricka, top, the Sisters of Mercy, volunteers, and physicians, above.

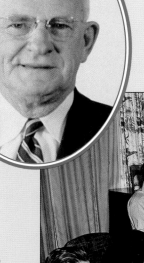

MODERNIZATION

Patient census soared as the 1950s began, and steady increases brought occupancy to an unheard of 95 percent. In March 1953, Sister Helen discussed the possibility of a new building program with the advisory board.[22] Advisory board chairman, Arthur Gormley, met with Mr. Pickworth of the Hospital Service for the State of Iowa who outlined details of the Hill-Burton Act, which allowed hospitals to seek funds for modernization or new buildings.[23] At the April 1953 advisory board meeting, Mr. Gormley asked that the board determine Mercy's needs, set goals, and apply for funds under the Hill-Burton Act.

In assessing hospital needs, the board first questioned whether or not to update present buildings. After touring Mercy's facilities, they found that the East Wing did not meet fire codes. It housed the chapel, milk laboratory, kitchen, dining room, and rooms for some ambulatory patients. A sprinkler system recently had been installed in the Central Wing, where two elevators transported patients. The pediatrics department had no isolation area for children, and the nurse in charge could not see all patients from her station. The obstetrics department was located too far from the nursery. With the great demand for obstetrical services, this department had only two delivery rooms and three progress rooms. Operating suites were equipped with new floors which safeguarded against the hazards of electric sparks. The West Wing was fireproof.

The consensus was that Mercy "although old...was very clean." [24] The board's task was to decide whether to improve existing structures or build new ones as they reviewed Mercy's history and noted that Des Moines needed additional hospital beds.

Since the opening of Mercy in 1893, more than 200,000 patients had been served.[25] By 1953, a city-wide survey conducted by the Iowa Department of Health determined that Des Moines needed 264 additional hospital beds. From January through April 1954, Mercy's daily occupancy averaged 104 percent. Mercy provided more than 240 days of charity care during 1954, at an average daily cost of $21.14. Mercy's administrators knew the value of Mercy Hospital to the Des Moines community, recognized the bed shortages, and determined that above all else, they must continue to minister their comforting care to those in need.[26]

After many surveys and discussions, Mercy leaders unveiled plans for a new building at the February 1954 advisory board meeting. Mr. Brooks of the architectural firm of Brooks, Borg, and Skiles presented drawings of the proposed new building which would be located south of the hospital on what was at that time the physicians' parking lot.[27] Final plans called for Ascension Street to be closed to traffic and the South Wing to be built on that site. An all-out fund-raising campaign took place. The South Wing and other Mercy expansions took place during the 22 months between June 1957 and May 1959.

In 1953, plans began developing to modernize Mercy Hospital. Advisory board chairman, Arthur Gormley, top, worked closely with Sisters Pauline, left, and Anita, right, to begin a building campaign for the hospital. Plans were presented in February 1954. They included the South Wing expansion and other improvements to existing areas of the hospital. ❧ In 1955, Mercy displayed statistics in the kind of factograms shown below. ❧ Opposite: In July 1956, Mercy experienced another baby boom when 186 infants entered the world.

ADMISSIONS	BIRTHS	SISTERS	PHYSICIANS	OPERATIONS
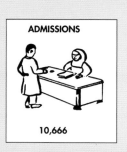	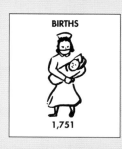	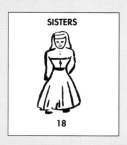	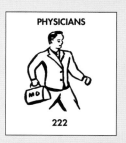	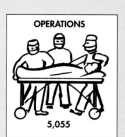
10,666	1,751	18	222	5,055

MERCY'S BABY BOOM

Comforting patient care never wavered during the planning and building of the South Wing. Mercy's maternity department bustled with activity, breaking all records in July 1956 when 186 babies entered life at Mercy. The greatest number of births occurred on July 16 and 17, when ten infants made their debut at Mercy Hospital. On July 19, Sister Mary Zita and her hard-working crew squeezed 41 mothers into an area with a normal capacity of 31.

Part of this influx of maternity patients came as a result of a misfortune at another Des Moines hospital. An outbreak of a gas bacillus infection caused Iowa Methodist Hospital to close its maternity wing for a few days. Mercy graciously opened its doors to care for the extra patients. Sister Zita remembered receiving a letter from the administrator of Iowa Methodist, thanking Mercy for its help.[28]

A very special feature added to Mercy's maternity department about this time was the "six-pack" of formula given to new mothers as they left for home with their babies. The Mercy milk laboratory prepared enough formula to put into six eight-ounce nursing bottles, complete with nipples and caps, in a convenient carrying carton. Processed using terminal sterilizing methods, this baby formula was safe and convenient for the first 24 hours after the new family went home.

IN CHARGE OF OBSTETRICS WARD

Nun 'Loves to Hear Babies Cry Quiet Ones Worry Her

By Staff Writer.

Sister Mary Zita has bathed and diapered, fed and cuddled more than 20,000 babies since she took charge of the obstetrical ward at Des Moines Mercy Hospital 16 years ago.

It's easy to see she cherishes the little mites in the nursery from the gentle way she snuggles them in her arms, from her deep concern over the welfare of the tiny crew in the incubator room.

Thus, it was surprising to hear her say: "I love to hear them cry."

'Good' Baby.

Most people don't like to hear a baby cry. It's a sound that worries, distresses or even irritates young mothers. But the hospital nursery ...

Mercy Hospital
Premature Nursery

Dear Mommy and Daddy

Good morning. Its me, your little Julie Ann sending you greetings on Valentines Day. The Nurses have been teaching me to write. I hope you like it. I am also learning how to say my prayers. and I can say God Bless Mommy and Daddy and everybody. I heard the Doctor telling the Nurse today that if I keep on gaining I will soon graduate from the Isolette. You see I am 3 lbs 3 oz to-day, and am eating all they give me so I can grow up and come home soon. We had a Valentines party in our room and it was lots of fun, the Nurses sang with us and no one had to keep the tune. Oh here comes my bottle, which means its time to eat - then take a nap. Good Night Mommy and all

Julie Ann

Come, see me soon and bring my Daddy

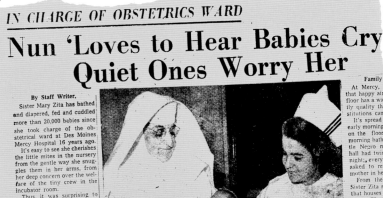

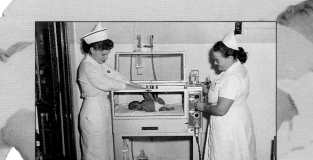

131

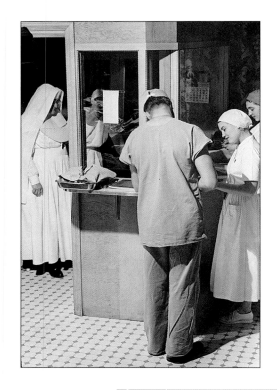

FOR THE INTERNS

Mercy had sponsored an active intern educational program since the early 1900s. At the end of their Mercy service, early interns were awarded a special key (an ornament to hang on their watch chains) decorated with Mercy's name and engraved with the physician's name. During the 1950s, Mercy tailored the intern training program to the needs of the general practitioner, a move which strengthened the overall program. Mercy began offering pathology residencies at this time, and added surgical residencies in the 1960s. Mercy's intern training program was first accredited by the Council on Medical Education and Hospitals of the American Medical Association in 1956.[29]

Mercy was fortunate to have an enthusiastic medical staff to train interns. An Intern Committee regularly reviewed and supervised the program and the students to maintain quality standards. The educational staff worked diligently to help foreign interns who came to Mercy.

In 1951, Mercy received approval from the Bureau of Immigration and Naturalization to allow foreign physicians "to pursue training in their respective fields in the United States and to promote the general interests of international exchange."[30] These students faced obstacles of language barriers and differences in levels of training. The interns became more fluent in English by taking classes several nights each week. This enabled eight out of nine to pass their board examinations. Mercy was quite proud of this record.[31]

Mercy's first medical education coordinator, Dr. Floyd Woodard, was named in 1953. Dr. Julius Conner, an intern in 1957, remembers Dr. Woodard as: "The one responsible for setting up schedules and all the monthly rotations. Any problems we had, we came to him."[32] During the 1950s and 1960s, Drs. Frank Coleman, Noble Irving, and John Bakody formed a medical staff "triumvirate" dedicated to improving Mercy's intern and residency educational program.[33]

The most important phase of intern training at that time consisted of daily, organized ward rounds, with bedside teaching by mentor physicians. Clinical presentations, films, conferences, rotations through outpatient and emergency, and journal review presentations, rounded out training for the new physicians. A special television link to the University of Iowa Medical School allowed interns a firsthand look at their programs. The cost to Mercy for the service was $700 per month.[34]

The Mercy Medical Staff sponsored the fledgling physicians, assuming the serious responsibility of preparing them for their roles in community service. Mercy paid their interns a stipend of $175 per month. Apartment accommodations for all students were provided at Wakonda Village. Free laundry, meals, hospitalization, and paid vacation were welcome benefits for the interns. For the six years between 1953 and 1959, twenty-five interns pursued residencies for specialized training. By 1959, Des Moines benefited from this when nine physicians established practices in the city after completing internship at Mercy.

In 1956, a four-year pathology residency began through Mercy's laboratory. By September 1959, nine pathologists had completed residencies at Mercy, and three

Sister Pauline, *top,* **supervised the surgical nurses' station in the 1950s.** ❧ **A special television link between Mercy and the University of Iowa Medical School allowed interns a firsthand look at the school's programs.**

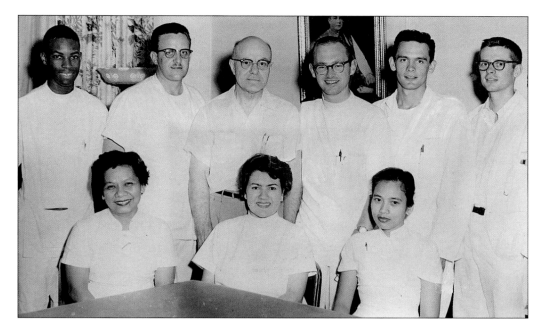

additional students were in training. The course of study was divided into three-month rotations through many areas, including medical technology, cytotechnology, and nursing.

Mercy Medical Day

The first Mercy Medical Day was inaugurated on September 23, 1959. The medical staff and the Sisters of Mercy used this medium to introduce Central Iowa physicians to Mercy's newly expanded facility. A luncheon in the new hospital cafeteria was provided by the Sisters for 200 area physicians. Three special guests presented scientific papers and a clinical symposium following lunch. Drs. Charles Mayo, Herbert Schmitz and Arnold Jackson were principal speakers, whose topics included: Diverticulosis and Diverticulitis and the Value of Preoperative Irradiation to Adenocarcinoma of the Endometrium. Drs. Neil McGarvey, Daniel Crowley, Jr., Noble Irving, Jr., and Frank Coleman, of Mercy's Staff served as a discussion panel for diseases of the thyroid gland. After the educational session, the visitors were treated to a tour of the new South Wing and remodeled areas with special attention given to new clinical areas in the laboratory, operating suites, and radiology. All agreed that Mercy had become "a center for the healing arts in this section of the country."[35]

Regular department head meetings, general information meetings, and new employee orientation programs evolved during the 1950s as well. The agenda for these meetings was published in the Mercy *Bulletin*.

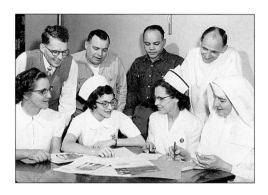

A Need To Grow

Mercy's staff embraced new changes as the result of World War II. Patient census soared, and all worked diligently to provide the best service with the latest technology. Mercy's gracious volunteers gave welcomed assistance to the sisters and staff. It became apparent that Mercy needed more room, and everyone eagerly looked forward to that possibility.

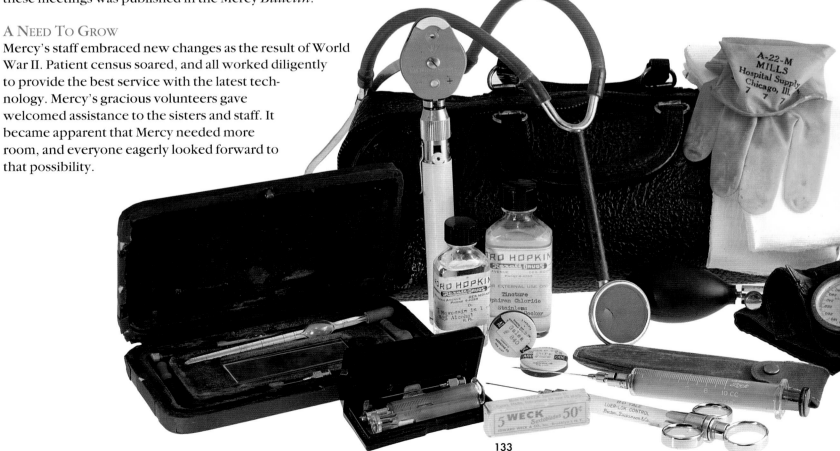

CHAPTER TWO
TOMORROW'S HOPE: STRUCTURAL GROWTH

The years 1947-1969 saw massive structural changes at Mercy Hospital which proved to strengthen it from the inside out. Physical changes to the hospital were extensive. Personnel moves and diversifications came about at an equally impressive rate. Strong educational programs set the pace for Mercy's future in a high-tech tomorrow.

In 1953, excitement filled discussions about the possibility of building Mercy's South Wing, expanding existing services and departments, and creating or modernizing others. At the same time, Mercy's administration experienced several changes. Sister Helen was re-assigned to Mercy Hospital in Council Bluffs, and Sister Anita Paul returned to Des Moines to serve as administrator for a second term. Sister Anita was the only administrator from the Omaha Province who served more than one term. After Sister Helen's departure, Sister Pauline Hammes became assistant administrator, and for the first time, Mercy hired a business manager, Donald J. Conroy.

AN AMBITIOUS BUILDING CAMPAIGN

Once the decision was made to build the South Wing and expand Mercy, the administration and advisory board embarked on the first major fund-raising campaign in Mercy's 61-year history.

Acting on the advice of the advisory board, the sisters hired American City Bureau of Chicago, a campaign firm, to direct the fund-raising.

Mercy faced stiff competition in its city-wide plans to solicit funds. The YMCA had just finished a major fund-raising campaign, the Catholic Diocese solicited funds for the Bishop's Campaign, and the annual United Campaign was just completed. Goals for all totaled $6,000,000.

Mercy's campaign and building plans received the support of Bishop Daly, although monies would not be solicited from Catholic parishes in a general campaign. The board of consulters of the diocese gave a gift of $250,000.[1] A grant of $124,000 from the Ford Foundation came to Mercy just before Christmas 1955. With this award, Mercy counted itself among the nation's fortunate colleges and hospitals to receive a share of $500,000,000 given by the Ford Foundation. Mercy qualified for this grant based on its number of patient days and births. These contributions boosted Mercy's building plans substantially.[2]

Supplied with funds from the diocese and the Ford Foundation, Mercy began its fund-raising campaign with confidence. The campaign

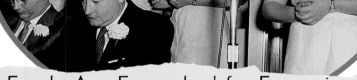

Funds Are Earmarked for Expansion
Mercy Hospital Given $917,000 Federal Grant

Des Moines.—The Iowa Hospital in federal funds to Mercy Hospital construction and expansion program

Diocesan Hospitals Presented $325,100 By Ford Foundation

Des Moines.—The four Catholic hospitals in the Diocese of Des Moines were listed last week as eligible for grants from the Ford Foundation totaling $325,00.

The southwest Iowa Catholic hospitals named, with their proposed grants, are Mercy Hosptial, Des Moines, $124,000; St. Bernard's Psychiatric Hospital, Council Bluffs, $101,800; Mercy Hospital, Council Bluffs, $86,800; and Rosary Hospital, Corning, $12,500.

No final determination for the use of the funds has been made by local hospital authorities as yet. Mercy in Des Moines is planning a new multimillion dollar wing and St. Bernard's has already announced plans for a new nurses' home.

The hospitals are among the 3,500 voluntary, nonprofit hospitals in the United States, its territories and possessions, which will share $200,000,000 in aid from the foundation.

A special appropriation of $500,000,000 was approved by the foundation to be distributed among colleges and hospitals across the land. The foundation gift is the largest single appropriation in the history of philanthropy.

In 1954, Mercy embarked on the most extensive building campaign the hospital had ever undertaken. The goal was to raise money to build the South Wing and improve and modernize existing facilities. Fund-raising efforts were set at more than $2 million.

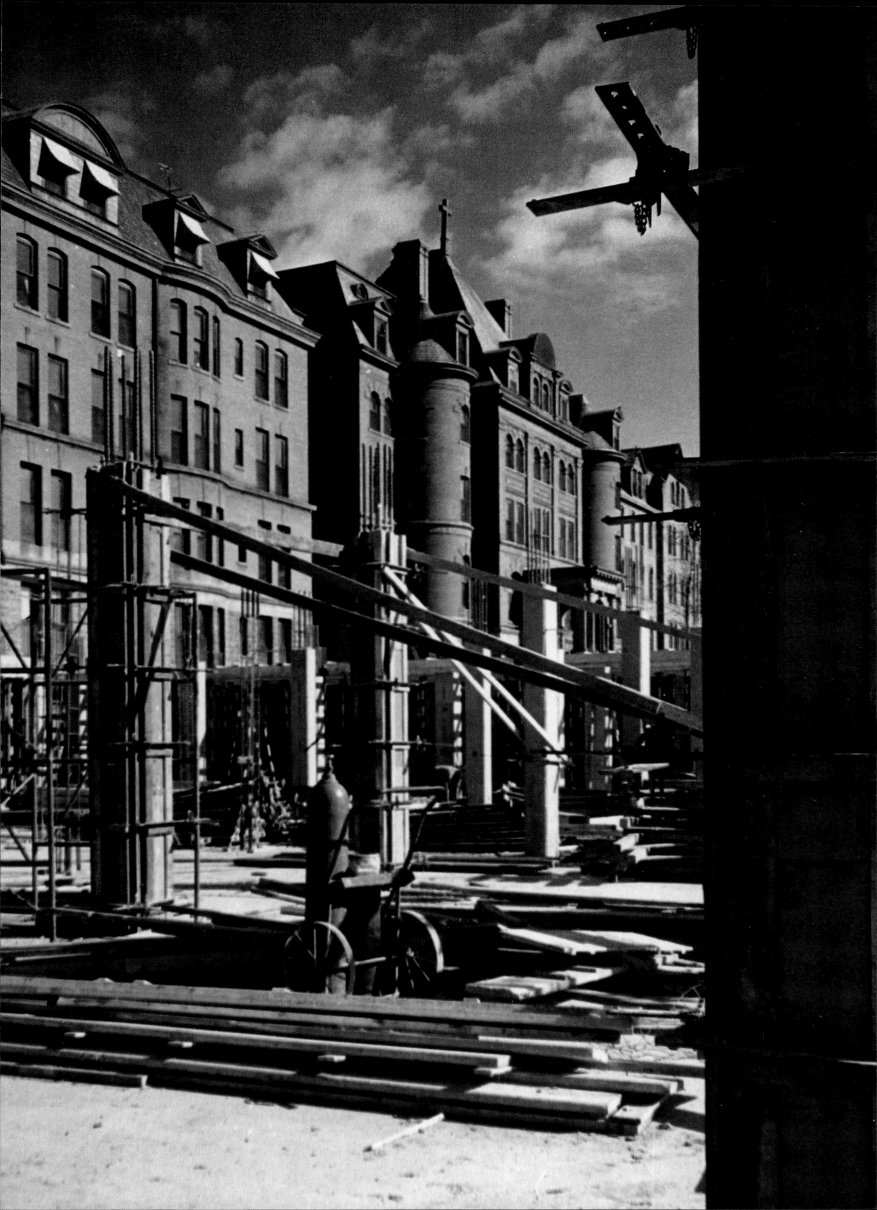

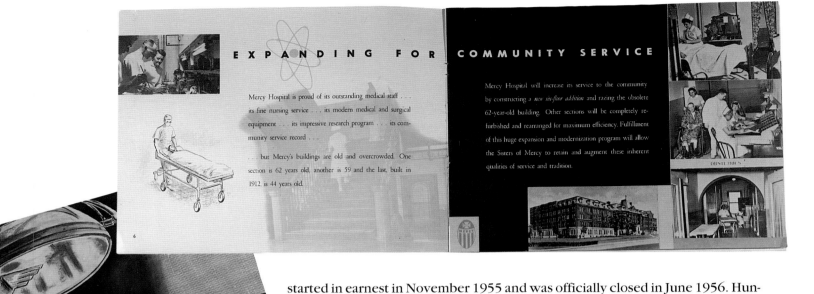

started in earnest in November 1955 and was officially closed in June 1956. Hundreds of hours of planning, organizing and motivating kept the project on target, ensuring a successful attainment of goals. When the campaign ended, director Bob Curry, spoke about the success of the program, giving credit in this way:

> *"...It may have been the excellent leadership provided by the Medical Group; it may have been the challenging pace-setting gifts of our large corporations; it may have been the activity of the Mercy Hospital employees; it may have been the aggressiveness with which the organization moved after delays; it may have been the exciting enthusiasm of the 'Catholic Participation' gift to the program. Summing it all up, credit for [the campaign's] success is due to the timely participation of certain groups, and the fine leadership supplied by the community."* [3]

In the end, $2,347,460 was raised through this ambitious campaign. Federal monies received from the Hill-Burton Act totaled $917,000, bringing the amount raised to $3,264,460. This outpouring of support for Mercy's efforts prompted Sister Anita to write:

> *"No matter where you are, or in whatever manner your interest in our expansion program was demonstrated, whether by labor, by financial help, by prayer or perhaps only by an expression of concern that we succeed in our efforts to obtain more area for patient care, we want you to know that we are sincerely grateful for your assistance...[This will be] a building which for years to come will stand as a memorial to your kindness and generosity. May God bless you, and keep you friends of Mercy Hospital."* [4]

EXPANSION AND RENOVATION

It took two years and $4,750,000 ($1,100,000 more than anticipated) to complete the South Wing and modernizations at the hospital. Remodeling in other areas and the future demolition of the East Wing enlarged Mercy's bed capacity to 300. Bids for the expansion were approved on June 21, 1957, and six primary contractors were chosen for the job.

The renovation was divided into five phases: Phases I and II created the new wing and expanded the boiler room and laundry building. Phase III began after the new

Hundreds of hours of planning and motivating kept Mercy's building program vital and on track. In the end, the outpouring of support was so great that the hospital raised $3 million. Sister Mary Anita gave credit for the successful effort to the kindness and generosity of the Des Moines community.

wing was completed. It consisted of remodeling the West Wing which included a new delivery room suite and a newborn nursery area, lavatories and oxygen piped into each patient room, as well as a new x-ray unit for the first floor. Phase IV involved the demolition of the East Wing, the destruction of which paved the way for Phase V— the construction of a new chapel.

SOUTH WING CONSTRUCTION

The groundbreaking for the new South Wing was held at 10:30 A.M. on Thursday, June 27, 1957. In spite of a gentle rain, all were smiling when Sister Anita turned over the first shovelful of dirt. Charles T. Cownie acted as master of ceremonies.

Mercy petitioned the Des Moines City Council to close Ascension Street between Fifth Avenue and Fourth Street to accommodate the new six-floor structure that would connect at the southwest corners of the West and North Wings. The South Wing would house a basement and a penthouse that contained the air conditioning, heating, electrical, and pneumatic tube communication systems. The surgery area would be expanded to 10 operating rooms, with a 12-bed recovery area. New supply and delivery and dietary areas were planned.

As a result of this expansion, the main entrance to the hospital moved from the Central Wing front stairway to the ground-floor level in the South Wing. The new entrance was covered by a canopy to ease the arrival of patients during bad weather.

Construction on the South Wing began just after the groundbreaking. A large shade tree that had graced the entrance for many years felt the blow of the workers' axe. Openings were cut into five patient rooms, the chaplain's bedroom, and the autopsy room on the basement level to make a connection to the new wing on each floor. Plans called for the South Wing to open for occupancy by January 1, 1959.

A DOOR THAT NEVER CLOSES

Work on the new wing proceeded closely on schedule, delaying the grand opening by only three months from the original projection. Religious dedication ceremonies for the South Wing were held on Friday, April 10, 1959. Father Lloyd Connolly, Mercy's chaplain at that time, blessed the new facility during a ceremony for church and civic dignitaries. Members of the medical staff were hosted at a special reception that same evening. For the next two days, more than 6,000 visitors were treated to hour-long guided tours. Mercy's cherry-garbed Guild members acted as gracious hostesses,

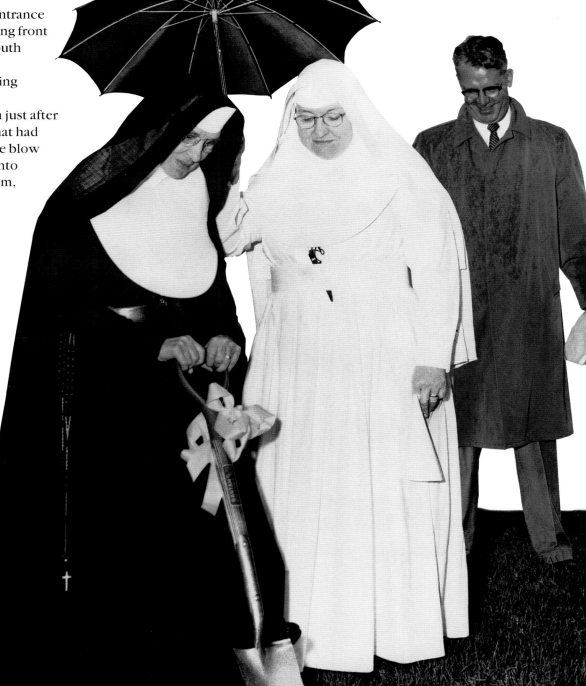

The South Wing groundbreaking was held on June 27, 1957. *Left to right below:* Sisters Anita and Pauline and Master of Ceremonies Charles T. Cownie were on hand to turn the first shovelful of dirt.

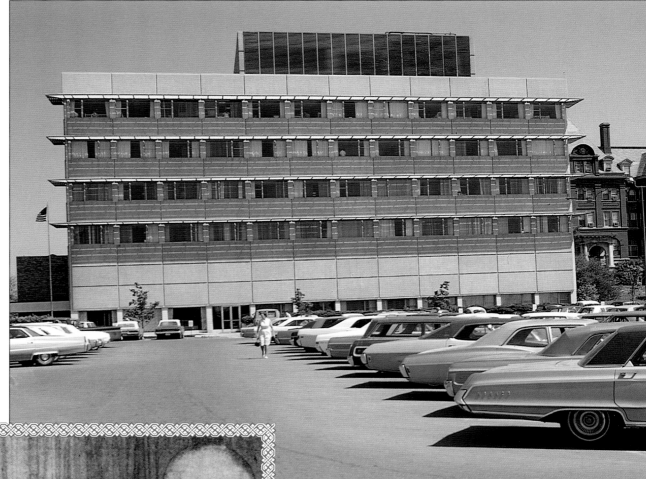

The South Wing, *right,* was ready for occupation in spring 1959. 🔔 Religious dedication ceremonies were held in April when Arthur Gormley presented Sister Anita a key to the new wing, *below.* The move into the facility began on May 2, 1959.

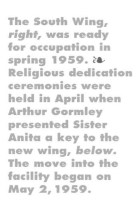

walking countless miles through the new facility. When Arthur Gormley presented Sister Anita with a key to the new wing, she responded:

> *"What shall I do with it, because a hospital door never is closed?" Then, in answer to her own question Sr. M. Anita said: "It shall be a symbol of our pledge to the people of Des Moines to give the best patient care."* [5]

SOUTH WING OCCUPATION

Occupation of the new wing officially began at noon on Friday, May 2, 1959. By late afternoon, 72 adult patients and 48 newborns were settled securely in the new rooms. The babies were bundled up and carefully carried by student nurses to their mothers' new rooms for feeding.

Once patients were safely in their rooms, everything on wheels became a carrier to move supplies and equipment into the new wing. Wheelchairs and beds were loaded with linens, supplies, footstools, charts, and whatever else needed to be transported. There were the inevitable bugs in the system. Elevators and telephones did not work smoothly, but Mercy's maintenance team stood ready to straighten out problems as they arose.

Sister Mary Therese Bannon, supervisor of the medical-surgical department, worked throughout the day, sorting supplies, checking equipment, dusting furniture; doing whatever needed to be done. "Talk about the Exodus...I was so tired at the end of the day," recalls Sister Therese. These sentiments mirrored the feelings of Mercy's staff as they assembled in the new cafeteria for an evening meal. They had put in a long, hard day, and anticipated more of the same on the following day. The Sisters of Mercy graciously announced that this first meal in the new facility would be "on the house."

When the move to the South Wing was completed, new room rates were set. Private rooms cost $28 per day and rooms with two beds were priced at $16 per day. Prices in the older building varied: Two-bed rooms in the West Wing cost $14.50 per day; in the Central Wing, $13.50. A fee of $30 was charged for the delivery room.[6]

A New Dietary System

Mercy began experimenting with a new type of patient tray delivery system a few months before the opening of the South Wing. This made a smoother transition to the new facility. Special carts containing divided sections for cold and hot foods transported meals to the floors. No longer was food prepared in bulk in the main kitchen, put on the dumb-waiter with stops on each floor, re-heated in the special diet kitchens, loaded onto patient trays, and distributed to the patients.

In the new system, patient trays were portioned and set up within the new kitchen, loaded into special hot and cold sections on the food trucks, moved to the floors, and delivered to each patient's door. At that point the cold and hot foods were assembled according to the patient's diet, combined with an appropriate beverage, and delivered to the patient. Approximately 1,600 meals were prepared in the new kitchen each day.

Plans were in the works for the first "selective" menu to be distributed to each patient who then would choose from a selection of foods appropriate for their diet. This variety would give "the poor fellow who doesn't like calves' liver [the opportunity] to choose a second meat (at long last)."[7] This selective menu became a reality in February 1961.

In 1963, Mercy set aside a special area in the new dietary department for the preparation of kosher meals. Mercy invited Rabbi Irving A. Weingart to supervise setting up and maintenance of the kosher kitchen.[8] Mercy continues to prepare kosher meals four to six times each year. Special knives are kept just for this practice, and meat is purchased from a local kosher delicatessen.[9]

Two new eating areas located in close proximity to the new dietary unit also made their debut during this time. An employees' cafeteria, designed to comfortably seat 150 persons, was located adjacent to the new kitchen. A conveyer belt placed on one end of the cafeteria facilitated the return of soiled dishes to the kitchen. A large-capacity dishwasher waited at the end of the conveyer.

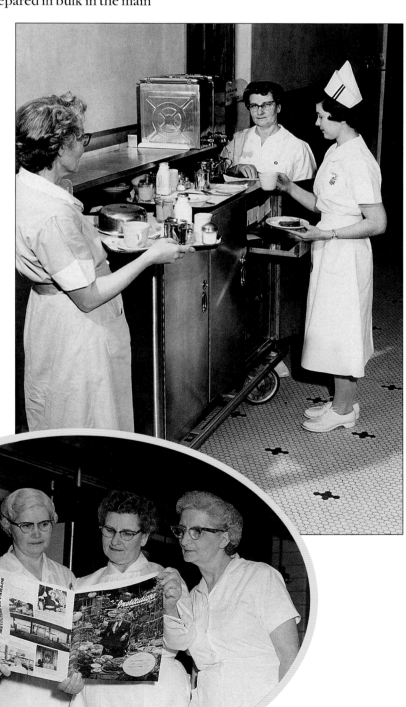

Mercy began experimenting with a new type of patient tray delivery system a few months after the South Wing opened. Food was taken directly to each patient's room. ❧ *Left to right bottom: Sister Mary Lucia, Lucy McLaughlin, Mildred Torrence, and Irene Tonsi read a copy of Institutions magazine.*

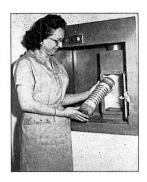

One of the most modern devices to be installed in the South Wing was a pneumatic tube system that served as a communication network for the hospital. Carriers, *below,* were designed to be large enough to deliver small instrument bundles, medical records, and more to all units connected to the system.

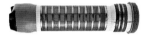

A SPECIAL TOUCH

One special feature of the South Wing caused considerable debate before it became praised as an intelligent foresight. Several members of the advisory board opposed the addition of air-conditioning in the new wing: "Why should we burden the sisters just to make [the physicians] comfortable?" [10]

Approval to go ahead with this expense was given after much deliberation. Mercy was the only Des Moines hospital to have this luxury for a time, and everyone who had worked or been a patient in the older areas of Mercy appreciated this special touch.

Another device representative of the era's technology was the central dictation network. This shortened the amount of time needed by physicians to vocally record their patients' progress. Twenty dictation stations, located throughout the new area of Mercy, allowed physicians to dictate medical records before leaving the hospital. The telephone-like instruments sent messages to be stored in the medical records department for later transcription. It was hoped that the ease of operating this new device would encourage physicians to complete their reports before leaving the surgery suite.

THE MEDICAL RECORDS DEPARTMENT

The medical records department was located on the first floor between the Central and West Wings, close to the doctors' parking and the ambulance entrance. Mercy began keeping records and statistics in 1921, when Mabel Burch was hired as the first medical record librarian. Three Sisters of Mercy directed the medical records department between 1922 and 1969: Sisters Mary Louise Owens, Raphael Murphy, and Agnes Klein.

A former employee, who worked in the medical records department during Sister Agnes' time, remembered:

> "Sister Mary Agnes was the one who taught me which saint you should pray to when you couldn't find a record. She often told Dr. Abbott to go to the chapel and pray to St. Jude. She wanted me to learn how to do the legal work, so she took me to court with her a couple of times. I carried her shawl and gloves." [11]

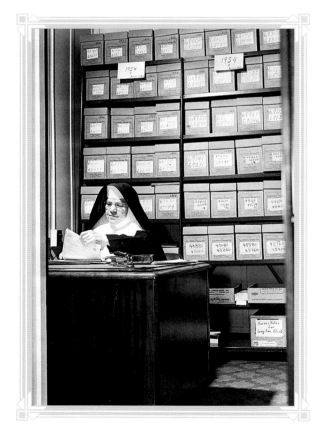

SISTER MARY RAPHAEL

Sister Mary Raphael Murphy directed the work of the medical records department from 1951 to 1959. A native of Connecticut, Mary Murphy entered the Sisters of Mercy in Council Bluffs in 1911. For the next 30 years, she taught primary grades in Imogene, Iowa; Grass Valley, California; Council Bluffs; and at St. Peter's, All Saints, and Holy Trinity Schools in Des Moines. Sister Raphael was a co-founder of St. Peter's School and served as its principal for many years. [12] Several students remember her as a tiny but strict educator.

During the 1940s, Sister Raphael made a career change from teaching to hospital work. She served in the records rooms of hospitals in Valley City and Williston, North Dakota. Sister Raphael came to Mercy in 1951 and stayed until 1969. In ill health at that time, she moved to Mercy Hospital in Council Bluffs where she died on October 27, 1974.

SISTER MARY THERESE

Many of the young women who joined the Sisters of Mercy in Omaha were born in Ireland. Sister Mary Therese Bannon is one of these delightful women, who brought her charming accent and twinkling blue eyes to the United States.

Mary Bannon was not out of high school when she came to North Dakota in 1925 with her sister, Kathleen, and three other girls. A Sister of Mercy, who was a relative of Mary's father, came to visit the Bannon family in Ireland. Mary and two of her sisters planned to join the Mercy order in America, but the family thought Mary was too young. When one of her older sisters decided not to go, however, Mary went in her place.

Mary became Sister Mary Therese and entered nurses' training in Valley City, North Dakota. For several years, Sister Therese nursed in Omaha, where she received her bachelor's of nursing for Creighton. Her next assignments took her to Joplin, Missouri; North Dakota; and Roseburg, Oregon before coming to Des Moines in 1954. Sister Therese's first position was in the school of nursing as instructor for

one year. She then became supervisor in medical and surgical orthopedics. Sister Therese continued in nursing until 1969, when she received a new challenge at Mercy Hospital.

In the late 1960s, the Des Moines Catholic Diocese made the decision to establish a citywide Pastoral Care and Counseling Service Program. Mercy's administration felt that the hospital's needs could be best met through a coordinating internal department. Sister Therese and Sister Concepta worked with Father Duane Weiland to establish the department of ministerial services, which eventually became the pastoral care department.

When the public relations department was created in 1973, Sister Therese and Sister Concepta wanted to work there. They received permission to do so, and Sister Therese worked in this capacity for many years. Today, Sister Therese continues to volunteer, spreading her Irish cheer to Mercy's patients.

In 1959, Sister Therese's Irish eyes became the artist's inspiration for one of the figures in the South Wing mural. Artist, Stan Hess, recalled: "Sister Therese came by the mural when it was half done, looked at the brown-eyed figures and said, 'Don't you like blue eyes?' So, I painted the nun's eyes blue, like Sister Therese's."

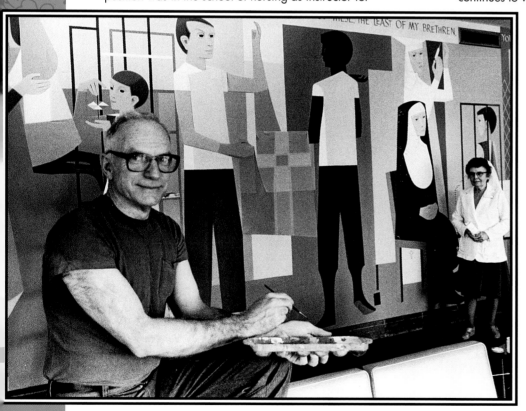

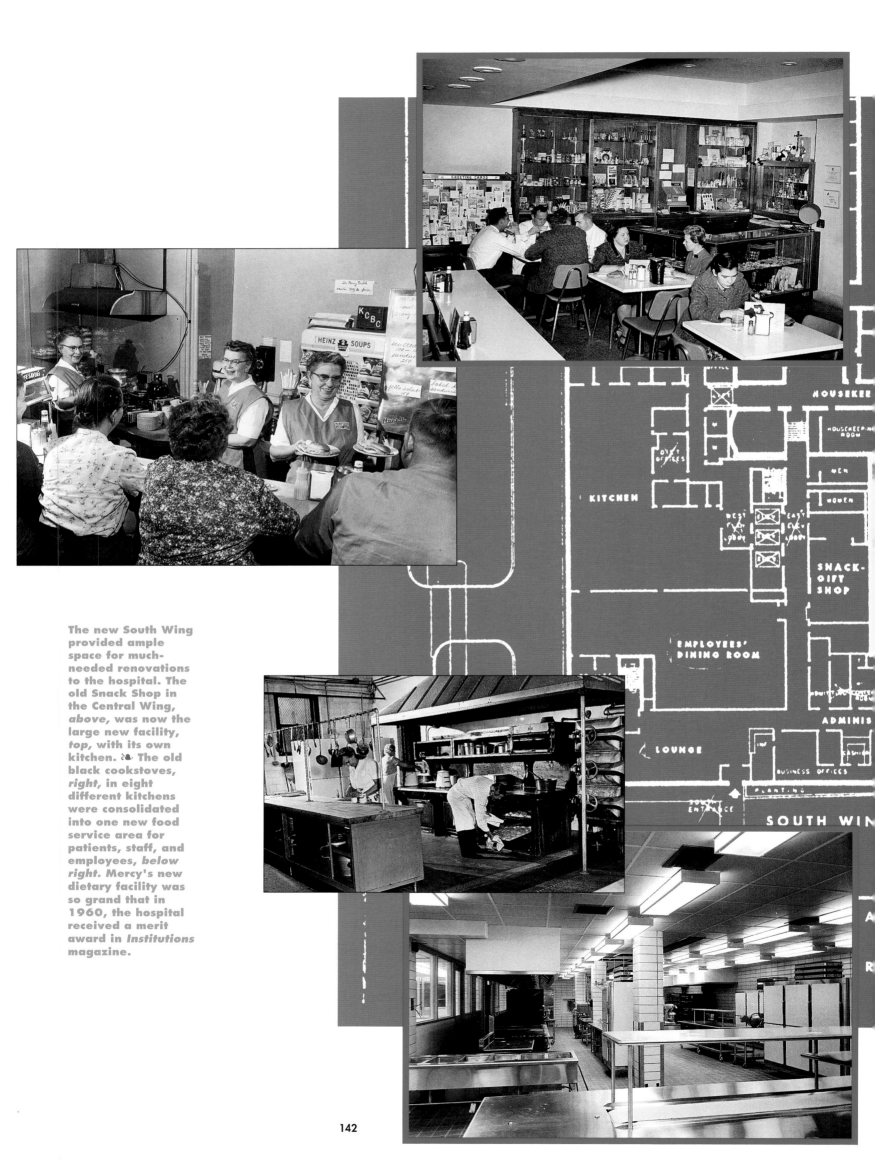

The new South Wing provided ample space for much-needed renovations to the hospital. The old Snack Shop in the Central Wing, *above,* was now the large new facility, *top,* with its own kitchen. ❧ The old black cookstoves, *right,* in eight different kitchens were consolidated into one new food service area for patients, staff, and employees, *below right.* Mercy's new dietary facility was so grand that in 1960, the hospital received a merit award in *Institutions* magazine.

142

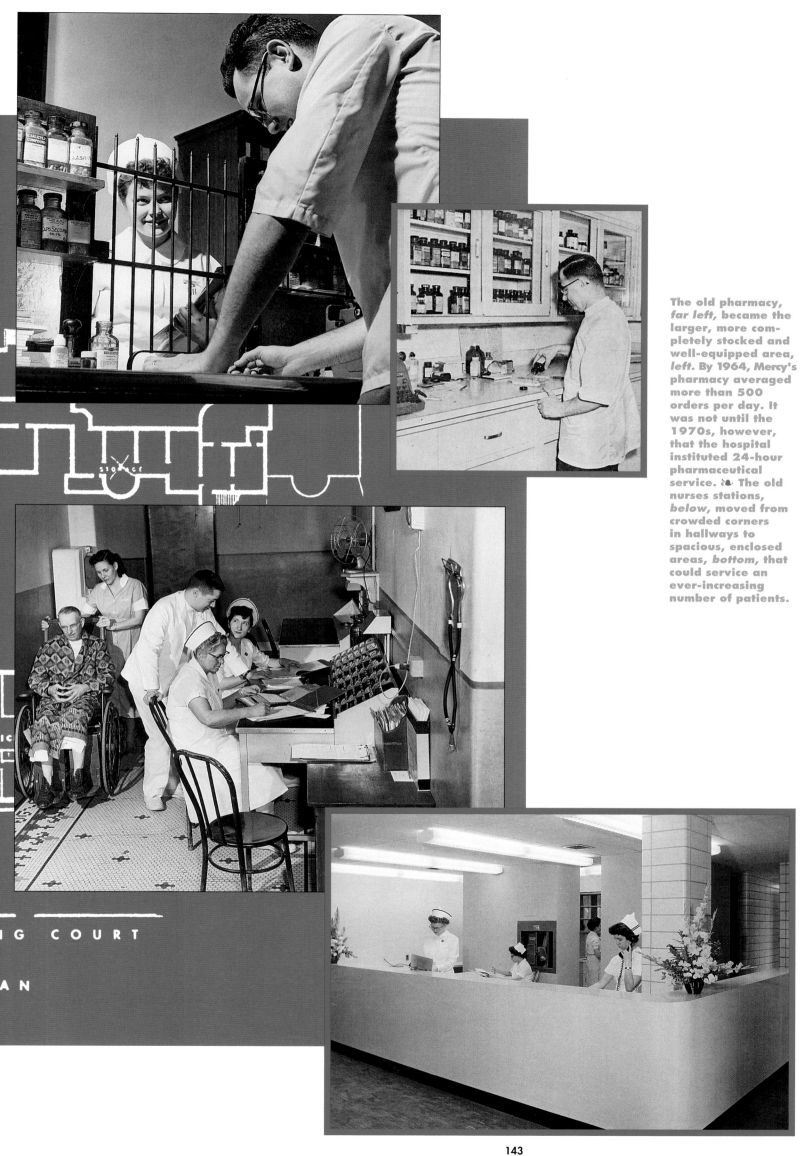

The old pharmacy, *far left,* became the larger, more completely stocked and well-equipped area, *left.* By 1964, Mercy's pharmacy averaged more than 500 orders per day. It was not until the 1970s, however, that the hospital instituted 24-hour pharmaceutical service. ❧ The old nurses stations, *below,* moved from crowded corners in hallways to spacious, enclosed areas, *bottom,* that could service an ever-increasing number of patients.

EVOLUTION

Other departments relocated to the South Wing included the laboratory, surgery rooms, radiology, pediatrics, and emergency.

Laboratory improvements had been frequent over the years, but this facility promised to be the "creme de la creme" in the new wing. In addition to being relocated to the first floor of the South Wing, the laboratory took on a new name—Mercy Hospital Pathology Department. The name better represented the many functions being utilized in this modern clinical setting. The variety of laboratories incorporated under the department were: chemistry, exfoliative cytology, microbiology (bacteriology and parasitology), hematology, urinalysis, blood banking and serology, surgical pathology, and research. New autopsy and animal rooms relocated to the basement level of the South Wing.

Because of the newly expanded facility, Mercy's laboratory staff were able to increase the kinds of services they provided. The laboratory was the first in Des Moines to begin regular PKU (phenylketonuria) testing of newborns. This simple blood test detected a genetic factor responsible for a rare form of mental retardation. If the disease was detected during the baby's first month, with proper dietary therapy, brain damage could be avoided. This procedure began as a result of a grant from the Iowa Health Department and Mercy, which provided staff, materials, equipment, and time for the project.[14]

A SURGICAL SUITE

Ten state-of-the-art operating rooms formed the new surgical suite, also housed on the first floor of the South Wing. Six major operating rooms comprised the hub of this facility, part of which is now Beh Auditorium. Two rooms were equipped for EENT (eye, ear, nose and throat) procedures. Two additional rooms were furnished with equipment used for cystoscopic procedures, containing urological tables with built-in x-ray units. Special terrazzo flooring reduced the possibility of anesthetic explosions. Oxygen and vacuum outlets were installed in each room to facilitate the use of these vital elements. Each room had a different color of ceramic tile, making this new suite "one of our most colorful departments."[15]

For the first time in Mercy's history, a recovery unit opened adjacent to the surgical suites. All recovering surgical patients were moved to this unit for observation following their surgeries, instead of being returned to their rooms to recover. The new unit was capable of handling 12 to 15 patients. Central supply was located conveniently next to the surgical unit, making the movement of surgical supplies easier for the staff.

RADIOLOGY

The radiology department stayed in the same location in the West Wing. However, the department took over all the space formerly occupied by physical therapy, outpatient and emergency, and the cystoscopy and fracture rooms. Several rooms were set aside specifically for patient care: Two rooms were designated for radiographic procedures; two for fluoroscopic procedures; two for therapy and dressing. Other rooms were set aside for offices, reception space, viewing and consultation. The newly expanded area also contained specially equipped facilities for the use of radioactive isotopes.

HOUSE OF GLASS

Part of the pediatrics department relocated to the fifth floor of the South Wing and was designated for the specific care of newborns and children below the age of six. The area had four nursing stations labeled "the House of Glass" which provided a

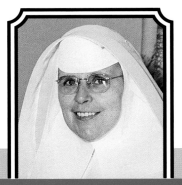

SISTER MARY FRANCIS

Sister Mary Francis Hunt followed Sister Anita as administrator in Des Moines in 1959. Sister Francis was born Anna Marie Hunt in 1904 in Mosca, Colorado. She entered the Council Bluffs Sisters of Mercy in 1929.

After becoming a Sister of Mercy, Sister Francis served as bookkeeper, first at St. James Orphanage in Omaha, and later at Mercy Hospital in Denver. She decided to study nursing and received her bachelor's degree in nursing at St. Louis University in the early 1940s. Sister Francis spent the next 17 years in Denver and Durango, teaching and supervising. She served as administrator at Mercy Hospital in Durango prior to coming to Des Moines.[13]

Sister Francis guided Mercy through many milestone events, including the final phases of urban renewal and the construction of the chapel, convent, and the intern apartments. In 1961, she was named president of the Iowa Conference of Catholic Hospitals. In 1963, Sister Francis was reassigned as administrator for the new Archbishop Bergan Mercy Hospital in Omaha. She died in 1983 in her beloved Colorado.

ADMINISTRATOR 1959-1963

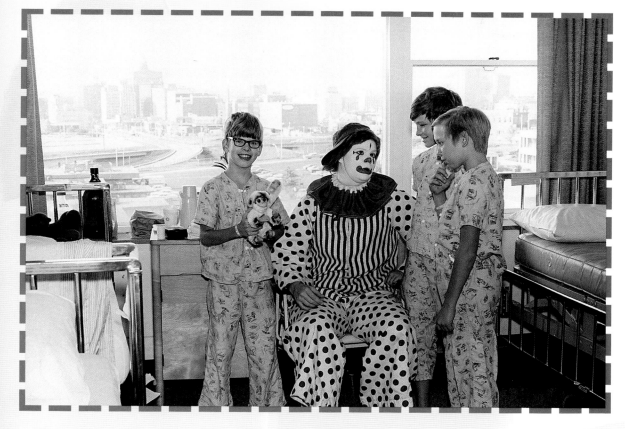

panoramic view of all patients. A nursery to care for sick infants was outfitted with 14 bassinets. This area incorporated its own charting station, examination rooms, and work rooms. A special isolation section contained three cubicles and a separate work area. Two additional rooms served as treatment and admission rooms. A total of 23 pediatrics patients could be accommodated in addition to the patients in the nursery and isolation areas.

A huge, brightly decorated playroom generated the most excitement. The tile floor came complete with a checkerboard built into it. A fresh-air play-deck was included on the east side of the building. Sister Patricia Clare helped plan this new pediatric department, although she was transferred before the new building was ready for occupancy. "Designing was really fun," she says. "We put the windows halfway down [the wall], and there were bathrooms in each room."

Up to 30 pediatrics patients, those aged six through teenage years, were cared for in the remodeled West Wing pediatrics area.

No Longer Just A Room

The emergency and outpatient entrance relocated from the northwest corner near the school of nursing to the first floor of the Central Wing. Mercy opened the remodeled outpatient area on December 7, 1960. This revamped facility was made possible by a $50,000 pledge from Mercy's Guild.

Carved out of old laboratory facilities, the new area was conveniently located near the ambulance entrance in back of the Central Wing. Seven examination rooms, a waiting room, a canteen, and a storage area for equipment enabled Mercy to care for more patients in need of this immediate service.

Two registered nurses, one practical nurse, and a receptionist were under the supervision of Sister Mary Sarto McMahon. The staff proudly displayed the new area, announcing it was no longer the "emergency room," but a department.

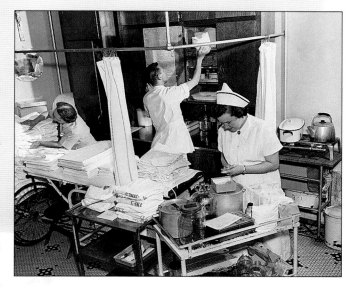

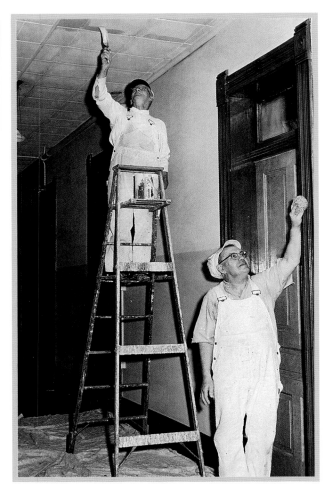

WEST WING REMODELING

Mercy's dream of a hospital with a 300-bed capacity came closer to reality in March 1960 when the second floor of the West Wing reopened after remodeling. It was the last section of the wing to undergo a face-lift in Phase III of Mercy's expansion. This floor accommodated 30 medical and surgical patients. Sister Mary Concepta continued as supervisor and Rachel Doyle was head nurse.[16] Father Paul Connelly conducted a special blessing service on each floor of the newly remodeled West Wing, dedicating the facilities to "alleviate pain...a work for the honor and glory of God."[17] By the end of April 1960, Mercy had 300 adult and pediatric beds and 50 bassinets. Hospital employees numbered more than 630.[18]

EDUCATIONAL ADVANCEMENTS

The 1950s forecasted the need for improved education for healthcare professionals. Mercy's staff took advantage of many educational opportunities offered through professional organizations to which they belonged. Catholic Hospital Association (CHA), American Hospital Association (AHA), Iowa Nurses' Association, National Council of Catholic Nurses, Iowa Hospital Association (IHA), Iowa Conference of Catholic Hospitals, and many others offered seminars and additional training for members of Mercy's healthcare team. Staff members were encouraged to take advantage of educational offerings outside of Des Moines.

Mercy strengthened its own in-house educational efforts by beginning training programs in the laboratory, in radiology, and for interns and residents. Three schools evolved from the laboratory: medical technology, cytotechnology, and histology.

Mercy's School of Medical Technology came alive in 1954 with a four-year program that combined liberal arts and medical technology in affiliation with Drake University.[19] The program provided three years of liberal arts with a strong emphasis on the sciences and a year of full-time clinical training at Mercy.

Dr. F.C. Coleman, Mercy's pathologist, became director of the school. After completion of the program and upon earning certification from national boards, students were awarded bachelor of arts degrees from their sponsoring colleges.[20]

Mercy's cytotechnology program began in January 1959 when six students enrolled in a six-month program. Under the direction of Drs. Coleman and Denser, students who had completed at least two years of college, with 15 hours in biology and three hours in chemistry, could begin study in cytotechnology. The first classes met in a room at Drake. In May, the class moved to Mercy. Students completed their studies in July.

In October, 1961, Cathy (Barton) Wintermantel was named instructor of the second cytology class. This new program was designed for twelve months. Three students graduated in October 1962. From this point on, classes were conducted at the Clinical Pathology Laboratory, located across the street from Mercy, and clinical studies were performed in Mercy's cytotechnology area in the basement of the South Wing. In 1965, the program changed its name to the Des Moines Medical Center School of Cytotechnology, and in 1966, another Mercy-sponsored cytotechnology training school opened with four students. Janet Sams was appointed instructor of the program.

Shortly after the relocation of the laboratory to the South Wing, Mercy began training histology technicians. Eileen Lex became the instructor for the one-year program. Offered to high school graduates, the course included lectures and hands-on training. After passing Mercy's course, graduates took a national exam and were certified by the American Society of Clinical Pathologists, if they passed. This training continued at Mercy into the late 1970s.[21]

Fond Hails And Farewells

Almost two years to the date after the first shovel of dirt was turned for the South Wing, the East Wing was demolished. For 65 years, this wing served as the proud cornerstone of Mercy Hospital in Des Moines. Over those years, the building sheltered countless patients, nursing students, Sisters of Mercy, employees, the chapel, dietary facilities, and medical records. It was a sad day in 1959 when the building came down, but everyone was excited about the prospect of a new chapel, Mercy Hall, and the garage facility that would rise in its place.[22] Excavation and construction began on the chapel before the South Wing was finished.

In 1959, Mercy experienced another change of administrators. Sister Anita was appointed administrator of Mercy Hospital in Council Bluffs. Sister Anita had served in Des Moines for many years, guiding the hospital through myriad changes. During her last administration, she spearheaded projects at Mercy such as the revamping and expansion of the physical plant, acquiring accreditation for the school of nursing, improving the internship program, creating new methodology in administration, encouraging growth in all departments, and fostering the formation of the Mercy Guild. Sister Mary Francis Hunt became the new administrator in 1959.

Nearly one year to the day after the world's attention focused on the tragic assassination of President John Kennedy, the citizens of Iowa were shocked by news of the tragic deaths of Bishop Edward Daly and Monsignor Joseph Sondag. After attending a session of the second Vatican Ecumenical Council, the two prelates were flying out of Rome on November 23, 1964, when their plane crashed, killing 44 of the 73 persons on board. The grief expressed by all Iowans was profound. During his 16 years as the spiritual leader of the Des Moines Diocese, Bishop Daly endeared himself as a "friendly and gracious man with a quiet humor, an agile wit and an enjoyment of other people."[23]

George J. Biskup became Des Moines' fifth bishop in February 1965. Bishop Biskup was a native Iowan whose Czechoslovakian name "Biskup" translated as "a bishop." Bishop Biskup's term encompassed 32 months, before he was reassigned to Indianapolis as archbishop in October 1967. Many of his flock never got to know this quiet man, but the Sisters of Mercy praised him.

An old Mercy friend became Des Moines' sixth bishop, Maurice J. Dingman. He brought to Des Moines skills learned as chancellor of the Davenport Diocese, teacher, superintendent of schools, and most importantly for Mercy, hospital chaplain. Dingman was chaplain for Mercy Hospital in Davenport from 1953 until 1967. The sisters in Des Moines were fond of Bishop Dingman, who remained bishop of the diocese until an incapacitating stroke forced his early retirement in 1987. He died at Mercy Hospital in Des Moines on February 1, 1992.

Never To Waver

The period after World War II found Mercy caught up in mercurial changes evolving in health care. This time marked the biggest challenges in medical education and technological advancement in Mercy's history. Medical professionals and hospitals found this to be an era of growth in education, skills, and technological advances, filled with seemingly limitless possibilities. As Mercy's skyline changed, the famliar comforting care given by Mercy's family never wavered, and the hospital became an even stronger influence in the lives of Central Iowans.

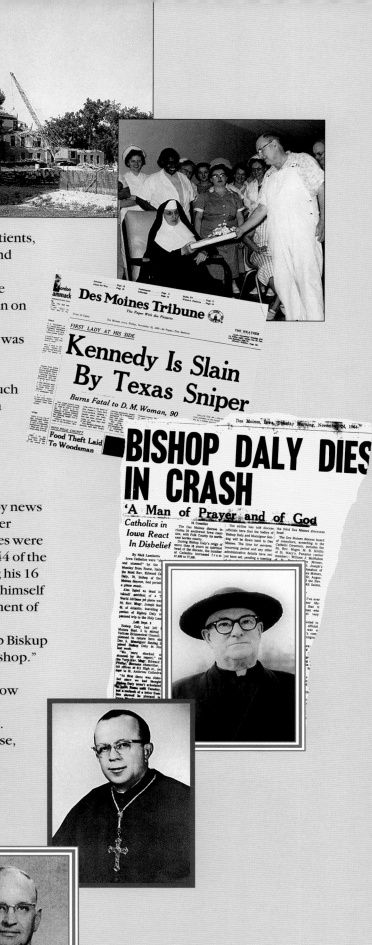

CHAPTER THREE
SCHOOL OF NURSING: 1947-1969

By the time World War II was over, the status of nursing had undergone changes and growth which permanently altered the image and duties of the profession. National organizations formed committees to examine the current developments in nursing. One product of this scrutiny was the "Brown Report" which studied nursing education and projected sociological health needs.

Sister Mary Kieran, *below,* taught three student nurses in Mercy's School of Nursing library. The Brown Report, produced after World War II, studied problems in nursing education and had a lasting impact on Mercy's school of nursing programs.

While the recommendations of the Brown Report were debated for many years, the study had a lasting impact on nursing education in the United States. The report defined "professional" nursing, recommended accreditation for schools, and advised affiliation of those schools with colleges and universities.[1]

A NEW AFFILIATION

Early in 1948, Sister Mary Helen Mackenzie attended a meeting of four Des Moines hospital administrators to discuss new directions in nursing education. The hospital administrators recognized that the quality of nursing education must keep up with the demand for better trained nurses, and the new expectations designed by the professional nursing organizations. Out of this discussion it was decided that a series of courses would be taught at Drake University to student nurses from all of the hospitals. The administrators expressed concern that this new program would be expensive, but Sister Helen and Sister Sebastian felt that Mercy could not let this essential educational opportunity slip away. The advisory board appointed a committee of five members to raise $10,000 for needed increases in scholarship amounts used to pay Drake tuition and fees. Within three months, the scholarship fund received $18,900 in pledges, and the committee set a goal of $25,000 based on the response they had received so far.[2]

By the mid-1950s Mercy was able to offer an expanded scholarship pool. In addition to the original fund established by the advisory board, other sources of scholarship and loans were provided by: the American Cancer Society, American Legion Auxiliary,

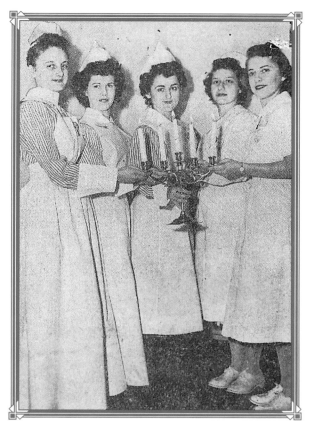

Women's Auxiliary of the Iowa State Medical Society, Rotary Club, Order of the Eastern Star of Iowa, P.E.O. Sisterhood, J. B. Sax Charity Fund in Ottumwa, Polk County Tuberculosis Association, United Food Markets Foundation, and other fraternal and charitable sponsors. During 1958, scholarships were given to 16 students.[3] Additional funding for students was available through direct loans from the school. These loans often were forgiven or pro-rated if the student began working at Mercy Hospital after graduation.

THE 50TH ANNIVERSARY

Mercy's School of Nursing observed its 50th anniversary in November 1949. Catherine Callahan and Mrs. E.J. Kelly chaired the event. A two-day celebration held on November 19 and 20 opened with a solemn High Mass at St. Ambrose Cathedral. On Saturday evening, a banquet was held at Younkers' Tea Room.

Emma Tyrell and Christine Hoffman, two Des Moines women who were among the first graduating class were honored at the evening banquet. Mrs. Tyrell reminisced about her short, but active nursing career as "something I've always been proud of, and it has been useful many times over the years."[4]

Christine Hoffman holds the distinction of being the first Des Moines Mercy graduate to be licensed in Iowa. Also honored during this celebration as the oldest member of the Mercy Medical Staff, Dr. E.B. Walston told about early days at Mercy.

An open house was held in the nurses' residence on Sunday. Several students conducted tours of the building dressed in the five different styles of Mercy nursing uniforms worn since the school opened. Students from St. Joseph's Academy provided special music. More than 600 persons attended the two-day celebration.

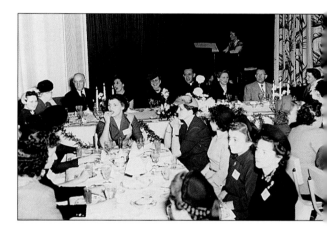

SISTER MARY SEBASTIAN GENESER

Sister Mary Sebastian Geneser became the new school of nursing director after Sister Mary Helen Mackenzie was promoted to Mercy administrator in 1947.

Sister Mary Sebastian Geneser was a native of Des Moines who grew up in the shadow of Mercy. Her family belonged to St. Mary's Parish located at Second and Crocker Streets until it was torn down to make room for I-235 during the River Hills revitalization. Sister Sebastian remembers passing by Mercy as a child to catch the Sixth Avenue streetcar.

Sister Sebastian entered the Council Bluffs Sisters of Mercy in 1923. She worked for a few years in dietary at Council Bluffs and Centerville. In the mid-1930s, Sister Sebastian returned to Council Bluffs where she received her nursing diploma and began further study at Creighton while working.

Sister Sebastian first came to Mercy in 1938. Her good friend, Sister Helen, asked for Sister Sebastian's help training students in the school of nursing. She instructed the students in Nursing Arts, Professional Adjustments I and II, Anatomy, and other subjects. Sister Sebastian was assistant director of the school from 1943 to 1947 when she became director. She served as director until 1960, when she

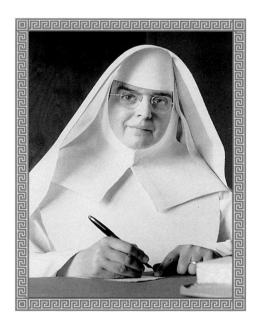

was re-assigned to Coos Bay, Oregon. Sister Sebastian currently resides in the Bishop Drumm Retirement Center. Student Barbara Paul's memories mirror the sentiments of many Mercy nursing students:

> *"When I entered the Mercy School of Nursing in 1948, I was frightened. I was from a small town, was not Catholic, and had never been associated with Catholic religious sisters. Sister Sebastian was the director of the school of nursing at that time. She was very professional, and strict. I later looked back and realized that she was not only professional, but was a caring, fair person, teaching students what was important in nursing and in life—respect for all individuals."* [5]

MERCY GUILD'S COMFORTING CARE

As the shortage of nurses became more critical in the late 1940s Mercy's School of Nursing received immeasurable help from the new Mercy Guild. The primary goal of the newly formed Guild was to stimulate interest in Mercy Hospital and its school of nursing.

The Guild sponsored social events for the students, many of whom suffered from homesickness in the "big city" of Des Moines. These Guild-sponsored activities gave the students something to look forward to besides school and hospital work.

Mercy's Guild purchased equipment for the dormitory and provided home-like touches, such as a well-stocked cookie jar. Members of Mercy's Guild became actively involved in student recruitment by traveling throughout Central Iowa, visiting high schools, and introducing students to a nursing career at Mercy.

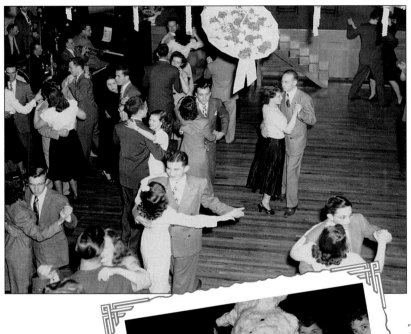

THE MAJOR LABOR FORCE

The 1950s were not much different from previous decades in one way: Nursing students still provided most of the labor force in the hospital. When Mercy experienced a nursing deficit, students filled in. They juggled clinical training, college classes, and floor duty. "It was not unusual to work as many as 60 hours in a week between floor duty and classes. That was still during the time when nurses were working five and one-half days each week." [6] A particularly hectic time forever stands out in the memories of one Mercy graduate:

> *"There was a terrible blizzard and many nurses could not get to work. Some of the seniors were asked to work. The hospital called to ask if I would work 7:00 P.M. to 7:00 A.M. and I said, 'Yes.' They said I would be in the OB nursery, and I said 'Oh no, anywhere but the nursery.' Several minutes later, Sister Zita called and said, 'You will work the nursery.' I said, 'OK Sister.' There were 27 babies, six newborns, myself, and an aide. It was warm in the nursery, and I had a 12-hour sweat. Two days later, Mrs. Callahan informed me that I had forgotten to measure one of the newborns."* [7]

By 1957, there was a gradual relaxation of the heavy use of nursing students as the main labor force in the hospital. Nursing students already enrolled found it much easier to handle the lowered level of 40 hours of work and classes: "I can honestly say I had less responsibility as an upper classman....We didn't put in any more than 40 hours a week with classes." [8]

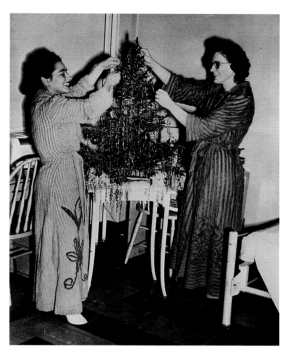

EXTRA-CURRICULAR ACTIVITIES

Rules and regulations abounded during this era. Curfew in the dormitory was 9:30 P.M., and there was no relaxation of this rule on Sunday evening. There was one 10:15 P.M. and one 11:30 P.M. late night allowed each week. Students still were required to stand up when physicians approached the nurses' station, and senior students carried charts while accompanying doctors on rounds.

After graduation in the 1950s, a Mercy student could expect to be hired at Mercy for $245 a month for a straight shift. A newly hired nurse received an additional $20 per month for accepting a rotating shift.

CLOSING THE GENDER GAP

Mercy's first male student originally was hired by Sister Pauline to run the elevator in the Central Wing while he still was in high school. Ronald F. Caulk initially did not

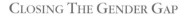

apply to Mercy's School of Nursing because he knew that they had never admitted a male to their program. At the urging of Sister Concepta, however, he finally applied and was considered a test case.

"I lived at home (nothing coed in those days)...used the recreation room at the dorm at certain approved hours and did not have to worry about being 'grounded' as I always made chapel. [Because of my prior Mercy experience] I was 'Ron' to everyone. I felt sorry for all of them when I became 'Mr. Caulk.' I am fortunate that all the women in my class accepted me without any reservations. I have a special love for all of them." [9]

Ronald Caulk successfully completed Mercy Hospital's nursing program and graduated with the class of 1959. He later became a nurse anesthetist, serving twice as president of the International Federation of Nurse Anesthetists.

ACCREDITATION

At the beginning of the 1950s, Mercy's School of Nursing began the process of accreditation. Since 1908, Mercy had gone through an accreditation review by the Nurses' Examining Committee of the Iowa Public Health Department.

During the 1949 review by the State Board of Nurse Examiners, Mercy's school did not meet minimum requirements for faculty because most classes were taught by part-time faculty. The examiner gave Mercy five years to correct the situation. Mercy's school faculty began to implement the necessary changes. One of the first moves by the school was to formally divide the faculty into two groups: faculty and associate faculty. The new organizational structure also established committee structures; some for faculty only, and others which included students. After long hours of planning and restructuring, Mercy was granted temporary accreditation status during the initial listing in May 1952.

Mercy's School was reviewed twice in 1954. The first review by the Iowa Nurse Examiners recommended that the school secure the services of a consultant from the

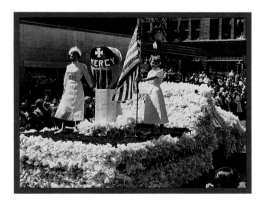

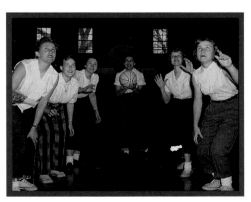

Two student nurses, *left,* decorated a Christmas tree for the nurses' dormitory. Mercy's students drew on their high school experience and formed a basketball team, *bottom,* in the mid-1950s. Trophies were won by this team often and by other nursing students for floats, *below,* designed for the Drake Relays Parade.

NURSING CAPS

Nurses are members of a proud profession which is rooted in the earliest Christian practices. A call to penance in early Christianity was a call to perform acts in social service and public health service. As a sign of self-denial, caps were worn at that time by women to hide their crowning glory—their hair.

As late as World War I, women rarely cut their hair. Wearing a cap lessened the need for frequent hair-washing. For those involved in the care of the sick, a cap shielded patients from the dangers hidden in unclean hair. Caps also protected nurses from the health-threatening conditions in which they often found patients.

The earliest nursing caps were made of book-muslin and organdy with many frills and pleats not easily laundered. Most styles completely covered the hair. Caps with fewer frills, covering only the top-knot of hair and requiring less laundering, were adopted by 1910. The addition of black bands on nurses' caps to signify graduate rank evolved from the military.

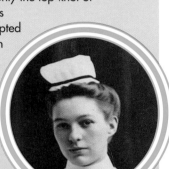

1901

When the first class graduated from Mercy's School of Nursing on June 17, 1901, the seven graduates wore a small organdy or muslin cap perched like a crown on the top of their heads. A simple narrow black ribbon drew the cap into a graceful puff. Mercy's graduates are pictured in this cap through 1908.

By 1915, the Mercy cap style changed and students began sporting a starched conical hat with a turned up brim in the front. The caps were one piece, white—with no additional adornment—and did not unbutton to lie flat. Some graduates from that time said that the caps closely resembled ice cream cones, turned upside down.

In the mid-1920s Mercy's nurses adopted the cap which became the distinctive Mercy shape for many years. The front turned-up edge did not encircle the student's head, but rested on the head and hung down to about ear-level. This style is reminiscent of a Pilgrim cap,

1915

Conference of the Catholic Schools of Nursing, at the earliest possible date.[10] Margaret M. Foley, R.N., from the Conference of Catholic Schools of Nursing, conducted a second review of Mercy in April 1954. Her report showed that the director had accomplished much to improve the school over the last ten years of reviews. Mrs. Foley further commented that these changes could only have been implemented because of the spirit of cooperation which existed between the administration and faculty. She complimented the school on being "modern and comfortable, and recommended that the faculty undergo additional reorganization, outlining 15 additional points for full accreditation.[11]

Mercy's faculty devoted much time and effort toward carrying out Mrs. Foley's recommendations. The application for full accreditation was completed and mailed in April 1957. The National League for Nursing granted Mercy's accreditation on July 9, 1958. Mercy was one of only two Des Moines schools to merit this distinction. The next review was scheduled in 1964.[12]

FACULTY CHANGES

Other important changes within the school during this time involved the creation of the position of educational director. Sister Mary Lorraine Daniels was the first to be appointed, relieving the school's director, Sister Sebastian, of responsibility for the educational program.

School administrators began looking at an innovative curriculum in 1960. Plans for a 27-month (three-year) program were developed and reviewed by the faculty and administrative committees for the academic year, September through May. The tentative starting date was set for September 1963, but Mercy's shortened academic year program began earlier than anticipated.

By the fall of 1961, the faculty and school administration decided to implement the new curriculum with the class entering in 1961. Several schools outside Des Moines had already adopted the academic year, but Mercy was the only hospital in Des Moines to do so.

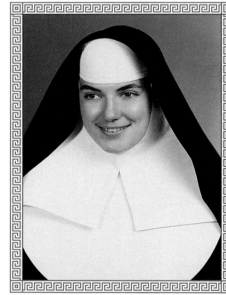

SISTER MARY TIMOTHEA SULLIVAN

After 13 years as Mercy's school director, Sister Mary Sebastian Geneser accepted the new challenge of establishing a school of practical nursing in Coos Bay, Oregon. In August 1960, Sister Mary Timothea (Patricia Clare) Sullivan was appointed school director. Sister Timothea had been involved with Mercy's School of Nursing during her first years in Des Moines, from 1955 to 1958.

A native of Cortland, Nebraska, Sister Timothea taught nursing to students in Des Moines, Durango, and Denver before returning to Des Moines in 1960. Her youth and physical vitality attracted the young students. She was considered fun-loving and always available to students. "The poor woman, she never got away from us."[13]

THE DECISION TO NURSE

Many times young people who were interested in becoming a nurse began working at Mercy as aides or as nursing assistants before entering nursing school. One Mercy graduate commuted from Stuart, Iowa, to work as a junior nursing assistant in pediatrics because she was sure she wanted to be a nurse. Judy Eldredge's summer job introduced her to feeding and bathing children, always under the direct supervision of a nurse.

> *"I remember the area was not air-conditioned, and it was very hot that summer. I remember assisting the nurse with a small infant who had suffered burns. We were all gowned and gloved and perspiration rolled off of us."* [14]

During the 1960s Mercy hired nurses' aides to ease the nursing shortage. More than 20 Des Moines high school girls over the age of 16 applied to work part-time during the school year for an hourly wage of 75 cents. Many planned to study nursing, and this was a good opportunity for them to experience nursing first-hand. Suzanne Mains proudly exchanged her pink nurses' aide uniform for the white uniform of the Mercy student nurse after her nursing aide experiences.

THE ROUTINE

Early-1960s freshmen students worked their clinical training in the hospital from 7:00 A.M. until noon, then attended afternoon classes at Drake beginning at 1:00 P.M.

Quiet hours for study were strictly enforced each evening in the dormitory between 6:00 and 8:00 P.M. Students signed in and out when leaving the dormitory. Curfew was 10:00 P.M. during the week and later on the weekend. No men were allowed in the dormitory, except to greet their dates in the lobby. Lights-out meant exactly that as Sister Timothea made rounds with her flashlight at 10:20. One student hid in a closet to keep from being discovered in a room other than her own.[15]

Tuition for nine months was $300, which included Mercy board and room and Drake fees. Students attended Drake during their freshman year. The second and third year of nursing school meant an increase in clinical hours and a decrease in didactic hours as nursing skills and confidence increased. Under the new shortened academic year, most students worked during the summer at Mercy filling in on the second and third shifts where there was a greater need.

DAYS TO REMEMBER

Graduation day 1964 was a triumphant day as the students were chauffeured from the dormitory to St. Ambrose Cathedral in special limousines provided by one of the local funeral homes. Forty-three women formed the proud "white line" of Mercy graduates. The graduation gift from the sisters to each of them was a pair of cuff-links that fastened the long sleeves of their formal graduation uniforms. The new graduates looked forward to passing state boards and a starting registered nurse salary of about $2.15 per hour.

FEDERAL AID FOR EDUCATION

Under the sponsorship of the Nurse Training Act of 1964, the Surgeon General's Consultant Group on Nursing offered federal aid to nursing schools and students. In addition to defraying the cost of initial education, this act encouraged nurses to stay in the nursing profession by offering a partial cancellation clause in the funding, based on their years of employment as professional nurses. It was estimated that a shortage of 70,000 nurses existed in the United States, and it was projected that at least 130,000 nurses would be needed before 1970.

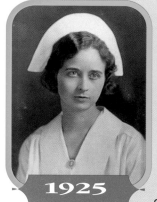
1925

without the flat back. The Mercy cap came to a point. This model unbuttoned in the back to flatten the cone shape for ease of laundering. It was white without any trim.

Mercy's formal capping ceremonies, to mark the end of the first semester for the newest nursing students, began as early as 1937. The first Mercy School of Nursing class to wear the distinctive black band of the graduate nurse in their graduation photo was the class of September 1948. By 1951, the school of nursing decided to distinguish students by attaching a narrow vertical stripe on the rim of the cap on the left side. One stripe represented freshmen; two stripes indicated juniors; and three stripes represented seniors. When men were admitted to the nursing program, they wore black stripes, on the left shirt-sleeve of their uniforms.

The 1960s brought changes to the nursing profession. Wearing nursing caps fell out of vogue, and the traditional capping ceremony was discontinued in 1967. In the late 1960s, Mercy's traditional starched, linen cap was replaced by a disposable model. Until the early 1970s, however, students were required to wear skirts and caps while on duty.

1960

The move away from wearing caps and uniforms has been seen by many as a move away from the professional image of a nurse. Those wishing to once again wear caps and uniforms are choosing to adopt a truly distinct symbol of the nursing profession. These symbols reflect the pride of generations of courageous women and men who have gone forth in the Christian tradition of service to give healing aid to those who come seeking their comfort.

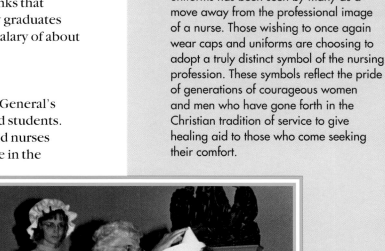
1990

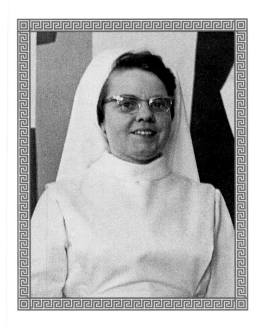

Above: Sister Mary Gervase Northup, Mercy School of Nursing director, 1964 to 1969. ❧ In 1969, three Mercy students, *below,* tested a newborn's hearing with a neo-meter— a gift from Mercy Guild members.

Mercy applied for the new money in 1964 to aid 34 students during the next two-year program. The average loan was $900. This new funding promised to relieve financial barriers for prospective nurses and to end what was described as the "most critical nursing shortage in history." [16]

This special federal funding continued for nearly 20 years. The cost of administering the funds and the heavy governmental regulations finally brought an end to Mercy's participation by 1984.

> *"It was an ideal opportunity for the students to borrow money at 3% for school. The interest raised to 6% by the end of the program, but that was still manageable for [students]. The money was repaid, or pro-rated according to the number of years the graduate worked at Mercy after her school years."* [17]

These federal monies and the shortened curriculum swelled Mercy's total student body enrollment to 138 by the fall of 1965. Also at that time, a man was hired for the first time as educational director for the school—Robert Olson. Sister Mary Vera O'Connor became medical-surgical instructor at the school in 1965.

SISTER MARY GERVASE NORTHUP

Another administrative change took place at Mercy's school in the summer of 1964. Sister Timothea was assigned to Williston, North Dakota, as director of nursing. Sister Mary Gervase Northup became the new director of Mercy's school during the fall term of 1964. Sister Gervase had been director of the school of nursing at St. Catherine's Hospital in Omaha. She received her master's degree in nursing at Catholic University in Washington, D.C.

MARRIED STUDENTS

A married student was admitted to Mercy's school for the first time in the fall of 1964. Pat Spurlock was the precedent-setting student:

> *"I think I had an easier time than the students living in the dormitory. I was very directed, and knew what I wanted. I was not distracted by the social life....It was harder for me adjusting to dormitory life when we went to Council Bluffs for psychiatric training my senior year."* [18]

Pat brought her young daughter into the hospital during pediatric rotation for observation by the rest of the students. It was hard to leave her with grandparents while Pat attended psychiatric rotation in Council Bluffs. By the time Pat finished nursing school, there were several other married students in Mercy's program.

LONGSTANDING TRADITIONS

The 1950s and 1960s proved to be a time of challenging change for Mercy's School of Nursing on many fronts. World War II imposed new expectations on women, as well as the nursing profession. Women's roles moved from the home to the work-place, as it became more acceptable for them to work while raising a family. Nursing presented an important opportunity for women seeking new challenges outside the home.

Changes in medical technology meant that more education was required for nurses to assume the role of confident, skillful care-givers. Mercy's nursing educators eagerly embraced these changes and instilled in their graduates a confident pride to meet the new challenges of providing the hospital's unique comforting care.

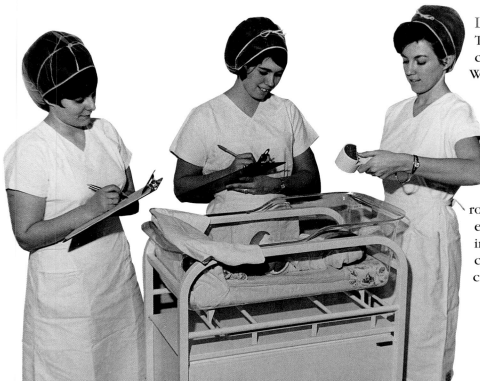

People Of VISION

1947-1969

SISTERS OF MERCY

Agnes Klein
Agnita Dutton
Angela Gilmore
Anne Mary Kelly
Anthony Bonen
Anton Lucius
Christina Weil
del Rey Ekler
DeLellis (Ruth Marie) Hotz
Eileen Moore
Francis Hunt
Francita O'Meara
Gervase Northup
Herbert Kaufmann
Innocentia (Mildred Ann) Zaver
Isabel Stack
Jeanette Brennan
Julia McKee
Kieran Harney
Kilian Clinton
Kurt (Patricia) Forret
Marla Heman
Martina Woulfe
Mary Anne Curran
Maureen Tracy
Nolasco O'Connor
Patrice Phelan
Raphael Murphy
Ricarda (Mary Ann) Bintner
Richard (Jean Marie) Gardiner
Rosine (Patricia) Scanlon
Rosita Goebel
Sarto McMahon
Sean Crimmins
Terrence (Terese) Tracy
Therese Bannon
Timothea (Patricia Clare) Sullivan
Vera O'Connor
Vidette (Regina Marie) Jacobson

MERCY SCHOOL OF NURSING DIRECTORS

Sister Mary Sebastian
Geneser, 1947-1960

Sister Mary Timothea
Sullivan, 1960-1964

Sister Mary Gervase
Northup, 1964-1969

CHIEFS OF STAFF

Walter D. Abbott, 1948
Bernard C. Barnes, 1949
Arnold M. Smythe, 1950
Lester D. Powell, 1951
Jesse H. McNamee, 1952
E. Thomas Scales, 1953
J. Fred Throckmorton, 1954
Clifford W. Losh, Jr., 1955
James W. Chambers, 1956
Daniel F. Crowley, Jr., 1957
Noble W. Irving, 1958
Bernard C. Barnes, 1959
Howard G. Ellis, 1960
Neil J. McGarvey, 1961
John T. Bakody, 1962
William J. Morrissey, 1963
Frank C. Coleman, 1964
Leo R. Pearlman, 1965
Marion E. Alberts, 1966
Marvin H. Dubansky, 1967
Dennis Walter, 1968
Austin Schill, 1969

CHAPTER FOUR
MILESTONES: CARING FOR ALL

As Des Moines approached the end of the 1950s, the new watchword for all citizens became urban renewal. Before Mercy finished the South Wing, city fathers began planning to change the look of Des Moines in response to a proposal for a federal interstate system on the northernmost edge of town.

Newspapers in 1958 described the area of the River Hills Urban Renewal Project, *below* and *opposite,* as a vast wasteland. Mercy Hospital committed to revitalizing this area at that time.

Two major interstate highways, I-80 and I-35, intersected in the city's western suburb of Clive. A major connection to the interstate roadways for Des Moines citizens was planned through the heart of downtown. City planners recognized a golden opportunity to harness the potential of this roadway system and revitalize targeted areas of the city. Mercy found itself almost directly in the middle of the primary area to be renewed—the River Hills Urban Renewal Project.

URBAN RENEWAL: A REVITALIZATION

Newspapers described this 178-acre tract as a vast area that was rapidly becoming a wasteland. Many vacant buildings gave the area a rundown and neglected appearance. Three years of planning, purchasing property, and demolition brought the Urban Renewal Board to the point of being able to offer 26 tracts of land for sale to developers. City officials envisioned parks, glass-fronted apartments, and offices gracing the Des Moines river-front instead of the "junk-strewn railroad tracks" and "grimey smokestacks."[1] Stretching right through the center of this large tract of land was the new, multi-lane I-235 interstate highway.

The River Hills tract was roughly divided into four sectors. The northwest sector included Mercy. This area was bordered by Sixth Avenue on the west, University Avenue on the north, the Des Moines River on the east, and the proposed freeway on the south. Nearly nine acres of land was available for development. Urban renewal

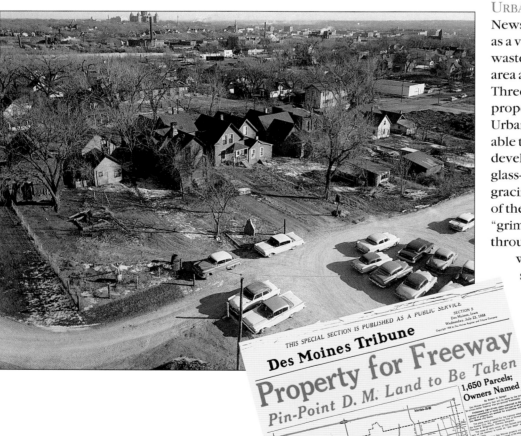

THIS SPECIAL SECTION IS PUBLISHED AS A PUBLIC SERVICE

Des Moines Tribune

SECTION 5
Des Moines, Iowa
Wednesday, July 23, 1958

Property for Freeway
Pin-Point D. M. Land to Be Taken
1,650 Parcels; Owners Named

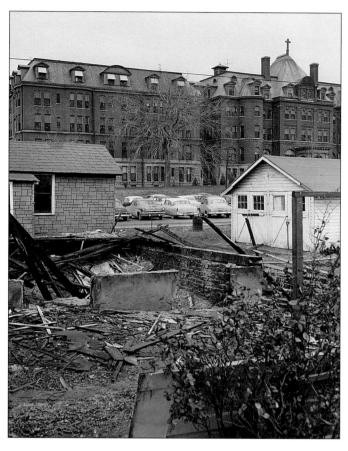

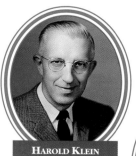

HAROLD KLEIN

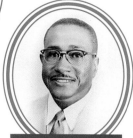

DR. E. THOMAS SCALES

officials, working with Mercy administrators, visualized a possible expansion for the hospital and related medical uses for the rest of the land. Mercy was given first choice to buy this tract.

Several members of the first Urban Renewal Board were close friends of Mercy, including the chairman, Harold P. Klein, a Mercy Advisory Board pioneer. Dr. E. Thomas Scales, a member of Mercy's Medical Staff and chief of staff in 1953, participated on the renewal board and developed an outstanding reputation for civic leadership. Before his untimely death in 1959, Dr. Scales urged the sisters on many occasions to ask for enough ground to accommodate whatever expansion might be envisioned for the hospital for the next 50 to 75 years. John Connolly, Jr., a prominent lawyer, actively promoted Catholic efforts in Des Moines. Charles T. Cownie, a member of Mercy's Advisory Board, played an active role in Mercy's 1959 addition. Connolly and Cownie agreed with Dr. Scales' recommendations and helped to position Mercy favorably during land acquisition for urban renewal. Other members of the community joined the Urban Renewal Board later and used their influence to aid Mercy: Ellis Levitt, John Hawkinson, and John McLaughlin.[2]

After much negotiation, Mercy submitted a bid to purchase almost eleven acres surrounding the hospital. In addition to the urban renewal tract, Mercy also asked to purchase five acres that included the area from Fourth Street, Mercy's east boundary, to Third Street and from University Avenue to Laurel Street. Mercy administrators hoped the Des Moines City Council would allow Fourth Street to be vacated. Mercy also hoped to purchase the property where St. Ambrose School was located.

The sale of the Urban Renewal tracts became final on Mercy Day 1962. The city council accepted Mercy's bid of $524,186 for nearly 14 acres of land. The St. Ambrose property was not part of the tract acquired by Mercy at that time, but the property eventually did become part of the Mercy campus in 1972.

As part of the business transaction, Mercy delivered a development plan to the Urban Renewal Board and the city. These preliminary plans called for the construction of an interns' residence, an addition onto the nurses' home to accommodate 100 extra beds, a convent, an ambulatory patient facility, an acute care wing, a new heating plant, and much-needed parking space. Overall plans for Mercy's development and expansion would not be formalized for nearly four years.

In the middle of the urban renewal plans, a change of administration took place for Mercy. Sister Mary Francis Hunt left Mercy in the summer of 1963 to become administrator of St. Catherine's Hospital in Omaha. Sister Mary Patrice Phelan became Mercy's new administrator.

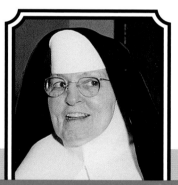

SISTER MARY PATRICE

Sister Mary Patrice Phelan served as administrator from 1963 to 1964. Annie Phelan was born in the town of Belmont, Massachusetts, in 1896. Her family migrated to Ferrar, Iowa, and she entered the Sisters of Mercy in 1922. Sister Patrice spent her early years caring for patients at St. Bernard's Hospital in Council Bluffs, Iowa, and St. Joseph's Mercy Hospital in Centerville. She came to Des Moines in 1957 as administrator of Bishop Drumm Home for the Aged.

Sister Patrice stayed at Mercy as local superior after Sister Mary Eileen Moore was appointed administrator in 1964. This was the first time since 1922 that the local superior and administrator positions were held by different Sisters of Mercy. After leaving Mercy in 1967, Sister Patrice again became administrator of Bishop Drumm Home. She remained there, serving in different ministries, until her death on July 12, 1989.

ADMINISTRATOR 1963-1964

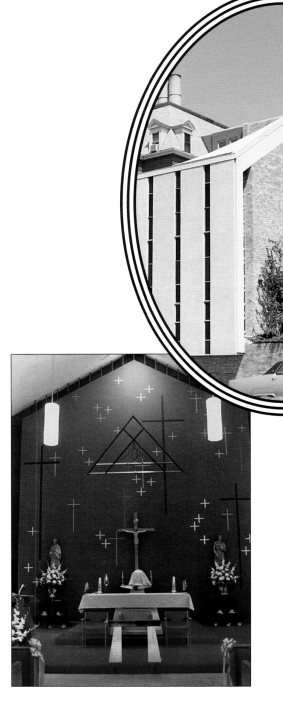

TENT OF GOD

The new Mercy chapel, the "pointy-topped" chapel as it was called, opened with a special liturgy by Bishop Daly on June 24, 1960, for the sisters and celebrated guests. Called the "jewel of the entire new setting," the chapel contained three stories. The top floor housed the chapel, the second floor contained an auditorium, and the lower level became a garage.

The most arresting feature of the new chapel was the roof-line and steeple. The chapel roof appeared as a tent-like drape, swooping up into a graceful point. The tent structure was quite evident from inside the chapel because eight-foot walls slanted upwards into a pinnacle 30 feet above the altar. The east face of the steeple had stained-glass that allowed light to cascade down onto the main altar area—especially beautiful during the morning hours. Light from the steeple shone through a bronze baldachin suspended over a green and white Italian-marble altar. The architectural inspiration for this design derived from the "Tent of God surviving from days when wanderers in the wilderness set up a tabernacle for worship." The technical term to define this particular style was "hyperbolic parabaloid."[3] The new chapel was constructed of buff-colored, precast concrete panels with red brick trim that was in harmony with the newly finished South Wing.

The design objective for the sanctuary was to have no more than 50 feet between the celebrant and the farthest seat in the chapel. Another attractive feature was the life-sized stations of the cross sculpted in bronze filigree and inserted into glass-divider walls between the interior and the hallway to the chapel.[4]

A TIME TO RECREATE

As the final phase of the building expansion drew to a close, the Sisters of Mercy announced that "all work and no play makes Jack a dull boy," and planned the first Mercy Hospital Employee Picnic in July at Riverview Park. A newly formed Recreation Committee planned the day's activities, including door-prize drawings every hour. Employees and their families were encouraged to attend by offering tickets for park activities at a reduced rate of seven cents per ticket. The sisters provided food prepared in Mercy's dietary department. More than 1,000 reservations were made for this special day. Everyone had such a good time that the Recreation Committee continued to plan other fun employee activities.

Along with well-rounded educational and recreational experiences for employees, the sisters planned days of recollection for the Mercy staff. The first of these were September 27–29, 1960. Employees were given a day off to use as a special time for retreat. Father Damian Crogan conducted the days of recollection in the chapel and in Our Lady of Mercy Hall. Homilies were supplemented by spiritual reading materials and discussion groups. Many employees used words such as "inspiring, wonderful," and "spiritually refreshing."[5]

THE CENTRAL WING REMODELING

The final stage of the renovation of the Central Wing drew to a close in the fall of 1960. The department of obstetrics and gynecology was

A new three-story, tent-like Mercy chapel, *above* and *top,* was blessed on June 24, 1960. The building was called the "pointy-topped" chapel because of its structure. ?& The first of many Mercy Hospital Employee Picnics was held at Riverview Park in July 1960, *right.*

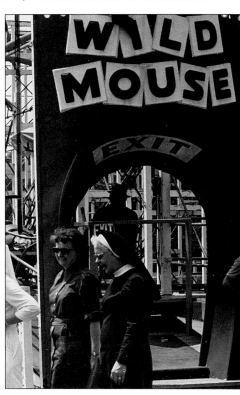

enlarged by including the Central Wing fourth floor space. Mercy's obstetrical areas were in closer proximity to one another after years of wheeling babies and mothers from one side of the hospital to the other. An improved premature nursery that could handle the care of 10 infants became a reality.[6]

THE HOUSE THAT HOPE BUILT

One of the first projects begun after the acquisition of the urban renewal land was a new convent. Although this new home had been in the dreams of the Sisters of Mercy for more than 40 years, it was only after the completion of extensive remodeling and expansion begun during the late 1950s and early 1960s that the sisters turned their thoughts toward a new convent. With the newly acquired property, the hoped-for convent could be placed conveniently close to Mercy's new chapel. This location was made possible by the closing of Fourth Street between University Avenue and Laurel Street.

With the exception of four years (before the construction of the Central Wing), the Sisters of Mercy lived on the upper-most, bat-infested, poorly air-conditioned, and drafty area of the hospital. Access to the chapel through the convent quarters afforded little privacy for the sisters. For years, they had pooled their savings, gifts from special friends, money earned from numerous bazaars and bake sales, and countless personal sacrifices into a special fund for a new convent. Dreams became reality for the Mercy sisters as construction began on a convent in the spring of 1963. The two-story structure provided living quarters for 20 sisters. The building contained a refectory (dining room), community room, utility and storage areas, and corridors that allowed direct access from the second floor living quarters to the chapel. Some of the sisters had lived in the old "loft" for as long as 40 years. Sister Pauline was a veteran attic-dweller who remarked dryly: "Yes, we will probably miss the old place, but after so many years of penthouse living we will enjoy a new home with lawn and flowers." The shrine of Our Lady of Fatima bordered the east side of the new convent. The sisters proudly displayed their new "house that hope built" in a public open house on Sunday, August 2, 1964.

TOWN-HOUSES

Mercy's expansion plans continued with the construction of apartments for interns facing Third Street. Ground was broken on the two-story town-house apartments in November 1964. Construction went smoothly at first but slowed due to labor troubles

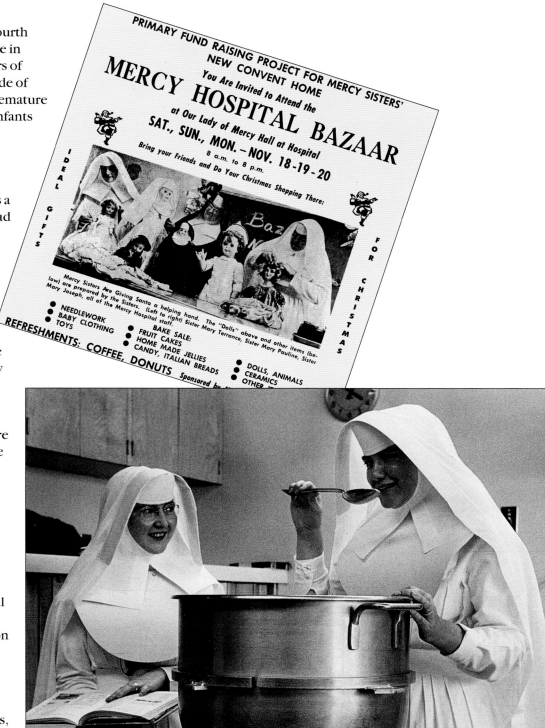

The Sisters of Mercy helped raise money to build a new convent through bazaars and other fund-raising efforts. Above: Sisters Sarto McMahon and Timothea Sullivan made fudge for one event.

and special underpinning reinforcements that had to be added to the lower complex. The apartments contained three levels. Construction on these units was made possible through a $265,000, long-term, 3.6 percent loan from the Housing and Home Finance Agency. To complete the project by September 1965, Mercy provided the remaining $45,000 .

TO BUILD OR NOT TO BUILD

As the urban renewal process gripped imaginations in Des Moines, Mercy's administration began to look at the hospital's role in this revitalization. Planned changes brought the promise that the area surrounding Mercy would continue to grow and the need for good hospital care would become even more necessary.

Mercy administrators wrestled with questions of whether to build, what to build, and where to build for several years. Early in 1963, it was announced that Mercy would undergo an $8.5 million dollar expansion program to take place over the next 15 years. The next step was to decide what form the expansion would take.

THE FRIESEN STUDY

Upon the advice of Mercy's Advisory Board, Gordon Friesen Associates of Washington, D.C., a prominent hospital consulting firm, was hired to review Des Moines' healthcare needs and to make recommendations based on their review.

The Friesen firm studied the Des Moines "hospital service area" by taking a look at the number and types of beds available, population changes, and medical care patterns, projecting Des Moines' healthcare needs for the next 15 years. The completed report indicated that Mercy was providing 20 to 25 percent of the hospital service in the surrounding area. If the current trends continued, the Friesen Company projected that Mercy would need as many as 700 beds by the year 1980.

The Friesen Company recommended that the Central Wing be replaced with a new facility. During February 1964, the patient census reached a high of 365, and another 15 beds were opened on Mercy's second floor Central Wing.[7] This overcrowding emphasized a need to expand the acute medical-surgical beds. In the 1960s, Mercy began to emerge as a major heart center. Friesen suggested that Mercy should increase the number of this type of bed by at least one half.

The Friesen Company projected the effect of the soon-to-be-implemented Medicare Plan on healthcare users. Too many elderly Iowans were unable to afford the price of good health care, but with the federal government picking up some of the cost of their care under the Medicare Plan, it was anticipated that a record number of patients now would be able to seek care which had been neglected. As Iowans aged, more beds would be needed to care for the chronically ill older patient. The Friesen study recommended that Mercy provide at least 150 such beds.

Additional outpatient and ambulatory diagnostic services held promise of keeping costs containable. Friesen recommended that Mercy would benefit from expansion of these services.

The result of all of this study was called the Friesen Plan. This plan recommended that a new building be constructed to house the acute medical-surgical beds and that the older buildings be removed or restructured to care for chronic disease and other less acutely ill patients.[8]

Mercy's administration took a long look at this Friesen Plan because of the expense incurred with any new building plan. Since beginning the South Wing expansion in 1957, the hospital had continued to build new facilities and remodel older buildings. The dust had never really settled, and the debt loomed larger than ever.

During the early, busy 1960s, Mercy operated in the red. In July 1961, the hospital had to borrow to meet the payroll for that month. Taking on more debt, even based on the best future projections, was intimidating, and Mercy administrators approached

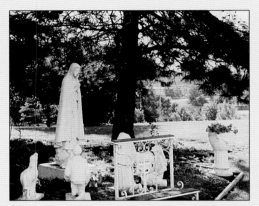

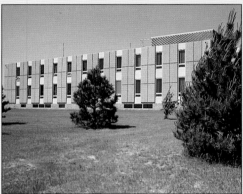

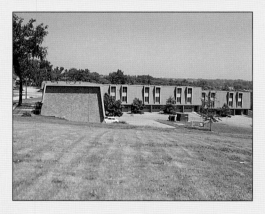

Mercy's shrine of Our Lady of Fatima, *top.* The Sisters of Mercy's new convent, *center.* The Mercy intern apartments, *above.* ‿ Reinforcing the need for further expansion, patient census reached an all-time high of 365 in 1964, which made it necessary to care for patients in hallways, *opposite.*

this decision with more than a little anxiety. Sister Patrice's Christmas letter of 1963 stated that the current debt was more than $1,000,000. [9]

A NEW MERCY SKYLINE

In July 1966, Mercy announced plans for a U-shaped tower expansion. The projected cost was $15 million. These initial plans were ambitious, extending over a 20-year period. The intent was to fulfill one of the suggestions that came out of the Friesen Study by increasing the number of Mercy beds to 700. These first plans never came about because Mercy spent an additional two years finalizing details for the tower expansion. Changes to these original plans accomplished the erection of the towers that are in place today.

In the middle of the tower planning, Mercy's administration changed for the fifth time during the period from 1947 to 1969. Sister Mary Eileen Moore became Mercy's new administrator in 1964. Sister Eileen was familiar with Mercy because she spent 1963 as an administrative resident in Des Moines. Sister Eileen came to Mercy from Mercy Hospital in Council Bluffs where she was supervisor of the radiology department. Sister Patrice remained at Mercy as superior and chairman of the Sisters' Governing Board.

The final plans were unveiled in July 1968 after hundreds of hours of meetings between the Sisters' Governing Board, the Planning Committee of the advisory board, the Planning Committee of the medical staff, Brooks-Borg Architects and Engineers, and Gordon Friesen Associates. Final approval for Mercy's plans came from the Health Planning Council, which also approved plans from three other Des Moines' hospitals. Although Mercy's plans called for adding 242 beds, there would be a gain of only 93 beds because 149 beds would be removed when the Central Wing was demolished. Mercy's new shape was represented in a 10-level, H-shaped tower.

This multi-staged project was divided into many phases which caused some head-scratching years later as old-timers struggled to remember what each phase meant. As soon as the decision was made to expand, events moved rapidly. By summer 1968, a new parking lot was completed, and work was beginning on the new emergency entrance and doctors' parking lot. This entrance was located just west of the staircase entrance to the Central Wing. The new doctors' parking lot was located right in front of the hospital. The design of this new approach made it necessary to remove the familiar stone steps leading up to the Central Wing—Mercy's front door until the South Wing opened. Numerous loads of dirt were hauled in to raise the grade of this front approach. The final asphalt coat gave an attractive appearance to the new emergency entry for its opening on October 14, 1968.

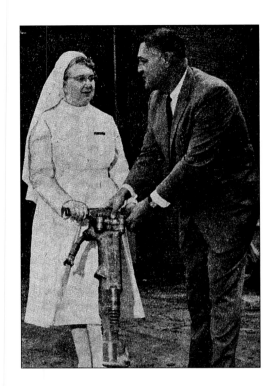

The groundbreaking for the new power plant and laundry facility was held in mid-October 1968. Sister Eileen used a jack hammer instead of the usual shovel to break the ground. Arthur H. Neumann and Brothers, Inc. and Des Moines and Iowa Sheet Metal Companies were awarded contracts that totaled $600,000.

By the following May, work was 50 percent complete, and the first firing of the boiler came on September 22, 1969, at 7:45 A.M.—a successful end to Phase 1-A just one year after the groundbreaking. This phase marked the beginning of the tower expansion program which would not be formally finished for nine years.

IMPROVING THE BEST

Mercy's educational programs grew by leaps and bounds during the 1960s. The School of Radiologic Technology began in the fall of 1960 with a two-year program. The roots of this program reached back to 1938 when Mercy's Sister Mary Jerome Burns began training radiology technicians. These students were encouraged to also enroll in a self-study program, sit for the exam, and take the test sponsored by the American Registry of Technologists.

Four students entered the first two-year program in 1960. Dr. Noble Irving, director of the radiology department taught the students with the help of the chief technologist. The students received clinical and didactic training in several different subjects. Upon completion of the program, candidates were allowed to take state boards to become certified by the American Registry of Radiologic Technologists.

One of the first graduates of Mercy's two-year program, Molly Hewitt, has fond memories of her time in training:

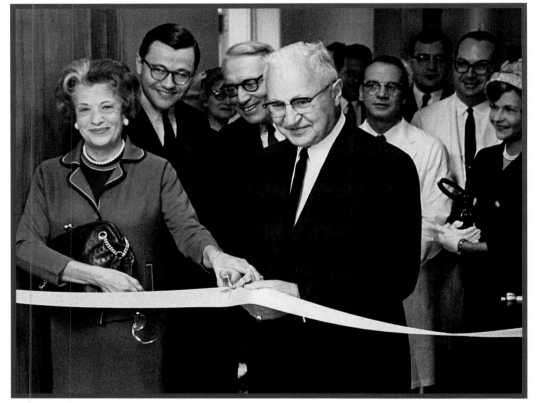

"It was a fun time....Everyone felt like they were part of a small family. Of course there were pranks. One stunt involved dunking a rather diminutive student in the huge wash tank in the darkroom. After she got out of the tank she put on a patient gown and hung her clothes in the film dryer cabinet to dry. Along came an unsuspecting Dr. Irving who opened the door of the cabinet to show certain films to a fellow physician. Imagine his surprise to find a young lady's undergarments drying in the cabinet among the films." [10]

NEW EDUCATIONAL OPPORTUNITIES

Under the direction of Dr. Howard Ellis, director of medical education and chief of surgery, a surgical residency program was initiated in July 1963. University of Iowa medical students were enrolled in a surgical residency program at Veterans Hospital in Des Moines. The dean of the College of Medicine, Dr. Robert Hardin, realized this program was not as well-rounded as it should be. Students were lacking exposure to surgery on women, children, and trauma cases. Drs. Ellis and Hardin established a more diversified program for surgical residents by offering Veteran's Administration students an affiliation with Mercy. Six residents went through the first year of training that ended in June 1964.

Walter H. Neumann, Jr. assists Sister Eileen, *top,* with a jack hammer at the October 1968 groundbreaking for Mercy's new power plant. ❧ Nellie and Ellis Levitt, *above,* cut the ribbon at the opening of Mercy's Medical Library in 1961. The Levitts provided funding for the new library.

A surgical technician program was started in 1964 by Sister Pauline Hammes. It was the only school for surgical technicians in Des Moines. Students who enrolled in the program were involved in a "earn while learn" program. For six months they attended lectures and did class and practical work. At the end of this time, they received certificates showing satisfactory completion of the course. Another six months, similar to an internship, was spent in training. Thirteen technicians graduated from the first session. Mercy's program continued through 1968. Karen Goodman graduated in the last class: "Certification was not an option at that time, but now it is. Those of us who graduated then became certified when it was made available." [11]

Mercy promoted another educational opportunity early in 1960 when the sisters hosted the annual meeting of the Catholic Hospital Association. More than 100 supervisory personnel from hospitals in seven states attended a three-day conference at Mercy. W.I. Christopher, director of Personnel Service for the Catholic Association of the United States and Canada, conducted the program for approximately 50 sisters and 60 lay persons. Four major fields of supervision were highlighted. [12]

Early in 1962, televisions were installed in each patient room. Two closed-circuit channels made it possible to broadcast educational programs and chapel services into the patients' rooms. [13]

A SCARCITY OF NURSES AND AIDES

In addition to the critical need for beds during the early 1960s hospitals faced an equally critical nursing deficit. Nationwide estimates projected that as many as 20 percent of hospital nursing positions were unfilled. An additional 70,000 nurses were needed. Mercy administrators approached the shortage in a typically tenacious way by launching several in-house training programs tailored to meet specific needs.

A new program to train hospital aides was begun in August 1963 by Sister Mary Ricarda Bintner, director of nursing services. This three-week training program taught basic nursing procedures. Plans called for the course to be taught four times per year and to employ aides certified through the course. [14]

One year later, Mercy offered a refresher course for registered nurses designed to help inactive nurses acquaint themselves with new nursing procedures, techniques, and drugs. Members of Mercy's nursing and medical staffs, under the direction of Sister Ricarda, taught the six-week course, twice a week for two hours, for a fee of $15. Forty-nine "retired" nurses completed the course that year, the only one of its kind offered in Central Iowa. This educational opportunity attracted inactive nurses from as far away as Grinnell. [15]

Expanding Mercy's existing volunteer pool, Sister Ricarda began a hospital aide

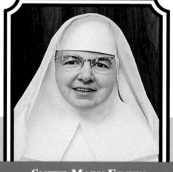

SISTER MARY EILEEN

Sister Mary Eileen Moore, Mercy's administrator from 1964-69, was one of a group of young women who migrated to Iowa as part of a recruitment trip to Ireland by the Sisters of Mercy. Sisters Mary Xavier Clinton and Clare Clifford went to Ireland from Council Bluffs in 1928 "in search of girls who may wish to offer themselves for missionary work in the faraway diocese of Des Moines." [16]

Fifteen Irish girls decided to leave their homes and families and go to America. From County Kerry through Nova Scotia to Iowa, these young women made a journey of faith to begin a new life with the Sisters of Mercy in Council Bluffs. One of these, Lena (Helena) Moore, finished high school with the sisters at Mount Loretto and entered the novitiate of the Sisters of Mercy in 1930. She completed nurse's training at Mercy in Council Bluffs with additional training in the radiology department and a bachelor's degree in nursing from Creighton. During the 1930s and 1940s, Sister Eileen nursed and worked in x-ray in Council Bluffs and Roseburg, Oregon.

In the early 1960s, Sister Eileen attended Xavier University in Cincinnati studying hospital administration. She spent 1963 as an administrative resident observing at Mercy Hospital in Des Moines. "I was supposed to study under Sister Mary Francis, but in the meantime, Sister Mary Francis was transferred to the new Bergan Mercy Hospital in Omaha, and Mr. Conroy took me under his charge. He was a real gentleman. I spent time in each department, which was most interesting. You really got practical experience there." [17]

After her internship, Sister Eileen became administrator of the hospital. She remembered that Mercy had a "very good advisory board...a progressive medical staff." [18] During her administrative tenure, Sister Eileen was admitted to the American College of Hospital Administrators. [19]

Sister Eileen left Mercy for a new assignment in 1969 to become administrator of St. Vincent's Home in Omaha. After a brief time spent in Red Bluff, California, she returned to Council Bluffs where she ministered at Mercy Hospital.

Sister Eileen currently resides in the Villa retirement home of the Sisters of Mercy in Omaha, volunteering two days each week in the day-care of Bergan Mercy Hospital.

ADMINISTRATOR 1964-1969

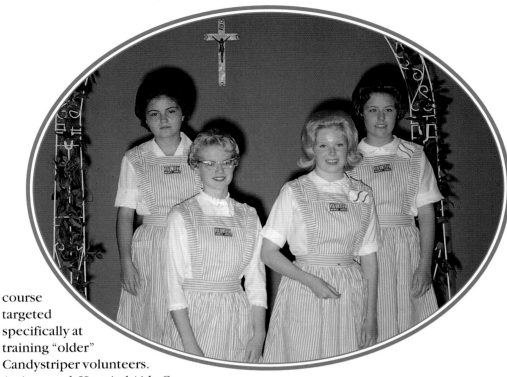

course targeted specifically at training "older" Candystriper volunteers.

A nine-week Hospital Aide Course covered topics such as: good service, flower arrangement, bed-making, linen-handling, personal relations between patient and worker, patient bathing, feeding and entertaining children, safety precautions within the hospital, and increased emphasis on hygiene.

This service expanded the duties of the Candystripers, and under the leadership of the Mercy Guild, the newly trained aides provided valuable service to the hospital as they performed simple tasks, easing the job for nurses.[20]

Adult education throughout the community became prominent during the 1960s. Beginning in 1961, Sister Mary Zita Brennan and Louise Brady conducted adult education classes in prenatal education .

A CITY WITHIN A CITY

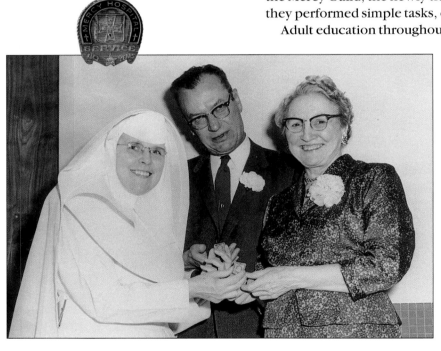

In gratitude to employees for their hard work, the sisters established the annual Employee Recognition Dinner. The first of these events was held in the new hospital dining room on February 23, 1960. Forty-four honored guests, representing more than 700 years of "faithful service" were entertained with a specially prepared meal, flowers, songs, and service pins.[21] In 1963 at this dinner, Master of Ceremonies. Dr. Walter Abbott saluted the honored employees in this way:

"I would like to compare Mercy Hospital to a 'city within a city' where, daily life comes and goes from the first bewildered cry of a newborn babe to the last gasp of the dying. Within the confines of this 'city within a city' are many personnel and there runs a gamut of emotions, from lust, greed, self-pity, to resentment, anger, defiance, fear, jealousy, and envy. All of these can only be overcome by forgiveness, charity and mercy....Remember your example may lend encouragement and perhaps be an inspiration to a patient to the extent you may be the only bible he or she may ever read. It is necessary for us all to daily take an inventory as each and everyone of us has a cross to bear." [22]

To recognize hard work, Mercy established an annual Employee Recognition Dinner in 1960. Sister Francis awarded 25-year service pins to J.W. Woods and Mae Wren, *above.* &. Mercy's Candystripers, *top,* volunteered many hours through the Mercy Guild. &. *Opposite: 1960s aerial view of Mercy's campus.*

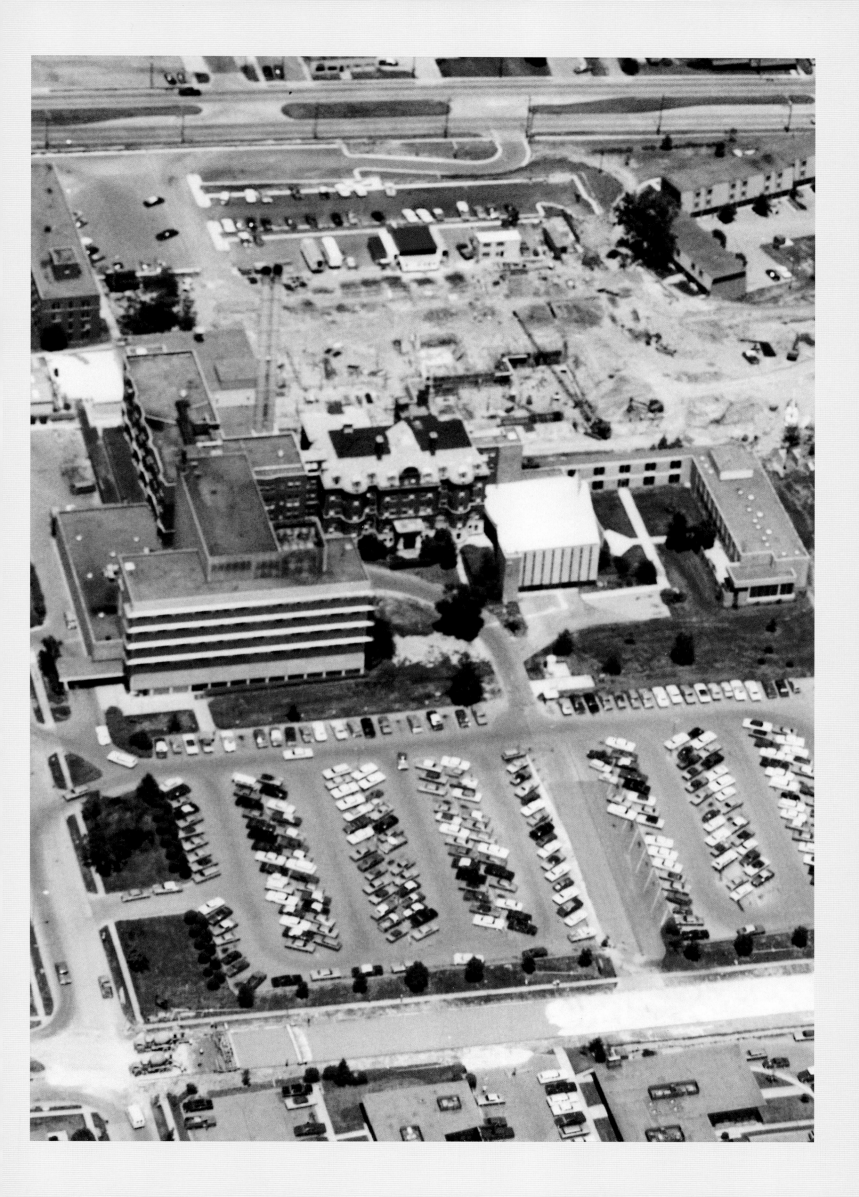

MERCY ADVISORY BOARD, 1957

Front Row, left to right:
Mrs. Charles B. Ritz
Mrs. E.T. Meredith, Jr.
Dr. James W. Chambers
Father Lloyd Connolly
Arthur T. Gormley
Paul T. Manning
Mrs. J.J. Kelly
Mrs. M.L. Northup
Sister Mary Anita Paul

Back Row, left to right:
Dr. Daniel F. Crowley, Jr.
James W. Hubbell, Jr.
Bernard D. Kurtz
Marvin F. Oberg
Carl J. Muelhaupt
William Poorman
J.W. Brooks
Charles Cownie

MERCY ADVISORY BOARD, 1966

First Row, left to right:
Mrs. J.J. Kelly
Mrs. J.R. Rowen
Mrs. E.S. Grask
Mrs. M.L. Northup
Sister Mary Eileen Moore
Mrs. E.T. Meredith, Jr.
Mrs. George Comfort

Second Row, left to right:
Dr. M.E. Alberts
Louis Norris
E.R. (Pat) Haley
S.R. Fisher
Bishop George J. Biskup
E.A. Boss
Arthur T. Gormley
W.B. Nugent

Third Row, left to right:
H.P. Klein
J.E. Olson
W.L. Lalor
G.A. Jewett
W.F. Poorman
C.J. Muelhaupt
S.L. Friedman
E.I. Levitt,
B.D. Kurtz
John J. McLaughlin
John W. Hummer

Fourth Row, left to right:
Earl Bucknell
M.F. Coonan
T.I. Veiock
S.F. McGinn
John Ringland
C.T. Cownie
J.W. Hubbell, Jr.
Father Harold Fischer

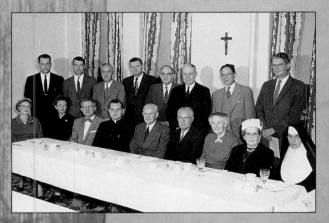

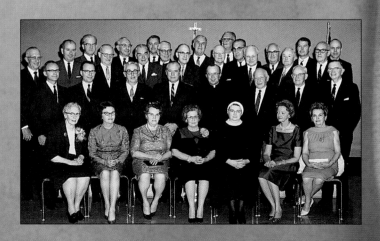

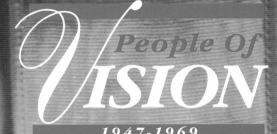

People Of

VISION

1947-1969

THE 75TH ANNIVERSARY

Mercy celebrated the 75th anniversary of the hospital in 1968. In the beginning of the tower expansion, the Sisters of Mercy celebrated this benchmark event, entitled "Caring For All."

There were many celebrations and the first was a "picnic in the park (actually Mercy Hall)" held on November 18, 1968, for all Mercy employees. Entertainment and refreshments were provided by the Employee Recreational Committee, who dressed in old-fashioned costumes. More than 680 present and former employees attended this party. Don Elefson of the laboratory served as Master of Ceremonies. Mrs. Ruby Aggers, a former employee, fashioned a five-layered pink and white cake for the festivities.

On December 9, 1968, Mercy hosted an anniversary dinner at Val-Air Ballroom. Tickets for the dinner were reasonably priced at $5 per person. Archbishop Gerald T. Bergan of Omaha and Bishop Maurice Dingman of Des Moines were the main speakers of the evening. The archbishop said of Mercy:

> *"The interest of the laity has increased tremendously over these many years. It is almost unbelievable on my return here to see the tremendous progress that has been made. All of the citizens can offer their congratulations to Mercy Hospital on the magnificent work very well done."* [23]

One of the special tasks of the anniversary committee was to track down the first baby born at Mercy. Records for the early days of Mercy's opening were gone, so an appeal for this information was made in the local newspapers. This request brought in some interesting information about Mercy's early past. One story involved a young man born at Mercy on July 18, 1910:

> *"[He] was born at Mercy before they had a maternity ward in the hospital. His crib was two chairs with a pillow, in a corner of his mother's room on the main floor to the left of the main entrance, first door, in what I always called the 'round room.' "* [24]

In response to this newspaper article, two earlier births were uncovered which won honors for first girl and boy. The oldest birth was Mrs. F. G. Appelquist, born on March 21, 1899. Mrs. Appelquist attended the anniversary dinner as an honored guest. Mr. F. Marcellus Wonderlin was born at Mercy on September 21, 1906.

Mercy ended the 75th anniversary celebrations with Sister Eileen's words:

> *"Looking at the history of the hospital, we learned that those who have preceded us must have adapted to change many times and must have accepted challenge with tremendous fortitude. This response to change and progress has encouraged us to proceed with our part in the present and future history of Mercy."* [25]

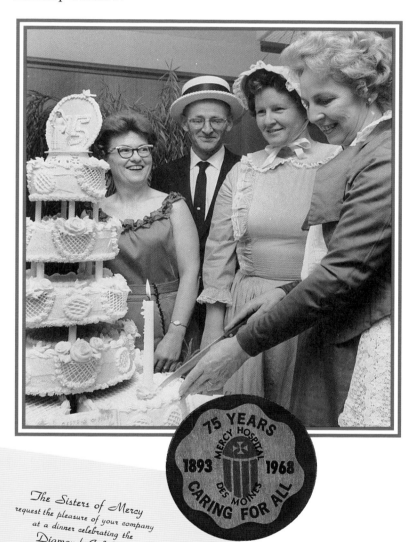

Mercy celebrated its 75th anniversary in 1968. Below left to right: Mary Rieff, Don Elefson, Jeri Rourke, and Dee Hogan, dressed in period costumes, cut the elegant cake at the November 18 party in Mercy Hall.

The Sisters of Mercy request the pleasure of your company at a dinner celebrating the Diamond Jubilee of Mercy Hospital Des Moines, Iowa Monday, the ninth of December Nineteen hundred and sixty-eight at 6:30 o'clock, Val-Air Ballroom Guest Speakers Archbishop Gerald T. Bergan, D.D. Bishop Maurice J. Dingman, D.D.

75 YEARS MERCY HOSPITAL DES MOINES 1893 1968 CARING FOR ALL

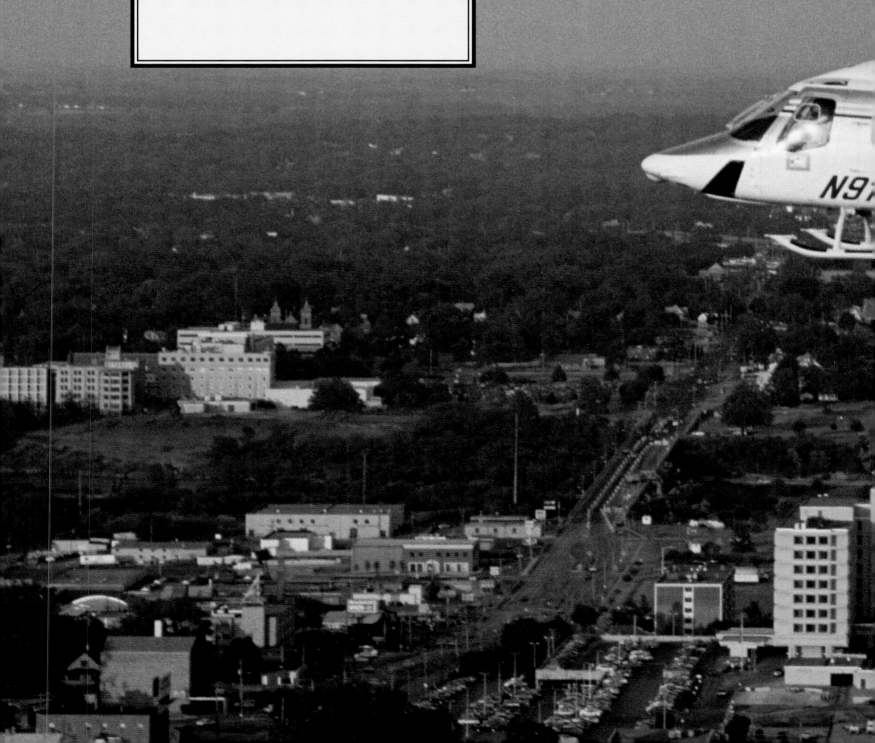

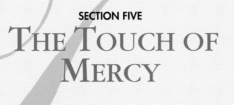

SECTION FIVE

THE TOUCH OF MERCY

1969 - 1993

That our leadership and compassion be dedicated to the healthcare needs of those we serve.

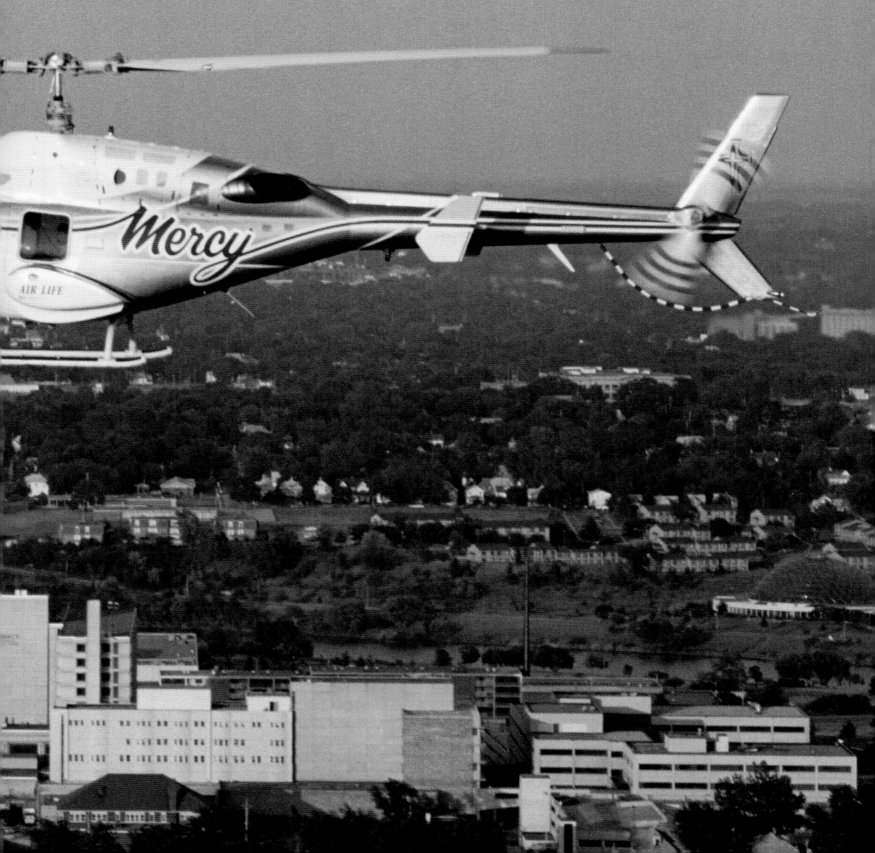

CHAPTER ONE

BRIGHTER VISTA: STRENGTHENING THE FOUNDATION

As the dawn rose on the 1970s, Mercy's sun-kissed hill changed completely. By the end of the decade the Mercy skyline featured unique H-shaped towers, and the hospital's bed capacity grew from 360 to 500.

New imaging modalities and diagnostic treatment procedures expanded Mercy's healing horizons, and the number of dedicated Mercy employees increased. When Sister Mary Gervase Northup took over the administrative helm of Mercy in 1969, the hospital was in the middle of two preliminary construction stages: Phase I-A and Pre-Phase I-A.

Phase I-A replaced the old power plant and laundry. Pre-Phase I included the demolition of two brick smokestacks and the extensions on the northern side of the Central Wing dating from 1912. Two parking lots, an addition on the western side of the West Wing enlarging the radiology department, and preparation of the site for the towers set the stage for Mercy's massive two-phase tower expansion.

PHASE I

Contracts totaling $11.8 million were signed in March 1971 for the tower expansion. Sister Mary Gervase, Mercy's administrator, said:

> *"This is an important milestone for us. We are grateful for the loyal support and hard work by our sisters, medical staff, hospital staff, advisory board, architects and the consultants who have brought us to this stage in the history of Mercy Hospital."* [1]

Bishop Maurice Dingman and Sister Gervase turned the symbolic first shovel on April 25, 1971. The ceremony was dedicated to the memory of Sister Mary Pauline Hammes, who had died unexpectedly on April 21. Sister Pauline had assisted in all phases of Mercy's changes during her 35 years of service.

Bids for Phase I came in under anticipated costs and Sister Gervase announced that it would be possible to "shell-in" the top four floors of the twin-tower structure. Work proceeded rapidly on the tower site, and by July, the walls of the below-ground level were in place. A crane, capable of rising 175 feet over the site, hovered in place early in August. In conjunction with the Phase I tower construction, an additional Phase X (ten) was completed: a new Cardiovascular Care Unit of ten beds.

By July of 1973, the outside of the tower structures was rapidly taking on a completed appearance as

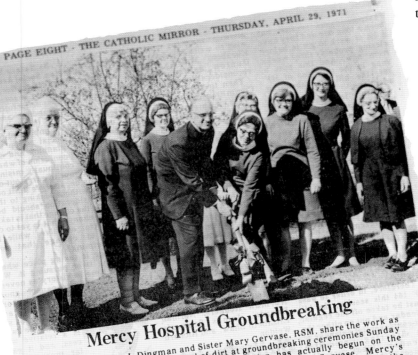

PAGE EIGHT - THE CATHOLIC MIRROR - THURSDAY, APRIL 29, 1971

Mercy Hospital Groundbreaking

Bishop Maurice J. Dingman and Sister Mary Gervase, RSM, share the work as they turn the symbolic first shovel of dirt at groundbreaking ceremonies Sunday at Mercy Hospital in Des Moines. Construction has actually begun on the nearly-$12 million addition to the hospital and Sister Gervase. Mercy's Administrator, announced Sunday that because construction bids were under the original estimate, the work will include "shelling in" of an additional four floors for the twin acute care towers. The dedication Sunday was made in memory of Sister Mary Pauline Hammes, RSM, was passed away April 21 after serving Mercy Hospital for 38 years. (See obituary notice this page) Members of the Sisters of Mercy community at the hospital present for this picture were: (from left) Sisters Mary Joseph; Mary Geraldine; Kathleen Mary; Mary del Rey; Elizabeth Ann; Mary Vera; Anne Mary and Mary Zita. (Not visible, dressed in white behind Bishop Dingman, is Sister Mary Concepta.)

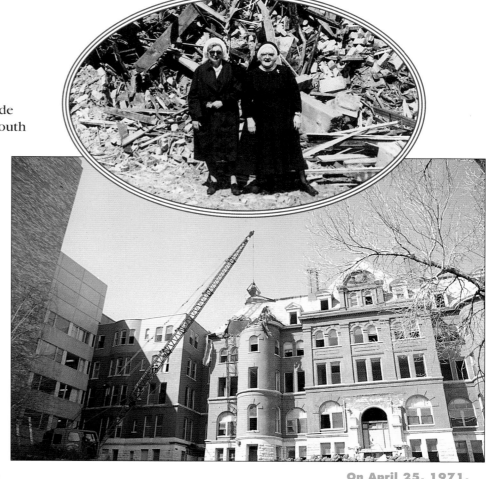

precast concrete panels were slipped onto the outside frame. The twin smokestacks were attached to the south tower leg and covered with matching concrete panels. A steel bridge linking the old North Wing with the south tower was put into place in the summer of 1973. This bridge linked the new nursery on South Four of the towers with the delivery rooms on old West Four.

The end of Phase I came in March 1974. Floors three, four, and five of the 10-level building were finished for patient care and the ground-level base or service chassis was completed. Costs exceeded $17.5 million.

It was especially appropriate that during St. Patrick's Day festivities, the daughters of Catherine McAuley should once again extend "a thousand welcomes" to the Des Moines community. Mercy hosted a dedication week, culminating in activities on three days, March 15, 16, and 17, 1974. Governor Robert Ray, Bishop Maurice Dingman, and Provincial Administrator Sister Maura Clark attended the formal dedication on Saturday, March 16. Rabbi Jay Goldburg gave the closing Benediction.

Mercy moved into the first step of Phase II with the demolition of the Central Wing. The removal of this wing was performed carefully to avoid damage to the chapel and West Wing.

A Painful Choice

The time between the two tower phases was delayed due to lack of funding and the required approval of the Health Planning Council (HPC). During this time, architects labored over four different plans. The accepted plan involved a radical and painful step: the removal of the beautiful tent-like Mercy chapel and meeting area known as Mercy Hall. This step was necessary to allow the service base to expand. The loss of Mercy Hall was to be filled by a new kitchen, cafeteria and meeting area. A new chapel, convenient to families and patients undergoing treatment in the new ancillary areas, was planned for the first floor of the hospital. Phase II called for the completion of three additional tower floors and a new two-level expanded service chassis on the southern side of the towers. The sixth floor remained empty, functioning as a buffer zone to keep noise and dust at a minimum during the completion of floors seven, eight, and nine.

In the summer of 1976, Mercy's front door changed for the fifth time in its history. The main entrance to the hospital was relocated to University Avenue. Construction for the new chapel began in September. Sister Gervase underscored the importance of the location of the new chapel:

> *"It is vitally important that, as a healthcare institution sponsored by a Catholic religious order, we make it clear that faith and worship are central to our lives and central to caring for the whole person."* [2]

The first Mass was celebrated in the new chapel on December 30, 1976, and the dedication ceremony for the new chapel was held on March 19, 1977, with Bishop Dingman officiating. In 1982, a portion of the chapel was designated as a Jewish Place of Prayer. [3]

On April 25, 1971, Bishop Dingman and Sister Gervase, *opposite below*, turned the first shovel at the ground-breaking of Phase I. ❧ Sisters Sebastian and Joseph, *top*, pose in front of the newly demolished Central Wing, in April 1974. ❧ Part of Mercy's chapel, *bottom*, was dedicated as a Jewish Place of Prayer in 1982. *Left to right*: Rabbi Jay Goldburg, Mrs. Wm. Friedman, Sister Patricia Clare, and Bishop Dingman.

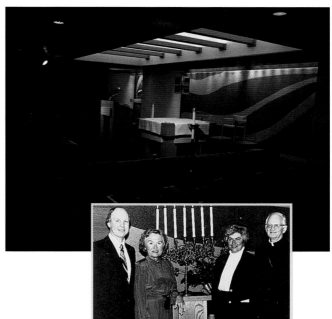

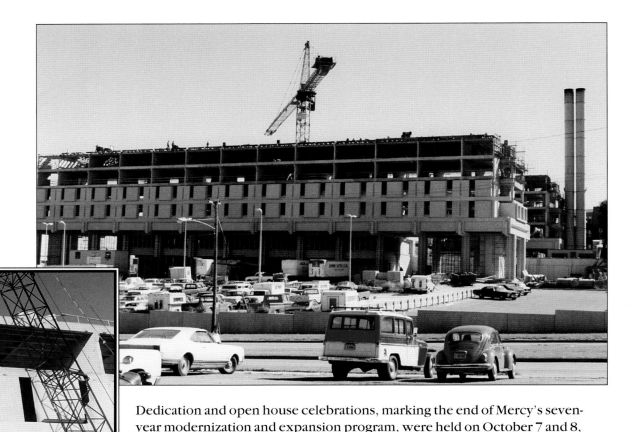

Dedication and open house celebrations, marking the end of Mercy's seven-year modernization and expansion program, were held on October 7 and 8, 1978. Governor Robert Ray complimented the Sisters of Mercy for completing such a comprehensive program under national average costs. Bishop Dingman blessed the newly opened areas in the hospital. Total cost for completion of the new facilities topped $37 million.[4]

FILLING THE TOWERS

The first Mercy patients were moved in early April from the South and West Wings to the newly finished floors in the towers. Two "old-hands" dusted off their moving skills to help with the patient relocation. Sister Concepta and Marie Bloomquist welcomed the first patient moved from South-2 to Main-7. Sister Concepta and Marie repeated a move they did in 1959 when the South Wing opened, and in 1974 when the first floors of the towers opened. Remembering this move, several people commented:

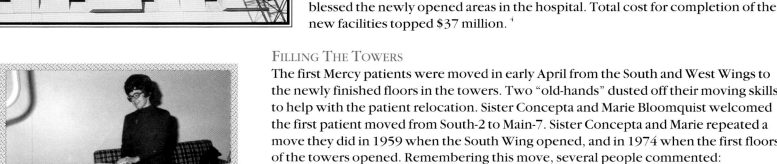

> *"The funniest things upset people, like they couldn't find the waste basket....I remember we had to lock the windows. No one had checked the windows. I worked from 11:00 til 7:00, and someone leaned against the window. No one fell out, but we had to get the key and lock the windows....I remember how much my feet hurt. Going from the old floors to the new carpet. It took us about two weeks to get used to that...and getting used to the beepers."*[5]

Construction of Mercy's H-shaped towers was completed from 1971 through moving day, March 4, 1974. Sister Gervase, *above*, welcomed Jo Nye to her room in the new towers.

Finishing touches continued on the entrances to the hospital. A new emergency entrance, located in the former personnel entrance, began in August 1978. This approach allowed ambulances to enter from the existing emergency drive into an enclosed garage. Another entrance for walk-in traffic was planned on the north side.

The large and complicated departments of surgery, laboratory, and radiology relocated during 1978. By February 15, 1979, all existing beds at Mercy were staffed and available for occupancy. Admissions were 407 and discharges were 405.

One of the last departments moved to the towers was the labor and birthing unit from West-4 to Main 4-N on July 17, 1979. Mercy initiated changes in the labor and birthing area during the early 1970s to meet the changing socioeconomic aspects of birth. The hospital began allowing rooming-in privileges in 1971. The baby and father stayed with the mother if she was in a private room. Fathers were permitted in Mercy's delivery room in 1972, if both parents had participated in childbirth education classes. The first "natural" childbirth with the father acting as coach occurred on May 19, 1972.

In 1974, Mercy began offering free candlelight dinners to new parents. Mercy's neonatal intensive care unit began in the mid-1970s.

BUILDING INTO THE 1980s

A two-phase program to improve visitor parking accommodations in front of the main entrance to Mercy began during the summer of 1979. This two-level parking area was made possible with the razing of the school of nursing building. Access to Mercy's front door was now possible directly from Sixth Avenue because of the extension of Mercy Drive through the former school site. A tunnel under Mercy Drive from the A-level of the north tower allowed access to the new lower level parking lot. A parking deck extending over the lower level, completed in early 1980, added accommodations for an additional 100 cars.

Other new construction contemplated for 1980 included a parking ramp on the southwest corner of the campus, a heliport on the former site of the school of nursing, and a newly expanded emergency department with two separate emergency entrances—one for walkup patients and one for ambulances.

NEW PHASES, NEW FACES

Several present-day departments began during this time: pastoral care, social services, utilization review and infection control, materials management, patient accounts, data processing, public relations, physical plant and construction, maintenance, security, personnel, and the Mercy Foundation.

From the time the hospital opened in 1893, Mercy's chaplain had been appointed by the diocese. This priest usually divided his duties between Mercy and other work assigned by the diocese. The goal was to provide a full spectrum of Catholic sacramental ministry and support services to Catholic patients and their families. Persons of other faiths were visited by their own pastors, but there was not a resident Protestant chaplain within Mercy.

During 1970, the chancery established a chaplaincy program for the Greater Des Moines area. Fathers Richard E. Gubbels and Joseph J. McDonnell were appointed co-directors of the program. In the fall of 1970, Mercy opened a department of ministerial services, with Sisters Mary Therese Bannon and Concepta Mullins as full-time staff members who worked with the diocesan team ministry.

Consistent with the move by the Sisters of Mercy to be leaders in holistic healing, Mercy began a formal pastoral care department in 1974. By November 1975, the staffing level of four full-time and one part-time chaplain had been achieved, including men and women, Catholic and Protestant. Father Paul Solomia joined the department in July 1975. He became director in 1980, and today, he coordinates 13 employees, providing 24-hour staffing.

Mercy head nurse, Louise Brady, *above*, conducted birthing classes for expectant parents in 1970. ❧ Mercy's Pastoral Care Department began in 1974. Father Paul Solomia, *below*, blessed patient, Sister Mildred Ann Zaver.

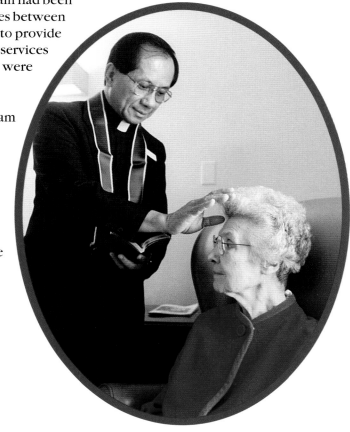

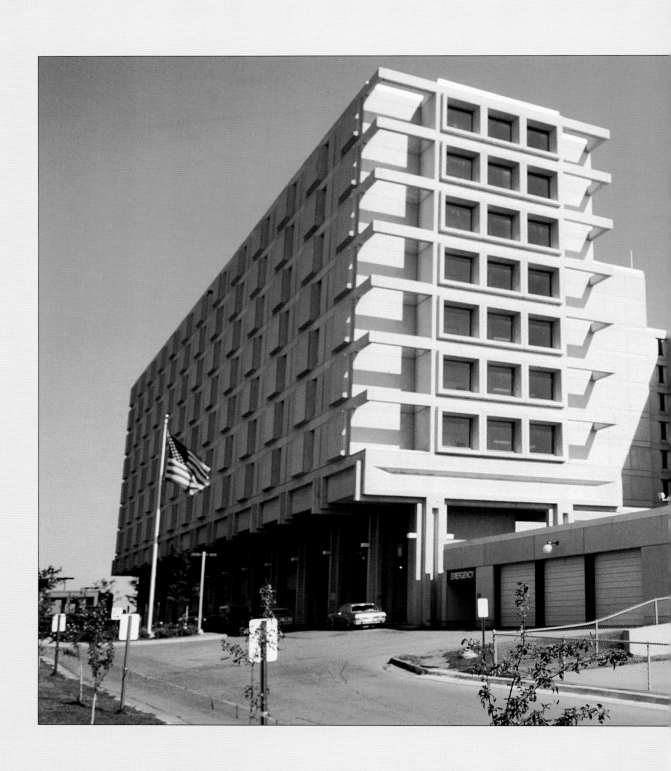

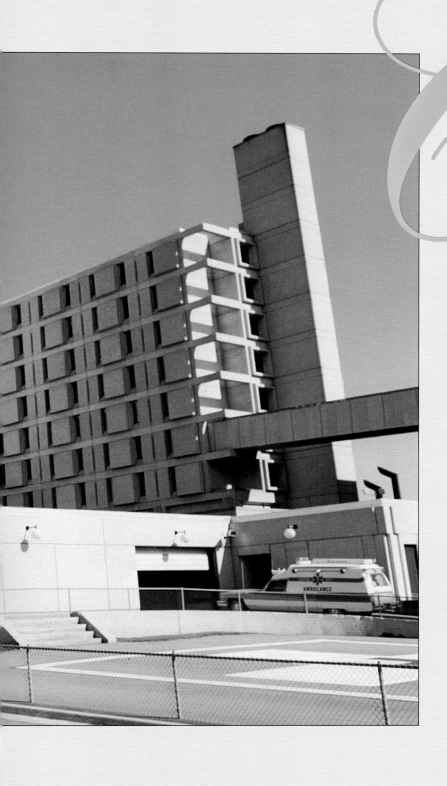

Construction on Mercy's towers began in 1971 and was finished in 1978. A new front door facing University Avenue and an emergency entrance from Sixth Avenue, through the old school of nursing site provided convenient access to the hospital. Dedication ceremonies were held in October 1978.

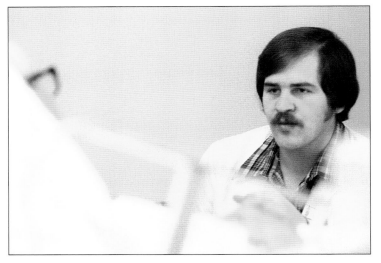

In the 1960s, Mercy's social services department opened on Central Two, near the chapel. Rosemary Brandstetter became director in January 1969. Sister Mary Charles Keane became director in 1971. Today, the department provides for discharge planning, protective services, in-services, transplant, consulting, and 24-hour on-call through the emergency department. Since the 1970s, the department has functioned as a clinical setting for students in degree programs in social work.

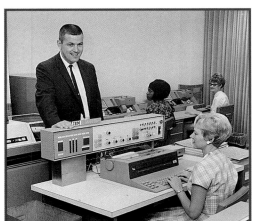

A utilization coordinator position was created in February 1971 with the hiring of Sandra Houts. This position was created to work closely with Mercy's social services, physicians, and the Utilization Review Committee of the medical staff. In 1972, Annette Bair became the utilization coordinator.

Hospital infection control evolved during the 1960s. This department later became part of utilization review. Sister Mary Elizabeth Ann Paul, a niece of Sister Anita's, became an infection control technologist. She continued in that capacity until her death in 1978. In 1992, Mercy employs two full-time infection control practitioners.

In 1964, Mercy began planning for its first computer.[6] The hospital's computer center started in the South Wing dietary area. By August 1972, the computer center moved to the basement of the convent, its current home. The first departments to go "on line" with terminals in their areas were admitting and housekeeping. Within a few months a customized system for admitting patients linked all ancillary departments.

Mercy's laboratory adopted an electronic record-keeping device with its MedLab computerized system. Medical records, patient accounts, credit, and cashier were added to the mainframe system in July 1975.

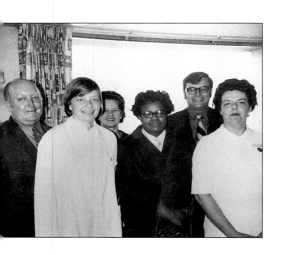
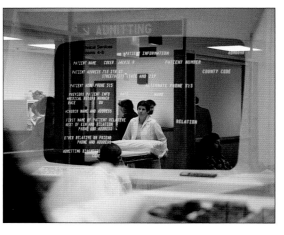
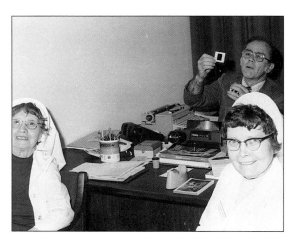

During the late 1950s, a Public Relations Committee was appointed by the medical staff. In June 1970, Robert Campbell was hired as the first public relations director. Today, the department coordinates Mercy's media relations and produces the *Bulletin, Journal,* and numerous other publications.

Art Dressler was appointed director of a new security department in the fall of 1970. By 1973, the security department provided round-the-clock hospital coverage. Today, the department provides services in security, safety, fire prevention, locksmith, parking, valet, shuttle, and courier.

The Mercy Foundaton began as a legal entity at the end of 1973. Its primary purpose was "the cultivation of gifts from people and organizations interested in supporting the healthcare mission of the Sisters of Mercy and Mercy Hospital."[7]

More Resources

Several of Mercy's existing departments expanded and changed names during the 1970s: personnel, maintenance, materials management, and patient accounts.

Joe Wilson became Mercy's first personnel director in 1967, when there were 950 employees. Today's human resources department provides employee services through: health education, employee health, personnel, and the Mercy Child Development Center.

Mercy's Board of Directors approved the development of a Child Care Center for children of Mercy employees in March 1977. The plan called for a full preschool program licensed by the state of Iowa. On August 8, 1977, the center opened in the former St. Ambrose Elementary School. Mercy's Child Development Center cares for 220 children with plans to move into the former LCM building in 1993.

In 1975, a new maintenance department was formed to combine buildings and grounds, painting, carpenter shop, signs, planning and scheduling, power plant, plumbing, electrical and electronics, and supply, processing and distribution. Ray Schneider was appointed director.

Other departments that combined functions appeared under new names in the early 1970s. Purchasing, stockroom, central services, and mail delivery evolved into materials management in February 1970. At the same time, insurance, credit and cashier duties combined into the patient accounts department.

Several specialized programs also began during the late 1960s and early 1970s as a result of new technology. Mercy was designated as the only Des Moines area hospital for cardiac care. This allowed Mercy to gain the superior status in cardiac care it enjoys today. New equipment such as the CAT scan expanded the imaging possibilities for cancer and special internal studies. Mercy also participated in a pilot stroke study. At the February 1969 medical staff meeting, Dr. John Bakody proposed that Mercy open a Stroke Study Center. In June 1969, the proposal became a reality.

Evolution Of New Structures

Until the 1960s, Mercy's governing body was the local Sisters' Council, composed of three Sisters of Mercy. As administrative systems became more complex, Mercy's structure flexed to fit the complexities. A board of directors, comprised of five resident Sisters of Mercy, replaced the Sisters' Council. New positions of department heads and managers evolved from the restructuring of jobs. By the end of the 1960s, three assistant administrator positions were added expanding Mercy's internal organizational structure.

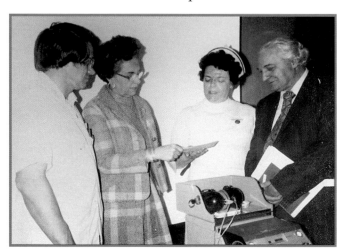

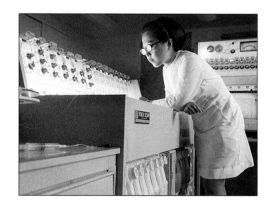

Two of the most elaborate and complicated areas to be relocated to the newly completed towers were the surgery, *top and above,* and laboratory areas. ❧ In 1973, the Mercy Stroke Project Committee received an MA-20 Maico audiometer to test hearing deficiencies. Mrs. Van Driel, *left,* presented a check for the equipment to Perry Bleadorn, Nurse Betty Hammes, and Dr. John Bakody.

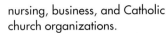

SISTER MARY GERVASE

Sister Mary Gervase Northup was born Harriett Therese Northup in Nodaway, Iowa. She entered the Sisters of Mercy in 1945 and studied nursing at the College of St. Mary in Omaha, where she received a bachelor's of nursing in 1952. Sister Gervase earned a master's degree in nursing from Catholic University in 1958. She spent 16 years in nursing at St. Catherine's Hospital in Omaha as a student nurse, floor supervisor, instructor and director of the school of nursing. In 1964, Sister Gervase succeeded Sister Timothea (Patricia Clare) Sullivan as nursing school director in Des Moines.

While she directed the nursing school, Sister Gervase was named to Mercy's board of directors. In 1969, she followed Sister Eileen as Mercy's new administrator.

Sister Gervase became administrator as Mercy embarked on its tower expansion program. She guided Mercy's building expansion and supported Mercy's developing cardiac program by positioning it to become the number-one cardiac care-giver in Des Moines. Sister Gervase led the way to forming a consortium of Des Moines' seven hospitals, known as the Hospital Association of Greater Des Moines.

During her administration, Sister Gervase served on the boards of: St. Catherine's; Archbishop Bergan Mercy Hospital; St. Joseph's Mercy Hospital in Centerville, Iowa; Iowa Blue Cross; Mercy Hospital at Devil's Lake, North Dakota; and Mercy Hospital Foundation of Des Moines. She held posts on several committees of the Omaha Province of the Sisters of Mercy, as well as in many nursing, business, and Catholic church organizations.

Sister Gervase received an honorary doctorate in 1973 from the College of Osteopathic Medicine and Surgery in Des Moines. In 1976, she received the National Conference of Christians and Jews award for distinguished leadership in the fields of human relations and community service.

In September 1976, it was found that Sister Gervase had a rare form of cancer. She suffered with this disease, bravely attending board meetings within the last month of her life. Sister Gervase was surrounded with loving attention during the final days of her illness. The tower construction for Phase II was particularly noisy, but contractors were constantly warned by loyal employees to keep the noise down. Another employee remembered sneaking Sister Gervase's dog, Pepe', up the back stairs to visit her.[8] After a brave fight, Sister Gervase died at Mercy on March 27, 1977. More than 700 people participated in her funeral Mass.

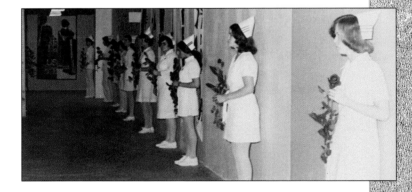

"A sense of sorrow and sadness, mixed with relief that [Sister Gervase's] suffering had ended, pervaded the hospital immediately following her death early last Sunday morning. But the wake service Monday evening and the funeral mass were occasions for celebration and praise...of her life here with us." [9]

Close friends of Sister Gervase remember her with quiet reverence, saying that "she was brilliant...very intellectual."

Sister Gervase's administrative term paralleled the tower expansion. It was fitting that her funeral Mass was celebrated in the almost finished laboratory of Phase II. Two lines of student nurses formed an honor guard, raising single red roses in salute, as Sister Gervase's casket left the makeshift chapel for burial in Glendale Cemetery.

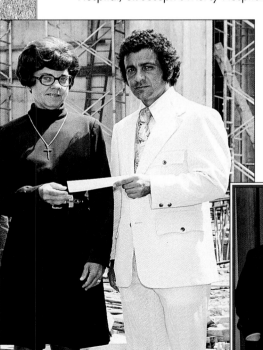

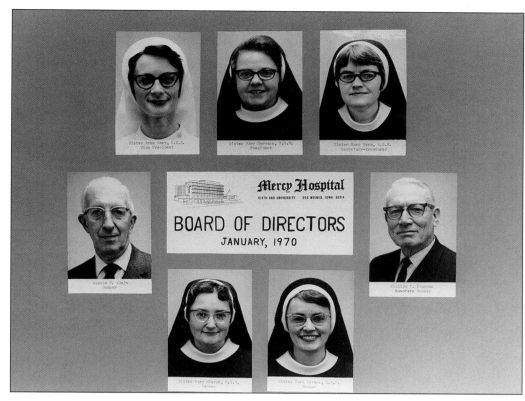

Mercy Hospital
SIXTH AND UNIVERSITY · DES MOINES, IOWA 50314

BOARD OF DIRECTORS
JANUARY, 1970

SISTERS OF MERCY

Alicia Gallagher
Bernadette Mulroney
Brian (Helen) Harty
Brigid Condon
Carlotta Clinton
Cecelia (Teresita) Zaver
Charles Keane
Claudia Robinson
Dolores Preisinger
Donata Landkamer
Elaine Delaney
Elizabeth Ann Paul
Francene Summers
Gloria Heese
Jane Reichmuth
Janel Sawatzki
Jeanine Salak
Jeanne Marie Christensen
Josephine Collins
Kilian Clinton
Lois Castelein
Margaret Ann White
Marie Elena Maldonado
Mary Ann Burkhardt
Mary Regina Selenke
Michaele McGuire
Monica Marie Reichmuth
Paula Radosevich
Rita Mary O'Brien
Rosalin Keane
Sally Smolen
Seraphia McMahon
Stella Lillie
Vidette Jacobson
Virginia Marie Kendrick

One of the biggest changes in Mercy's administration came at the beginning of the 1970s, when Harold P. Klein and William F. Poorman became the first lay members of Mercy's Board of Directors. At the same time, new Articles of Incorporation changed the main administrative body of Mercy to include a five member board, and non-resident Sisters of Mercy were added to the membership.

A precedent-setting change took place in Mercy's administrative structure in January 1978. The Mercy Board of Directors named two laymen to head the hospital governing body: Kenneth McCarthy, chairman, and Louis Norris, vice chairman. These men had been loyal supporters of Mercy for many years.

In September 1979, new corporate titles for administrators went into effect. The administrator became president and assistant administrator titles changed to vice presidents. Only two Sisters of Mercy have served Mercy as administrator/president and chief executive officer since 1969: Sister Mary Gervase Northup and Sister Patricia Clare Sullivan.

The Health System of Mercy was the governing body for all Mercy healthcare institutions, until the Sisters of Mercy of the Omaha Province joined with seven other religious congregations, forming the Catholic Health Corporation headquartered in Omaha, Nebraska. A. Diane Moeller is president in 1992.

STRENGTHENING FROM WITHIN

Shortly after becoming Mercy's administrator, Sister Gervase, as a delegate to the General Chapter of the Sisters of Mercy, participated in workshops designed to initiate long-range planning for sisters involved in healthcare ministry. As a result of her training, Sister Gervase was the first to ask the Health Planning Council of Central Iowa to begin similar planning on a local level.

"We were concerned with the quality of health care, with the rising costs to the public we serve, and with the prospects of expansion." [10]

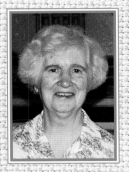

Sister Mary Kilian Clinton

The last Irish girl to join the Sisters of Mercy in the Regional Community of Omaha arrived in 1939. Cecelia Clinton was born in County Leitrim. She attended National Catholic School with her brother and five sisters. Her sister, Alice, migrated to America in 1928 with Sisters Eileen Moore and Josephine Collins to join the Sisters of Mercy.

In 1941, Sister Kilian received her nursing diploma from Mercy in Denver, and later, a bachelor's degree from St. Louis University. The majority of her career was spent supervising in pediatric nursing in Colorado and Council Bluffs. In the early 1960s, Sister Kilian worked with Sister Mary Charles Keane at the St. James Orphanage in Omaha.

Sister Kilian came to Mercy Des Moines as pediatrics supervisor in 1969. In 1974, she began working in pastoral care and later public relations. Sister Kilian and her sibling, Sister Mary Carlotta, are a familiar duo on the Mercy campus.

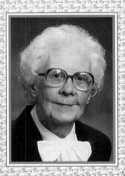

Sister Mary Charles Keane

Sister Mary Charles Keane was a native of Omaha. She was born Catherine Keane in 1907 as the second child in a family of seven. Three of the Keane daughters entered the Sisters of Mercy, and one of Sister Charles' sisters, Sister Mary Rosalin, lived in Des Moines with Sister Charles for several years.

Sister Charles entered the Sisters of Mercy in Omaha in 1924. She received her bachelor's degree in the classics, primarily Latin, from Creighton University. At the same time, she was teacher and principal of St. Peter's School in Omaha. After finishing her master's degree in social work, Sister Charles served as administrator of St. James Orphanage from 1944 to 1963. One sister remembered Sister Charles as "always kind and caring. She visited with the children, and always knew their names." [11] In 1963, Sister Charles was elected provincial administrator for 700 sisters in the Omaha Province. Following her two-term tenure as provincial, Sister Charles was invited by Sister Gervase to come to Des Moines as head of the social services department on May 14, 1971. She remained in this position until her retirement on January 13, 1978. "I was so happy at Mercy Hospital. The spirit is marvelous, compassionate, and kind." [12]

Sister Charles filled her retirement years as a member of various Mercy boards and as a gracious Sister of Mercy. She died peacefully at Mercy on September 16, 1990.

The Thread Becomes The Fabric

For every year of Mercy's history, more than one and one-half Sisters of Mercy opened their comforting arms to the people of Des Moines. Each of them stayed an average of ten years. The acts of unselfish giving these women have bestowed on the community of Des Moines in the last century from their house of healing on the sun-kissed hill are inextricable threads woven into the healthcare fabric of Des Moines and southwestern Iowa.

During the 1970s, four Sisters of Mercy came to give their comforting ministry to Mercy Des Moines, and they remained for more than ten years. They were: Sisters Mary Kilian Clinton, Charles Keane, Josephine Collins, and Francene Summers.

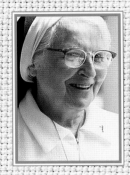

Sister Mary Josephine Collins

Another sister who came with the "famous fifteen" in 1928, was Briget Collins, born to a family of four on the Emerald Isle in County Cork. Briget entered the Sisters of Mercy in Council Bluffs, where she received the name Sister Mary Josephine. She graduated from nurse's training in Council Bluffs, with additional studies at Creighton and Catholic University. She worked at St. Bernard's Hospital until 1960 and was reassigned as pediatric supervisor at Mercy in Nampa, Idaho, from 1960 to 1965. Sister Josephine was twice administrator at St. Vincent's in Omaha and once at St. Catherine's in North Bend, Oregon. The early 1970s found her in Denver, and in 1975, Sister Josephine came to Mercy Des Moines.

There she worked in pastoral care and public relations as a patient visitor. Although she is retired, it is a rare day when Sister Josephine misses her rounds that begin in the chapel.

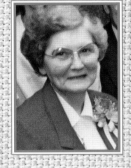

Sister Mary Francene Summers

In 1975, Sister Mary Francene Summers, a native of the "Show-Me-State," made her home at Mercy in Des Moines. This rosy-cheeked Sister of Mercy with a soft Missouri accent grew up on a farm near Shackelford, Missouri, with four older brothers. Her family formed close associations with the Sisters of Mercy who taught the Summers children in nearby Marshall, Missouri.

Catherine Summers entered the Sisters of Mercy in 1938, and after receiving her teaching degree from the College of St. Mary, she taught in Omaha and then became elementary school principal in the Kansas City area. During the 1960s, Sister Francene was appointed mistress of postulants at the Omaha provincial house. She returned to teaching as principal in Independence, Missouri, and as a teacher again in Kansas City. In 1972, Sister Francene began a new ministry in pastoral care at Mercy Hospital in Denver. She came to Des Moines with Sister Josephine in 1975 to join Mercy's pastoral care team.

Sister Francene extended her comforting service to Mercy in many ways. She made daily visits to cancer victims and their families for almost five years of her Des Moines service. Sister Francene retired to the Kansas City area in 1990.

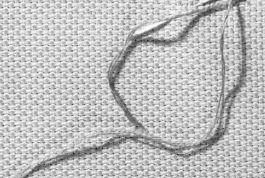

In the fall of 1973, Sister Gervase reinstated the policy of general information meetings in order to create a climate for questions and answers for Mercy's staff. Mercy continued its longstanding tradition during the 1970s of honoring and rewarding its employees for a "job well-done." In May 1970, a special employee appreciation dinner was served to 985 employees in the "Sisters Park" on the north side of the convent. Nearly 100 percent of the Mercy workforce attended the party.

Later that same month, the Sisters of Mercy recognized their long-time employees at the annual employee recognition celebration. Sister Gervase welcomed all with these words:

"This occasion points out dramatically that Mercy's employees, all of us, are a cohesive force and truly a 'family'....A dialogue of individuals who have been challenged by change, and have adequately met the challenge as a 'team.' " [13]

In the fall of 1973, Sister Gervase, *left*, reinstated general information meetings. Long-time employees, Mildred Walker and Nathan Betensky, shown, *bottom left*, with Sister Gervase, were honored along with others at a May 1970 employee recognition dinner, below. 🙿 Mercy's first whole-body scanner, EMI CT 5005, *bottom right*, became operational in January 1977.

Annual employee picnic celebrations continued at Riverview Park through the coordinated efforts of the Employee Recreation Committee. Beginning in the late 1970s, with the closing of Riverview, Mercy's annual picnic found a new home at Adventureland Park in Altoona, a tradition which continues in the 1990s.

In Loving Memory

Sister Gervase had been part of a team to acquire the first "whole-body" scanner or general computerized axial tomographic unit (CT). She, John Naughton, Dr. Irving, and radiology coordinator Don Kellen flew to Mayo Clinic in the winter of 1976 to see the CT in operation. Mercy requested permission and was approved by HPC to use the CT at the same time as Iowa Lutheran and Iowa Methodist.[14] "The entire Borough of Brooklyn had only one [scanner], and here Des Moines was going to have three. They [said] that all [three hospitals] had to start business the same day."[15]

Parts of Mercy's first scanner began arriving in November 1976, and the new CT—called the EMI CT 5005 whole body scanner— became operational in January 1977, two months before Sister Gervase's death.

As a touching show of love and support for their administrator's illness, Mercy's Maintenance Department spearheaded a campaign to collect money for the purchase of a whole body-scanner. A special fund was set up through the Mercy Foundation to help buy the scanner which was very close "to Sister's heart."[16]

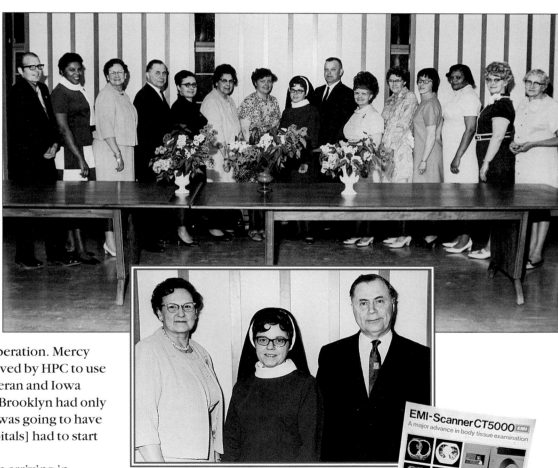

EMI-Scanner CT5000 EMI
A major advance in body tissue examination

THE SCHOOL OF NURSING IN THE 1970s

Sister Mary Gervase became Mercy's administrator in the summer of 1969. Mrs. Patricia Meintel succeeded her as school director. Mrs. Meintel had been an instructor, director of student welfare, and counselor in the school since 1961. She stayed at Mercy until August 1977. Mrs. Meintel remembered:

"In the fall of 1960, our family had just moved to Des Moines, and I was invited to attend a board meeting of the Guild. There I met Sister Mary Rosine, one of the sisters associated with the school of nursing. Sister Patricia Clare was director [of] the school at that time, and she and Sister Rosine took me to meet Sister Mary Zita. I had a cup of tea, and I was recruited." [17]

When Patricia Meintel became director of the school of nursing, there were 118 students enrolled. Mercy developed a six-week program in nursing skills, which prepared students to function immediately in Mercy's clinical areas as nursing aides.

The need for more nurses was urgent. For the first time, the school adopted open housing. Students could live at home or in unsupervised off-campus housing. More and more, non-traditional students became members of Mercy's student body.

Mercy's school began experimenting with learning packages specifically designed and tailored for each course by the instructor.[18] In 1969, the school received a grant of more than $8,000 from the Department of Health, Education and Welfare (HEW) to help with student loans and scholarships. Mercy continued to excel in its Continuing Education Unit program by becoming the first of three facilities in Iowa to win unconditional approval for its new CEU program for nurses.

The largest class in history enrolled in 1977. Seventy-five new students brought the total enrollment to 194. Seven men were included in this number, and 65 percent of the student body lived off campus.

Suzanne Mains, a graduate of Mercy's class of 1964, accepted the director's position in 1978. At that time, Mercy's total student body population topped 180 members, ranging in age from 18 to 58. In 1979, Mercy graduated its largest class ever when 69 students received their diplomas, and the number of Mercy graduates passed the 2,000 mark.

By the late 1970s, Mercy's educational program achieved a proud record when the school showed a low attrition rate and a high success rate on state board exams.

Patricia Meintel, *above*, became director of the school of nursing in 1969. Suzanne Mains, *below right*, became director in 1978. ❧ Mercy's School of Nursing, *below*, was torn down in 1979 to provide a new main entrance to the hospital.

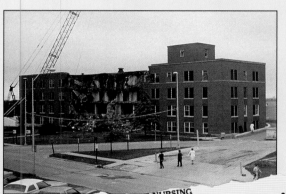

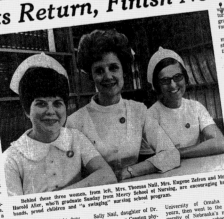

AT MERCY SCHOOL OF NURSING

Des Moines Tribune **Page** Fri., May 29, 1970

Dropouts Return, Finish Near Top

By Lillian McLaughlin

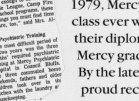

QUEST FOR THE BEST IN EDUCATION

In 1969, for the first time in Mercy's 77-year history, students of Des Moines College of Osteopathic Medicine and Surgery were allowed to study at Mercy. Mercy's Medical Staff voted to invite osteopathic students to Saturday morning conferences. By March 1970, Mercy's Board of Directors approved Mercy's acceptance of osteopathic students for extern and intern training. Clinical clerks began at Mercy in September 1970.

In the summer of 1976, Mercy became the first Iowa hospital to win accreditation for its continuing medical education program under a new, joint accreditation program of the American Medical Association and the Iowa Medical Society. The health education department was established in May 1978. This department began the Mercy Education Television on closed-circuit Channel Two.

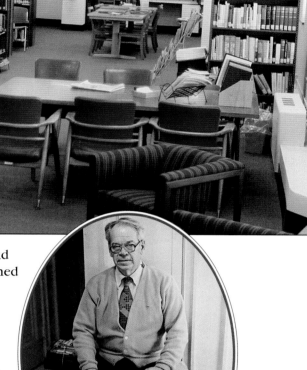

The library was moved several times during the 1960s and 1970s. In 1976, the Medical Library and the school of nursing libraries were combined and located on the second floor of the new towers. After a move to West Five in 1979, the library was renamed The Levitt Learning Resource Library in honor of Ellis Levitt, long-time supporter of Mercy's libraries .

A BEACON FOR HEALING

One month after Sister Gervase's death, Sister Mary Kieran Harney, chairman of Mercy's Board of Directors, announced the unanimous election of Sister Patricia Clare Sullivan to the position of Mercy's administrator. "We have every confidence that Sister Patricia Clare will do an outstanding job as successor to our late, beloved Sister Mary Gervase. Sister Patricia Clare brings a calm, deliberate spirit, an excellent education, and background experience to the task." [19]

Sister Patricia Clare took the mantle of leadership from Sister Gervase and positioned Mercy for the future. The hospital's familiar skyline and internal structure had changed completely during the 1970s. Now, towers gleamed above Des Moines as a beacon for healing. New procedures and technology expanded Mercy's care, and the number of Mercy employees had doubled.

Socioeconomic, political, and financial considerations affected Mercy during this era, but the hospital's Catholic mission to promote life and wholeness remained unchanged. New technology forced issues of competition, but in spite of it all, the hospital continued to extend its comforting spirit to the community. Even greater challenges were awaiting the hospital's healthcare team in the wellness-conscious decade of the 1980s.

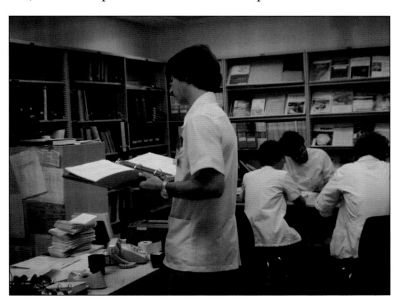

In 1976, the medical and school of nursing libraries were combined. After a move to West Five in 1979, the library, *top,* was renamed the Levitt Learning Resource Library. Dr. Daniel Crowley Jr., *above,* donated medical books to augment the library's collection. ◦ A group of pharmacy students, *left,* find time to study in 1973.

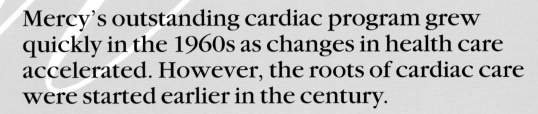

CHAPTER TWO
MERCY: LEADERS IN CARDIAC CARE

Mercy's outstanding cardiac program grew quickly in the 1960s as changes in health care accelerated. However, the roots of cardiac care were started earlier in the century.

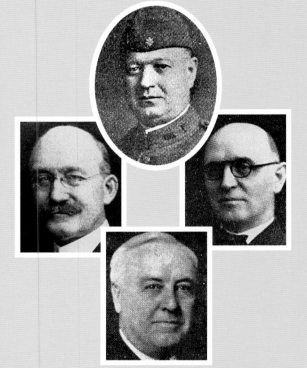

In 1905, a coal miner was brought from the edge of death by a heroic, pioneer Mercy surgeon. An argument between two employees of the Marquisville Coal Mine resulted in one miner being brought to Mercy for treatment. First reports said that the wound was fatal. While the surgeon packed the chest with gauze, the patient's heart stopped beating. Dr. W.S. Conkling, reached into the man's chest cavity and massaged the heart between his fingers. The heart resumed beating, and the patient recovered. The *New York State Medical Journal* printed an account of the incident in 1905.[1]

EARLY PREVENTION
The American Heart Association, known then as the Prevention and Relief of Heart Disease Committee, began in New York in 1915. The committee started as an outgrowth of concern for workers who could not keep up with their regular work because of diseased hearts. Committees in five other cities soon followed this lead. In 1924, Drs. Walter Bierring, J.H. Peck, John Russell, A.C. Page, and Merrill Myers formed the first committee "to benefit the whole community".[2]

Within 10 years, electrocardiograms were performed at Mercy by Dr. Bierring and Sister Joseph. The early monitoring device was very primitive, but it offered physicians the promise of better diagnosis for heart disease. When Mercy initiated the use of electrocardiograms, the response was favorable. Minutes of a medical staff meeting said:

> *"Anyone sending a patient in for this particular service will receive an official interpretation, or, if the doctor desires, the tracings will be sent to him. The total charge is five-dollars."*[3]

FOCUS ON HEART DISEASE
Dr. James Chambers served a one-year internship at Mercy in 1939 before leaving for military service. He returned to Des Moines to open a practice with Dr. Harry Collins. Dr. Chambers recalled:

> *"...the heart was inaccessible [during the 1940s] to any means of treatment other than Digitalis and maybe diuretics....Around the early 50s, I was on the committee who decided to have a cardiac care unit on the third floor of the Central Wing."*[4]

Discussion regarding patients with heart programs became a regular feature of the clinical portion of medical staff meetings in the early 1950s. Dr. Chambers was a regular lecturer for these discussions.

Shortly after the end of World War II, national attention focused on heart disease as the "silent killer." President Dwight Eisenhower's much-publicized recovery from a heart attack drew everyone's attention to the problems associated with heart disease.

The cardiac limelight focused on Mercy again due to the skillful and quick response of one of its physicians, Dr. Austin Schill. He was called back to the delivery area one day because a new mother's heart had stopped. Without waiting to put on a surgical gown, mask, or gloves, Dr. Schill immediately cut a five-inch incision in the woman's left side and massaged her heart until it began to function normally. The patient revived and was able to take her new son home ten days later.

Mercy was chosen as the site of a special research program sponsored by the Iowa Heart Association in 1957. A junior medical student from Iowa City studied lipid and cholesterol levels in some of Mercy's staff and patients known to have arteriosclerotic heart disease. Funds to continue this study were awarded again in 1958.

A Continuing Fight

In 1961, the electrocardiograph testing area was relocated to a room in the West Wing, close to the Central Wing. After the sisters moved into their new convent, part of the fifth floor of the Central Wing was remodeled for an area known as "special services." This was the beginning of the technical services department, offering inhalation therapy, electrocardiograms (EKG), and electroencephalograms (EEG).

Mercy continued to stay on top of the rapid changes occurring in cardiac care. In 1962, the hospital devoted part of a session to heart disease at its annual Mercy Hospital Medical Day.

During the mid-1960s, doctors became more aware that quick response to heart attacks increased patients' chances for survival. Dr. Paul From was in charge of a training program in cardiac resuscitation, using external cardiac massage. An outgrowth of this program was the monthly, noon-time educational session sponsored by the Major Diseases Committee of the medical staff. A better trained and educated staff led to the implementation of a new life-saving program known as Operation 77—a cardiac resuscitation emergency team on 24-hour call.

Under Dr. From's guidance, Mercy opened a new Cardio-Vascular-Pulmonary Diagnostic and Research Facility late in 1964. Dr. From, as president of the Polk County Division of the Iowa Heart Association, recognized the importance of this type of unit at Mercy. Startling statistics revealed that coronary disease was the greatest cause of deaths in men from the ages of 40 to 65. Chronic lung diseases were the second highest cause of disability in the United States. Development of similar diagnostic units throughout the country effected a recognizable 7.5 percent decrease in cardiovascular deaths during the previous 10 years.

A donation from Mercy's Guild defrayed initial expenses of $10,000 for the new unit. Mercy was the first hospital in Iowa to use a whole-body plethysmograph to measure resistance of air going through the bronchial tubes.

In addition to studying the lung and veins in the new unit, Dr. From and other staff members planned to perform circulation time studies of blood vessels by using radioisotopes. Their hopes and plans for beginning cardiac

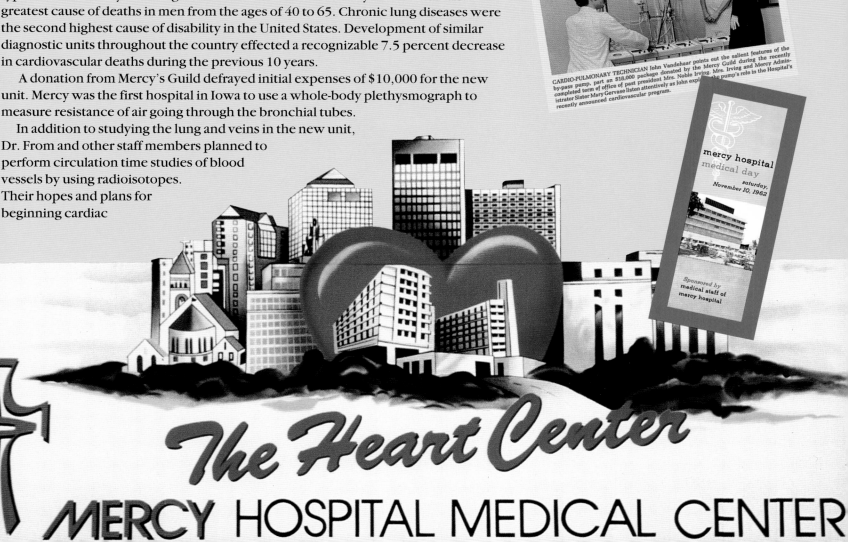

DOCTOR'S STORY
When Heart Stopped!
By Ronald Hart

Dr. Austin E. Schill (left) checks the x-ray as Timothy Aldi and his parents, Mr. and Mrs. Ro...

CARDIO-PULMONARY TECHNICIAN John Vandehaar points out the salient features of the recently by-pass pump, part an $18,000 package donated by the Mercy Guild during the recently completed term of office of past president Mrs. Noble Irving. Mrs. Irving and Mercy Administrator Sister Mary Gervase listen attentively as John explains the pump's role in the Hospital's recently announced cardiovascular program.

Mercy Guild Gives Heart Pump

mercy hospital
medical day
saturday,
November 10, 1962

Sponsored by
medical staff of
mercy hospital

The Heart Center
MERCY HOSPITAL MEDICAL CENTER

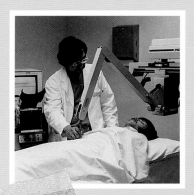

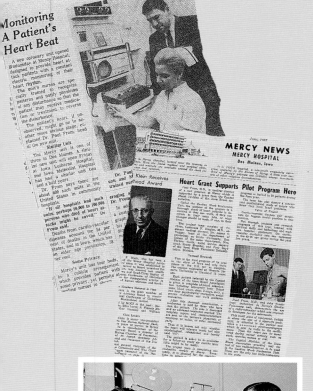

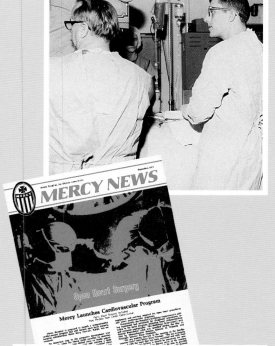

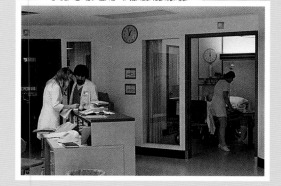

catheterization were far-sighted, and Mercy's first catheterization was performed within four years.

Before Mercy began performing catheterizations, new technology, utilizing sound waves, debuted in the radiology department, ultimately benefiting the hospital's cardiac care. Echocardiograms detected fluid surrounding the heart. Physicians were pleased with the relative ease with which this test could be administered and the five-minute turn-around-time on the test results.

Specialized cardiac monitoring devices came into use at Mercy during 1966. Continuous visual and auditory monitoring devices were installed to observe heart action on patients during and after surgery. Common usage of bedside monitoring devices led to the establishment of a special coronary care unit in late 1967.

This four-bed unit was equipped with $13,000 worth of sophisticated monitoring devices. It was designed with patient cubicles in full view of the nursing staff. Oscilloscopes were located at patients' bedsides, as well as at the nursing center, with patient status constantly displayed. A 30-hour lecture course was designed to train prospective coronary care nurses.

Mercy received a grant from the Capitol Heart Division of the Iowa Heart Association in 1967 to study heart disease patients and their ability to continue working when modifications were made in their lifestyles. Mercy was fortunate to inaugurate this program in Iowa, and to have one of only three of its kind in the United States. The program was patterned after an earlier study at Western Reserve University in Cleveland. Each patient received a physical examination, a two-hour psychological evaluation, social service evaluation, and work guidance evaluation. Each member of the team evaluated the patient and made recommendations to the patient's physician. Patients returned six months later for further evaluation. The October 1967 issue of *Hospital Progress* magazine highlighted Mercy's program. [5]

Cardiac Care Provider

In 1969, Mercy began performing angiograms. Drs. David Gordon and Noble Irving combined talents to conduct both right and left heart catheterizations. Specialized angiographic equipment with a price tag of $150,000 allowed physicians to diagnose cardiac defects and gave a tremendous boost to Mercy's cardiac program as the new decade dawned. When the 1970s began, the Health Policy Council appointed Mercy as the sole cardiac care provider for all Des Moines hospitals, and the hospital's cardiac program grew dramatically.

Mercy prepared to meet the challenges of the 1970s by announcing a comprehensive cardiovascular program in 1971. Sister Gervase outlined the new plan, which included open heart surgery. Mercy had been recruiting and training physicians, technicians, and other support personnel for several months. A cardiac surgery team under the leadership of Drs. Alexander Matthews and Joseph Torruella were preparing to meet the increased demand for cardiac care at Mercy.

Mercy's first coronary bypass was performed in August 1971. The young male patient entered the hospital complaining of chest pain. Coronary angiography discovered blockage in one of the main coronary arteries. Dr. Joseph Torruella performed a single bypass, and the patient recuperated in the hospital for 13 days.

In conjunction with the expanded cardiac service, Mercy inaugurated the initial stages of the tower expansion known as Phase X (ten), a ten-bed unit for specialized cardiac care finished in June 1972. The unit was located on top of the boiler addition—the three-floor structure located between the west end of the towers and the West Wing. The area currently contains part of the emergency department's treatment rooms and part of radiology.

The latest monitoring devices were incorporated into the new unit, and all four private, post-surgical beds could be watched from one nursing console. Another similar unit allowed nurses at one console to monitor the progress of up to six additional coronary care patients.

A program specifically designed to help hospitalized heart patients mainstream back into their normal activities began in April 1972. Called Operation Shape-Up, the

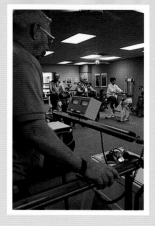

program provided patients with 14 steps of graduated exercises, education, and craft activities, ordered by their physicians. Patients began with passive exercises while still recuperating in bed and worked toward walking up and down ten flights of stairs.

A NEW CATHETERIZATION LABORATORY

By 1975, Mercy had performed more than 576 coronary angiograms, 161 cardiac catheterizations and 243 open heart surgeries. The rapid growth of Mercy's cardiac care program ensured approval for a new cardiac catheterization laboratory. Previously, all procedures were performed in the radiology department. Tentative cost for the equipment was $240,000.

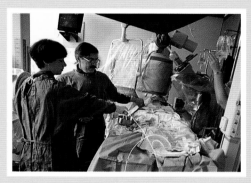

The new "cath lab" opened on the north end of West Two. The first procedure was performed on July 6, 1976. The new facility included rooms for: procedures, control, supplies, viewing and consultation; a staff office; and a four-bed recovery room. Dr. John Gay, pediatric cardiologist, was the interim director.

Mercy's cardiac program grew so rapidly that by the middle of 1976, it was ranked in the top ten percent of United States hospitals, based on numbers of procedures and quality of program. Mercy was one of three American heart teams to perform emergency open-heart procedures for the myocardial infarction patient.

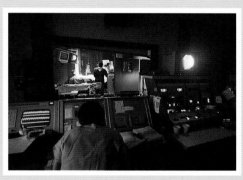

HEART DAY

Mercy's annual Heart Day began at the urging of Mercy cardiologists on April 21, 1977, in conjunction with the Iowa Heart Association and the Cardiovascular Medicine and Surgery Section of the Mercy Hospital Medical Staff. The first program was entitled "Spectacular Advances in Cardiac Surgery." One featured speaker was Dr. Adrian Kantrowitz, professor and chairman at Sinai Hospital in Detroit. In 1967, Dr. Kantrowitz performed the first United States heart transplant in New York. This operation followed three days after Dr. Christiaan Barnard performed the first transplant in the world. Mercy's Dr. Steven Phillips was a resident working with Dr. Kantrowitz at that time.

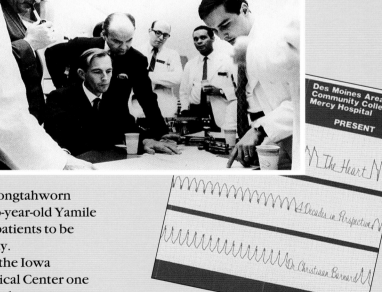

During the next year's Heart Day activities, entitled "The Heart—Four Decades in Perspective," Dr. Barnard gave two presentations on transplantation and cardiovascular surgery. Mercy continues to sponsor an annual Heart Day as a two-day program in May.

ARMS AROUND THE WORLD'S CHILDREN

Expanding their mission "to never turn away any person who needed heart surgery," the Sisters of Mercy in June 1979 began offering a program to mend the diseased hearts of the children of Yucatan. The Partners of the Americas program linked Iowa and Yucatan as "sister states." Drs. John Gay, Steven Phillips, and Cham Kongtahworn provided their unique skills at no charge to these needy patients. Two-year-old Yamile Suarez-Cuevas and 20-year-old Jorge Gongora were the first Yucatan patients to be given a chance for a longer life at Mercy. This program continues today.

In recognition of outstanding cardiac service to pediatric patients, the Iowa Chapter of Variety Club International designated Mercy Hospital Medical Center one of "two or three hospitals in the United States to help needy children who cannot afford heart surgery. Children from all over the world will be coming here. We feel Mercy is the finest institution in the Midwest for heart disease, and we wanted to be a part of it." [6] Sister Patricia Clare accepted $30,000, crediting the Variety Club with the foresight to choose Mercy which "will save and enrich the lives of many children." The program celebrated its 100th patient in November 1983, and eventually became known as the Mercy-Variety Club Children's Lifeline Yucatan Program. Mercy was honored for five years of charitable service to these young children in Los Angeles in 1984. Since then, the hospital has provided this tender care through Variety Club International and other philanthropic organizations to more than 375 youngsters from around the world.

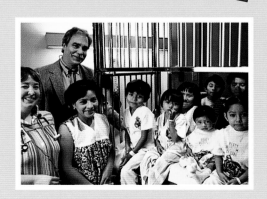

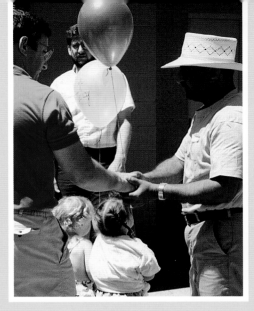

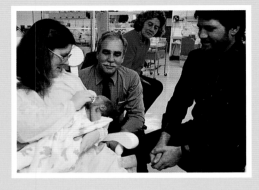

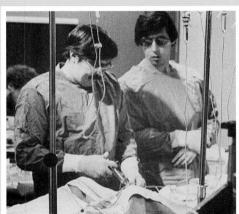

As a result of Mercy's outstanding services to Yucatan patients, the Gift of Life, Inc. and the Des Moines Rotary Club contacted Dr. John Gay about a joint program, extending heart care to children from Korea. Mercy began offering this help in the mid-1980s.

TENDER PIONEERS

Mercy's premiere cardiac capabilities were used many times to save the lives of the hospital's youngest patients. Early in 1981, Dr. Steven Phillips performed open heart surgery on an infant who was only 34-hours-old. The baby was born with a "total anomalous pulmonary venous connection below the diaphragm"— red blood routed into the abdomen instead of the left side of the heart. Using profound hypothermia and a heart-lung machine, the surgeon saved the baby's life.

In the late 1980s, a new ultrasound device (fetal echocardiography) enabled Mercy's pediatric cardiologists to monitor the heart of an unborn child. In November 1988, the life of a child was saved when ultrasound studies indicated that the child's heartbeat was too rapid. Physicians treated this condition with medications, and the baby was born normally.

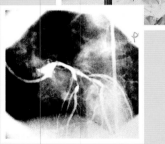 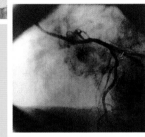

PTCA before   **PTCA after**

IOWA CARDIAC PATHMAKERS

Mercy's pacemaker program traces back to 1967. Drs. Paul From and Alex Matthews were the first to install this new cardiac regulating device. In 1982, a new "thinking" pacemaker called the "assistor" was used for the first time.[7]

Mercy made headlines on November 29, 1979, when the first percutaneous transcending angioplasty (PTA)—later called percutaneous transcending coronary angioplasty (PTCA)—was performed in Iowa by Mercy physician, Dr. Liberato Iannone. This non-surgical procedure allowed a plastic catheter equipped with a balloon to be inserted into a vein, threaded to a coronary blockage, and inflated to restore blood flow to the area. The procedure was hailed as a major healthcare cost-cutter, which also restored the patient to health more quickly than traditional cardiac surgery.

Mercy continued to pioneer in balloon-assisted cardiac procedures. In 1986, a balloon was used to open a valve of an adult patient for the first time in Iowa.[8]

Mercy's cardiac program scored another first for Iowa in January 1980, when the drug streptokinase was used on a patient who had suffered a heart attack. Mercy cardiologist, David Gordon, administered the drug, which dissolved a life-threatening clot. The patient went home without heart surgery.

HEARTS ACROSS THE SEA

In February 1983, Mercy began to establish an open-heart surgery program in Rome with Heart International. Mercy's involvement was best expressed by Sister Patricia Clare:

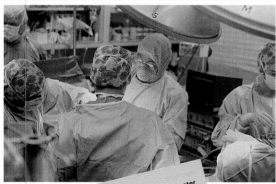

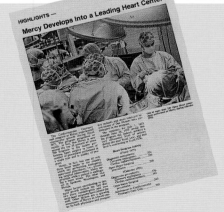

"It's exciting. Our world is becoming smaller, with more interdependence among countries. We have a tremendous resource among our staff and physicians, and we want to share that with others.[9] The goal of Rome, as far as mission, was to establish a Heart Center for educational opportunities for nurses from many third-world countries. We had places all lined up [in] Rome for training. We had already trained nurses from Trinidad, Bahamas, and Tobago. We brought nurses from

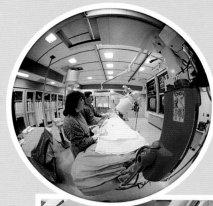

Colombia and Thailand to Rome. We had to have a hospital, modern equipment in that hospital, and permission for our physicians to work. We had the hospital. We had the equipment in the hospital. We could not obtain permission from the Italian government for our physicians to operate. So, by the summer of 1985, Sara Drobnich, the last of Mercy's staff in Rome, returned home." [10]

CATH LAB EXPANSION

Mercy's cardiac expertise expanded so quickly that the cath lab required equipment updates within a short time, and additional space was needed to facilitate these changes. The former radiology department was remodeled, new equipment ordered, and the cardiac care department moved from West Two to West One. Mr. and Mrs. Frank De Puydt donated money for a specialized procedure facility. It was reported that Mercy was the first in the world to use biplane equipment in the cath lab. [11]

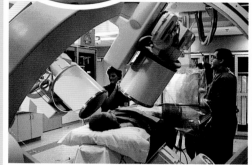

Mercy opened a Progressive Cardiac Recovery (PCR) unit for patients recovering from non-surgical cardiac procedures, located on Main Three. By May 1984, the new PCR unit recovered its 1,000th patient.

CARDIAC TRANSPLANTATION

By early 1985, Mercy's cardiac surgical team was ready to begin transplant surgeries, and on July 6, Paul Sarnecki became Mercy's first cardiac transplant patient and the second in the state of Iowa. Sarnecki proved to be a perfect candidate for Mercy, although he had been rejected by other transplant teams. His surgery was performed in three-and-one-half hours, and he returned home after 13 days. Mr. Sarnecki continues in good health in 1993 and is an active participant in organ donor awareness programs.

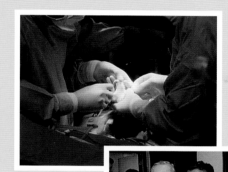

Three additional cardiac transplants were performed in November and December of the same year. Mercy's cardiac program continued to expand during the ensuing years. By early January 1993, sixty-four heart transplants had been performed. Forty-seven of these patients were men; eleven were women; four were children; and two were newborns.

JARVIK-7 ARTIFICIAL HEART

Mercy's cardiac teams took another giant leap when they initiated training on the Jarvik-7 artificial heart. The surgical team expected to use this device as a temporary life-sustaining bridge until donor hearts became available. Five members of Mercy's medical staff underwent training in Salt Lake City: Drs. Steven Phillips, Robert Zeff, Cham Kongtahworn, James Skinner and Richard Toon.

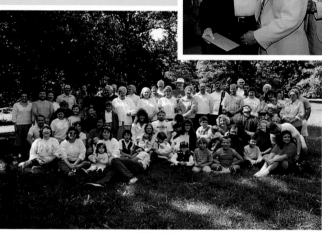

Mercy prepared for the eventual use of this machine by enlarging one room in the Cardiac Surgical Intensive Care Unit (CSICU) to hold the large "Utahdrive" needed to power the artificial heart. Final approval for Mercy to use the Jarvik came shortly before the pump was installed in a 40-year-old patient, Jack Green, on May 28, 1987. Mr. Green survived on the pump for 15 hours before a human heart was located. Dr. Phillips reported that the bridge "worked very well." The longest Mercy patient to survive with a Jarvik-7 was Gerald Smith who lived on the mechanical device for 81 days before receiving a human heart. Mercy used the Jarvik-7 for three years before it was recalled by the Food and Drug Administration (FDA), not for failure, but for procedures used by the manufacturer. [12]

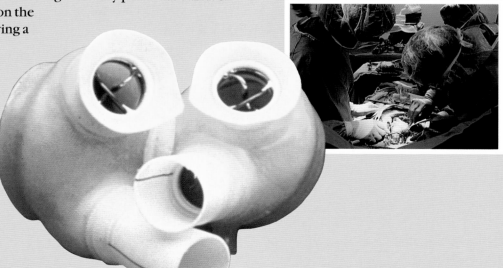

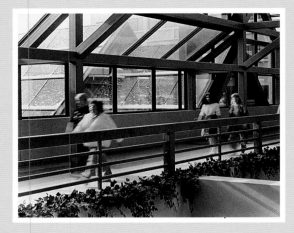

OTHER CARDIAC ASSIST DEVICES

Mercy used other creative ways to bridge the lives of their cardiac patients awaiting transplants. In May 1988, Mercy surgeons received permission from the FDA to use the Nimbus hemopump. Mercy was one of the first in the country to use this device. Surgeons used donor hearts in a "piggyback" procedure to assist patients whose hearts were weakened but still functioning. The first of these procedures was performed in January 1987. The donor heart was smaller than the original heart, so surgeons decided to leave the patient's heart in place and use it to boost the capacity of the transplanted heart. Mercy surgeons were the first in Iowa to perform this operation, and the patient still survives in 1993.

CARDIAC RISK PROGRAM

The Cardiac Risk Identification and Modification Program began in early February 1985. This program provided a comprehensive analysis of a person's physical condition, lifestyle, and nutritional habits and how those elements affected the heart.

In 1988, several Mercy cardiac rehabilitation programs moved from the hospital to the ground level of the Atrium. Cardiac prevention, cardiac rehabilitation, pulmonary rehabilitation, and health-assessment screens were based in the new facility. Cardiac Phase I continued on an inpatient referral within the hospital. In conjunction with the new rehabilitation programs, a circular walking track on the second floor of the Heart Center (Atrium) opened in June 1988.

Cordis 233D Pacemaker

KEEPING PACE

Mercy's Cardiac Surgical Intensive Care Unit and Catheterization Laboratory received much-needed updates during the late 1980s, to keep up with fast-paced changes in their services.

An expanded, 14-bed surgical unit, devoted solely to the care of the post-cardiac surgical patient, opened late in 1988. Within the new facility, Mercy's cardiac SICU nurses and staff were able to care for twice as many patients. Special bonding united patients and the CSICU staff:

> *"There's a strong bond between us because we work together in so many crisis situations. Heart patients can be anyone from infants to 85-year-olds. We're constantly evaluating how the patient is doing and giving physicians their status minute-by-minute. We give very intensive care."* [13]

In late 1988, Mercy's cath lab relocated above the MRI suite on Mercy's south side, between the hospital and the Atrium-Medical Office complex. The cath lab contained four procedure rooms. The new laboratory soon averaged more than 330 procedures each month.

Mercy's cath lab, as the busiest in Iowa, faced the need for further expansion in 1991. A new holding, waiting, and recovery area opened on the third floor of the old West and South Wings.

FIRST IN THE 1990S

Mercy led the way to being Iowa's first to perform directional coronary artherectomy; to install a combination pacemaker/defibrillator; and to perform radio frequency catheter ablation.

Nearly eleven years after performing the first Iowa balloon procedure, Dr. L. Iannone made Iowa medical history again by performing a similar procedure to clear a clogged coronary artery (directional coronary arthrectomy). Using a catheter equipped with a small rotary cutting tool, Dr. Iannone shaved through a blocked artery. This procedure removed the clogging material, whereas, the older procedure pushed the clogging material to the sides of the artery, with the possibility that the artery could reclose.

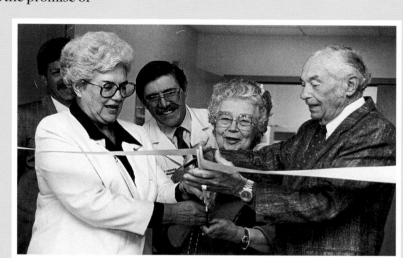

A combination pacemaker/defibrillator was used for the first time in Iowa history, when Mercy surgeons installed it in a patient in 1990. This unique device monitored the patient's heartbeat. If the heartbeat became too rapid, the defibrillator shocked the heart, slowing the beat down so the pacemaker kept the heart at a regular rate. In December 1990, another method of correcting an irregular heartbeat was used at Mercy for the first time in Iowa. Radio frequency catheter ablation directed radio waves, by means of a catheter, toward the part of the heart muscle that was misconducting. The radio signals destroyed the part of the muscle that changed the heart's electrical circuitry. Mercy's physicians felt this method held the promise of success because it cut down length of stay, and it cost 75 percent less than surgery. In 1991, sixty of these procedures were performed in Mercy's cath lab, with more than 600 electrophysiology studies performed during the year.

Mercy expanded this service by opening the John R. Grubb Procedure Room late in May 1992. Electrophysiology studies, including the radio frequency ablations which often take up to 12 hours, were performed in this new area. Other uses included heart biopsies and permanent pacemaker procedures.

PEDIATRIC INTENSIVE CARE UNIT

A new eight-bed Pediatric Intensive Care Unit, provided in part by the Variety Club International, enabled Mercy to step up to a higher level of critical care for children in the 1990s. According to Dr. John Gay, pediatric cardiologist: "This is the only pediatric intensive care unit in Des Moines and one of only two in the state that is equipped to provide cardiac care for children."

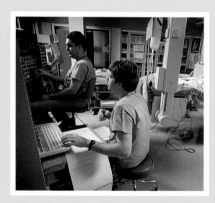

A SECOND MIRACLE

In 1991, one of the greatest feelings of success and fullfillment settled on the cardiac team, and all of Mercy, when one of its earlier stars, a cardiac transplant patient, successfully gave birth to her first child. Believed to be only the second or third cardiac transplant in America to give birth, Barbara Ostercamp delivered a healthy boy after a normal pregnancy. The event was billed as "a second miracle" for Barb. Her first miracle took place in September 1988, when she received a new heart. Barb continued to fight the potential of cardiac rejection with potent drugs. The second miracle took place in February 1991 when Scott Thomas Ostercamp was born. Barb's cardiologist through most of her life, Dr. B. Chandramouli, said: "I never expected her to survive, let alone have her own baby." Barb Ostercamp had a second son in August 1992.

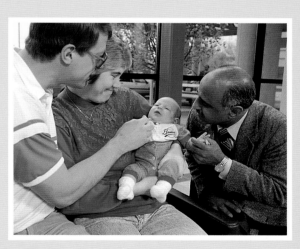

A BRIGHTER VIEW

Mercy was predestined to be a first-class cardiac caregiver from its earliest beginnings. Time and time again, Mercy's team is the creative and courageous innovator of the best cardiac care-ministry in Iowa. The hospital's patients can be assured that they will find no better place to mend an ailing heart.

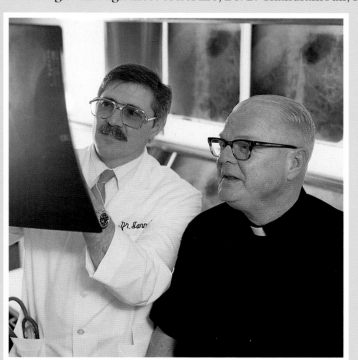

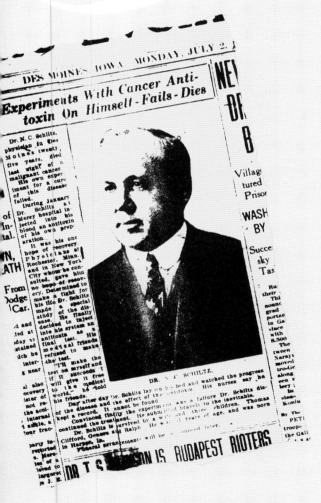

CHAPTER THREE
COMFORTING ARMS: CANCER CARE

Mercy's involvement in cancer care began in 1917 when Mercy physician N.C. Schiltz experimentally treated his own cancer in hopes of finding a cure. By 1922, Mercy physicians were treating cancerous tumors with radium.

In 1953, Mercy became the first hospital in Des Moines and the second in the state to begin using radioactive scanning. Radioactive isotopes of different sizes were injected or ingested by cancer patients and a photographic image was produced by a scanning device. Equipment in Mercy's isotope laboratory enabled physicians to isolate tumors in the brain, thyroid, liver, kidney, and occasionally in the bone.

Mercy's cancer research program actively began in the mid-1950s. The first cancer to be studied was breast cancer, and a joint effort for this purpose was established between Mercy and Nebraska Methodist Hospital. The partnership was funded by grants from the Iowa Division of the American Cancer Society, Drake University, the respective pathology departments of the two researching hospitals, and through personal contributions made by Drs. Coleman and Schenken. Research focused on two distinct problems with breast cancer. Pathologists studied the traditional method of obtaining cross-sections to see if it was effective enough to sight early stages of the disease. Then, they examined antibodies produced by rabbits that had been injected with breast cancer cells. Researchers hoped to find a better understanding of the antigen-antibody reaction of breast cancer.[1]

In 1956, a second grant of $5,500 from the Iowa Division of the American Cancer Society was awarded to Mercy and Drake University. This funding was given for research of the cytochemical relations in normal as well as cancerous cells.[2]

In the March 1957 issue of the *Journal of the American Medical Association*, Mercy physicians, Drs. Coleman, Irving, and Richards, published an article about the cure of a patient suffering from a giant-cell tumor of the bone, involving the fifth lumbar vertebra. These and other pioneering research efforts led Mercy Hospital toward becoming a first-class radioisotope imaging facility. Mercy began offering annual seminars to radiology personnel in order to educate technicians in the proper use of radioactive substances and specialized equipment. A Mercy radiology technician, Don Kellen, became one of the first registered nuclear medical technicians in Iowa.[3]

LABORATORY AND SCIENTIFIC ADVANCEMENT

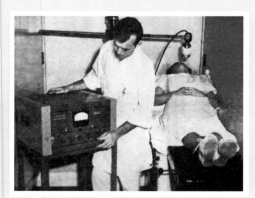

Mercy's first tumor registrar, Mary Jean Worthington, started in February 1963, and tumor registry became an important tool in the laboratory. Follow-up studies were done on all cases of cancer diagnosed at Mercy. By 1964, more than 1,000 active cases were being tracked by this registry. From January 1, 1973 through the end of 1991, Mercy's Cancer Registry entered more than 13,600 patients. More than 3,000 of these patients are currently followed. In 1965, Dr. Frank Coleman resigned after nearly 20 years of service, and Dr. Joseph Song became Mercy's chief pathologist. During this time, Mercy received a research grant from the American Cancer Society for more than $6,500 to study "Circulating Cancer Cells in Carcinoma in Situ of Uterine Cervix."[4] In 1968, Mercy's Pathology Department began receiving an annual clinical fellowship awarded by the American Cancer Society. The society gave an annual stipend of $4,800 to sponsor a student for one year.

Mercy first began using ultrasound devices in 1966. Pioneering a new technique called echoencephalography, Mercy's radiology experts used ultrasound equipment to examine intracranial abnormalities, pericardial effusions, and fetal head measurements. Mercy's Medical Staff began performing needle biopsies late in 1969. This procedure involved the extraction of tissue through a needle for microscopic examination. At the same time, Mercy began offering monthly in-hospital cancer clinics for medical staff members throughout Iowa. The latest developments in the diagnosis and treatment of cancer were presented.

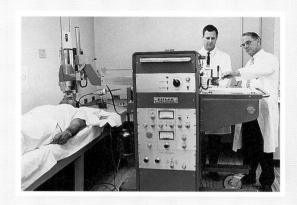

CHEMOTHERAPY

The year 1972 was a benchmark for Mercy's cancer program. During this year, the hospital began an experimental chemotherapy program, making it the first healthcare agency in Iowa to become involved in chemotherapy and research. A special cancer research laboratory was built to accommodate information generated as a result of this program. A new foundation, the Mercy Cancer Research Foundation, was formed to secure research grants and other funding from the United States Government and the American Cancer Society, as well as private organizations and individuals. Soon, Mercy was able to treat gastro-intestinal and ovarian cancers, testicular tumors, osteogenic sarcoma, brain tumors, and lung cancer with these chemicals.[5]

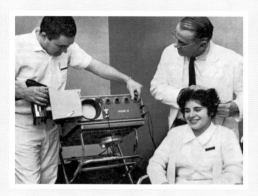

When the hospital began its early efforts to administer chemotherapy, patients were referred by family physicians. Much of the blood work and patient contact was performed by Mercy's pathology residents. One young resident felt the experience deeply:

> "Normally, in a pathology residency, there is minimal patient contact, if any at all. It was impressive for Mercy to get this program going in Central Iowa. I would have patients come to me in tears, because someone felt they couldn't help them and turned them away. Some of those people felt so cut off. The experience changed my life."[6]

In 1974, Mercy received recognition as one of only two Des Moines hospitals to have its cancer program approved by the American College of Surgeons (ACS). Veterans Hospital was the other.[7]

A PLACE OF HOPE AND LOVE

By 1975, Mercy's cancer program had tracked 5,226 active patients, necessitating the opening of a new oncology treatment center on the fifth floor of the West Wing. This new unit provided continuity of care for cancer sufferers, both inpatient and outpatient. Treatment center professionals established close, strongly supportive relationships with patients and their families. First-year statistics showed that the new 21-bed unit served 200 inpatient and

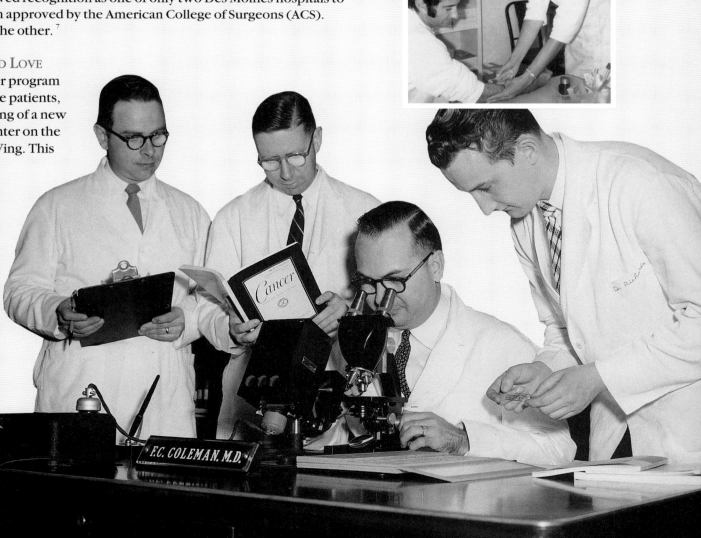

E.C. COLEMAN, M.D.

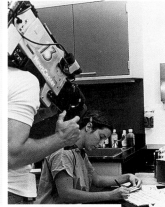

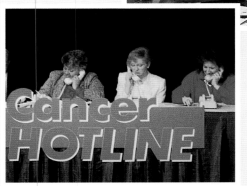

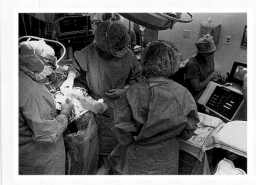

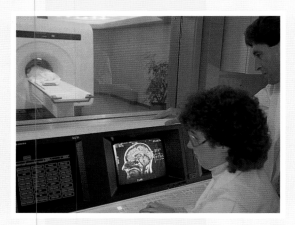

90 outpatients. A student from Des Moines Area Community College spent three days in the Oncology Unit as part of a class assignment. She recorded her experiences:

> *"I feel these three days were a true privilege and a rare experience in the human kindness of nursing. Science unlocks many doors, but hope, desire, and the love for life and family also play a major role in their struggle to live."* [8]

In 1975, Mercy received recognition as the sole institution from Iowa participating in cancer immunochemotherapy by the International Registry of Immunotherapy . In September 1978, Mercy became affiliated with the Iowa Oncology Research Association (IORA). IORA is associated with the North Central Cancer Treatment Group and the Eastern Cooperative Oncology Group. Specialists actively accessed the new discoveries or protocols from this information.

ELECTRON MICROSCOPE

In June 1980, Mercy became the first hospital in Des Moines to utilize the electron microscope. Within two years, the hospital was processing more than 450 studies annually. The specialized microscope magnified objects up to 100,000 times, allowing for a much more definitive diagnosis. Most of the studies performed by Mercy's staff pathologists were for cancer.

CANCER EDUCATION

For persons who wanted to learn more about living and coping with cancer, Mercy began offering weekly, two-hour classes in October 1981, under the guidance of the American Cancer Society.

In an effort to heighten cancer awareness through community education, Mercy began providing free home tests for colon cancer to the public in the summer of 1982. Statistics showed that 2,200 new cases of colon cancer would be detected in Iowa during that year, with a projected mortality of 950. By September, Mercy mailed more than 12,500 tests. Nearly 3,000 were returned for analysis, and two percent tested positive. Mercy continued the program in the fall of 1983, and another 23 people were diagnosed with the cancer.

Mercy finished its initial colorectal cancer screening on October 11, 1985. More than 34,000 Central Iowans requested the home tests. The hospital's microbiology department became a busy place, where more than 1,800 tests were processed in a single day. In 1985, the hospital began a 24-hour telephone hotline service within Mercy's oncology unit.

Cancer pain-management classes began at Mercy in 1985. Patients enrolled in a program that had a holistic approach to treating cancer. They were taught that exercise, relaxation techniques, imagery, counseling, and nutrition were important elements in managing pain. The pain-management staff encouraged the families of patients to attend classes as well. In September 1985, a series of eight programs were offered through the cancer registry to employees and staff to assist them in educating patients about ways to reduce the risk of cancer.

NEW PROCEDURES

Near the end of the 1970s, Mercy installed the first generation of its computerized tomography scanners (CT Scanners). This unit was made possible by the work of Sister Gervase, and after her death, by many donations given in her memory. CT scanners provided valuable assistance for visualizing tumors. By 1983, Mercy installed a new generation of scanners which would perform faster and give more detailed information. This new scanner was particularly useful for diagnosing brain tumors.

In 1982, Mercy began the delicate art of laser surgery. Mercy surgeons used a Sharplan CO_2 Laser to remove brain and spinal cord tumors. In 1985, Mercy's surgeons began using another important tool to remove tumors. This ultrasonic device, called the Cavitron Ultrasound Surgical Aspirator (CUSA), gave better

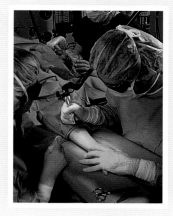

observation for the surgeon, caused less damage to healthy tissue and resulted in less blood loss.

Mercy continued to minister to its cancer patients, offering the most up-to-date equipment and trained personnel with another important tool in 1988. In the new office plaza building, a powerful radiation therapy unit called a linear accelerator was installed. Dr. James McNab, an oncologist trained in radiation therapy, painstakingly planned each patient's therapy.

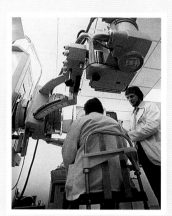

> *"The course of treatment we use is custom-designed for each patient. Radiation kills the cancer. It might also be used in conjunction with surgery, or chemotherapy. It can save lives, it can prolong lives, and it can offer those with terminal cancer a better quality of life by easing the pain many experience."* [9]

HOSPICE CARE

Mercy's mission to promote the quality of life and death prompted the hospital to open a Hospice program within Mercy. In February 1986, under the direction of the home care department, physicians, nurses, social workers, chaplains, and volunteers united in a total team effort. "We want to make the patients as comfortable as we possibly can, give them the best possible quality of life that they can have at this stage of their lives, and at the same time, provide support and help to their relatives." [10] Mercy's Social Services Department established a group to give emotional support to family members of Mercy cancer patients. During 1991 and 1992, Mercy's hospice program provided more than 3,065 days of care to terminal cancer patients.

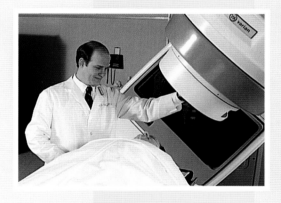

STAYING ON TOP

By 1987, Mercy was one of six Iowa hospitals providing a cancer treatment program approved by the American College of Surgeons Commission on Cancer, extending the most complete cancer care program available. Earlier diagnosis, more definitive treatment, better education, and supportive networks enable Mercy's patients to face their cancers in a more positive manner. One patient underwent a mastectomy with a year of chemotherapy and added radiation treatment: "It really hasn't been terrible," she said. "A lot worse things could have happened to me. I think there are probably a lot of people like me." [11] Mercy's comprehensive program made it possible for patients to receive the most definitive care available close to home. Dr. John Maksem became Mercy's new chief pathologist in December 1988. Dr. Maksem received his medical training at the Washington University School of Medicine in St. Louis.

Mercy's linear accelerator was the first of its kind in Central Iowa. According to Dr. James McNab, radiation oncologist, the linear accelerator provides physicians and technicians with greater capabilities to treat cancer patients. As a result, many cancer patients who formerly had limited treatment options, can now be offered an effective alternative.

HOPE FOR A CURE IN THE 1990s

At the opening of the 1990s, Mercy began adding new services to help cancer patients. Mercy Network received $750,000 in federal grant monies to fund a cancer control project among Iowa farmers. This grant was renewed in 1992.

Mercy added another new service in February 1992 with the addition of a cancer coordinator. Victoria Smith became the first Mercy coordinator who provided a single source of information to every cancer patient about programs and services. With so much information available about cancer, patients and families are struggling to deal with their illness. One Mercy oncologist reflects on prospects for cancer care:

> *"The field is continually going through evolution and change with treatment improvements and breakthroughs coming almost every month. We're finding the causes and better ways to treat the diseases all the time."* [12]

In the 1990s, Mercy continues to lead the way in bringing hope, comfort, and tender care to victims of cancer and their families. Mercy's team-centered healing constantly reaches out to support, to surround, and to give solace with ever-open comforting arms.

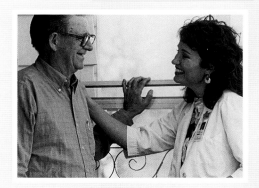

GROWTH THROUGH THE CENTURY: THE BUILDINGS

1894

On July 3, 1894 Mercy broke ground on the present campus. That first building, the East Wing, opened in a gala celebration on April 23, 1895. Tours of the new Mercy facility revealed a four-story structure that was 50 feet by 100 feet long with accommodations for 50 beds. Two hundred twenty-one patients received care during the first year of operation.

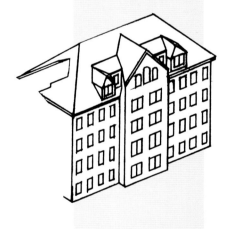

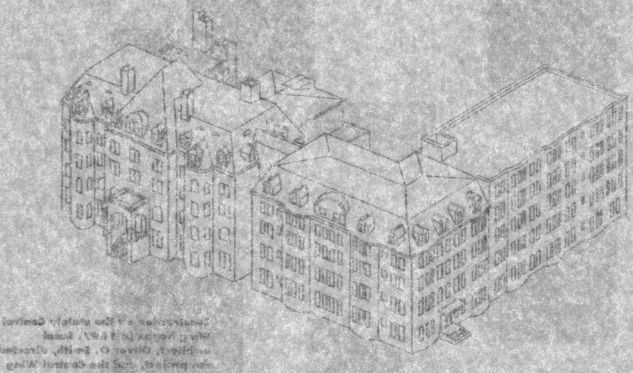

1910-1913

Mercy remodeled and added two attachments onto the back of the Central Wing during this time. A four-story addition improved the dietary areas. It was blessed by Des Moines' new bishop, Austin Dowling on December 12, 1912. A second structure also attached to the rear of the Central Wing, was called the "Red Wing." It housed rooms for surgery, laboratory, radiology, and physical therapy.

1914

An endowment from Des Moines' Polk family enabled Mercy to build the North Wing. This addition and a small part of the earlier West Wing are the only original structures still standing. The North Wing is now known as the West Wing.

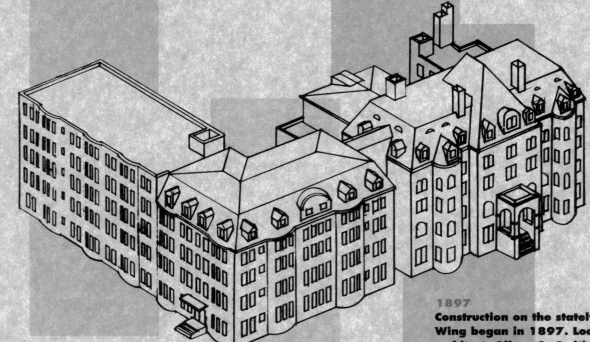

1897

Construction on the stately Central Wing began in 1897. Local architect, Oliver O. Smith, directed the project, and the Central Wing opened on November 15, 1899, providing a turret-flanked main entrance to the hospital for many years. The Central Wing cost $75,000 and created space for 150 additional patients.

1908

The third Mercy structure faced Ascension Street. The West Wing was built during the years 1907-1909. This addition increased Mercy's capacity by one-third. The West Wing cornerstone remains intact today in Mercy's Beh Auditorium.

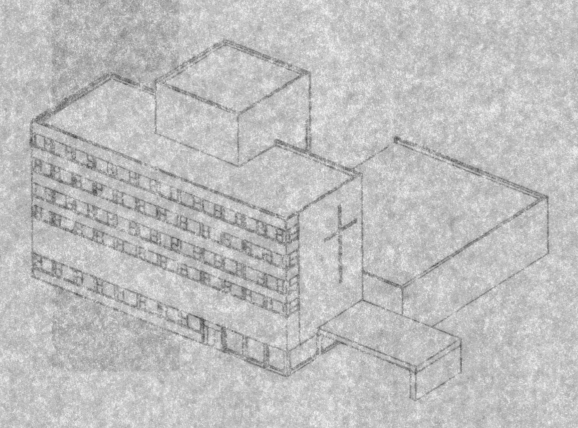

1959

Mercy opened its third front door in 1959 with the completion of the South Wing. More than 3 million dollars aided the construction of this wing and remodeling of older structures. The South Wing contained modern features of air-conditioning, a central dictation system, and a pneumatic communications network.

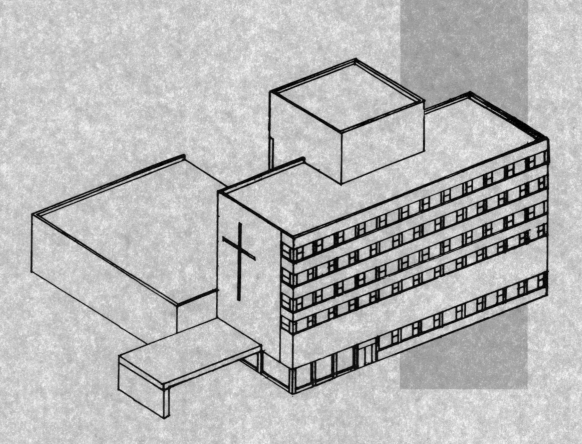

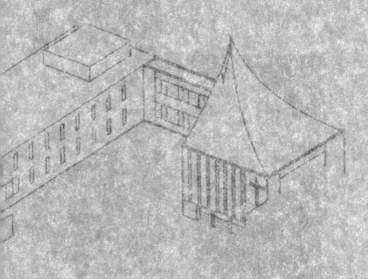

1964
After 40 years of living in drafty, far-from-private quarters, the Sisters of Mercy built a modern convent with accommodations for 20 sisters. Today, the facility is the hub of Mercy's data processing department.

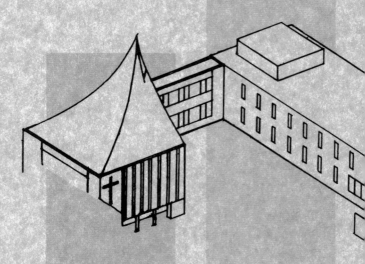

1960
The "pointy-topped chapel," as it was known, was completed in 1960. This three-story building served as Mercy's prayer center, meeting hall, and garage storage, until it was removed in 1977.

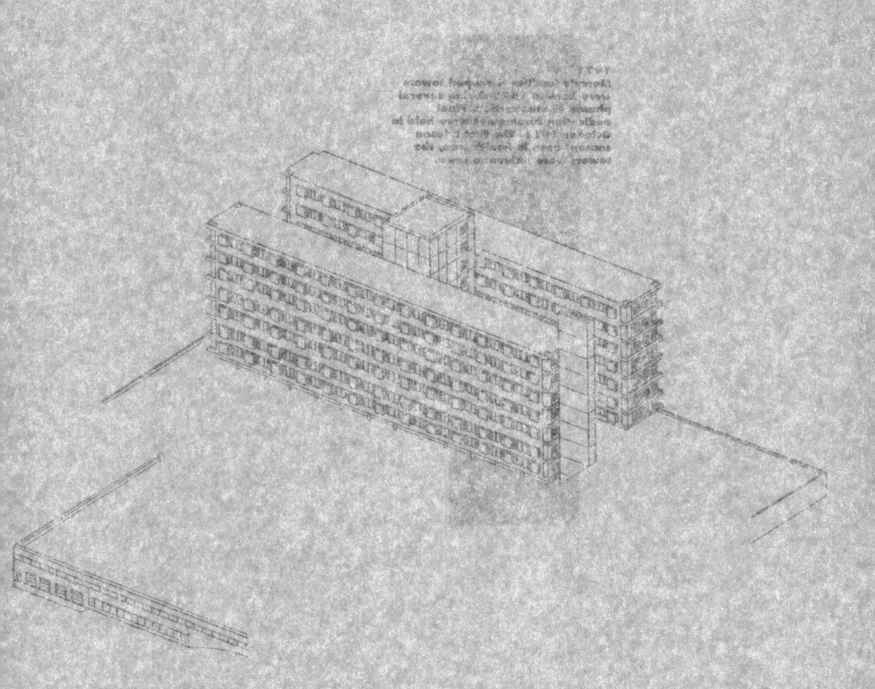

GROWTH THROUGH THE CENTURY: THE BUILDINGS

1971-1978
Mercy's familiar H-shaped towers were born in 1971 during several phases of construction. Final dedication ceremonies were held in October 1978. The first Friesen concept used in health care, the towers were unique to Iowa.

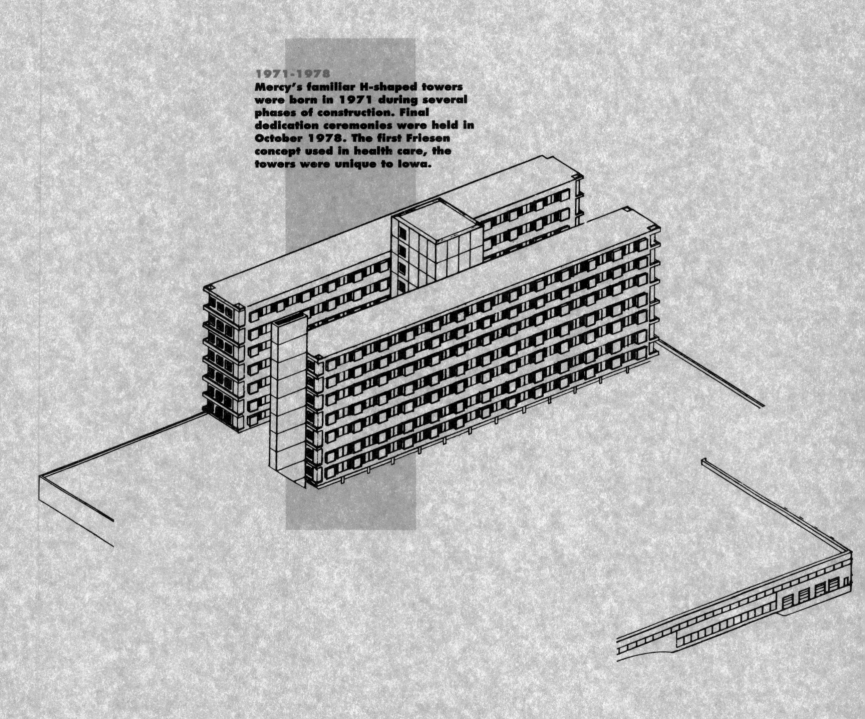

Mercy Firsts

1927 - First in Des Moines to have a traveling library within the hospital.

1941 - First in Iowa to have a hydrotherapy tank.

1953 - First in Des Moines to use radioisotopes.

1967 - First in Iowa to study cardiac patients determining their ability to resume work.

1969 - First in Des Moines to allow students of the College of Osteopathic Medicine and Surgery to be interns.

1972 - First in Des Moines to begin rehabilitation of cardiac patients while in the hospital. This was called "Operation Shape-up".

1973 - First in Iowa to purchase the intra-aortic balloon pump.

1976 - First Iowa hospital to win accreditation for its Medical Education Program.

1978 - First Friesen hospital in Iowa.

1979 - First in Iowa to perform a PTCA. Mercy physician, Dr. Liberato Iannone, used the balloon procedure to clear a patient's clogged coronary artery.

1980 - First in Des Moines to use electron microscope.

1980 - First hospital in Des Moines to provide adult day care service.

1981 - First hospital in Iowa to used Streptokinase.

1982 - First in Iowa to open a fully-accredited Pain Center for persons suffering from chronic pain.

1982 - First in the United States to operate an Occupational Evaluation Center to determine an injured worker's ability to resume work.

1983 - First catheterization laboratory in the world to use bi-plane equipment.

1984 - First Des Moines hospital to offer home care program.

1984 - First in Iowa to use a YAG laser for the follow-up treatment of cataracts.

1985 - First in the United States to use intermittent "piggyback" IVs.

1985 - First Beta site for new barcode system introduced by the Standard Register Company for the supply, distribution, and purchasing department.

1987 - First in Iowa to use a laser for clearing an artery in a patient's leg.

1987 - First in Des Moines to use mitral valvuloplasty to open a closed heart valve.

1987 - First in Iowa to use a "piggyback procedure" for cardiac transplant.

1988 - First in Iowa to open a hyperbaric oxygen chamber.

1988 - First in Iowa to perform a single lung transplant.

1989 - First in Iowa to use the Jarvik-7 artificial heart.

1990 - First in Iowa to install a pacemaker/defribrillator.

1990 - First in Iowa to use directional coronary artherectomy.

1990 - First in Iowa to perform radio frequency catheter ablation.

1991 - First in Des Moines to have a Pediatric Intensive Care Unit fully equipped to provide cardiac care for children.

CHAPTER FOUR

FOR MERCY'S SAKE: THE GUILD

Volunteer efforts during the second World War produced a lasting impact on the growth of volunteer services in American healthcare. Two years after the end of the war, Mercy began an organized volunteer service. The Guild started as an offshoot of the Mercy Advisory Board.

On October 22, 1948, Mr. Ralph Branton, advisory board chairman, called together Mercy leaders: Sisters Mary Helen and Sebastian, Mr. E.H. Mulock, Mr. Harold Klein, other members of the Mercy Advisory Board, and Dr. F.C. Coleman, Mercy's Pathologist. Also invited were: presidents of Catholic women's organizations, wives and women members of Mercy Medical Staff and Advisory Board. This group agreed that Mercy needed a unit of Des Moines women to stimulate interest in Mercy Hospital and in its school of nursing. "This was to be accomplished by promoting the educational interests and social activities for the student nurses in a variety of ways." [1]

Advisory board member, Mary Northup, assumed temporary chairmanship of the new auxiliary at the initial Mercy meeting. On November 5, 1948, officers were elected: Mary Northup, president; Mrs. John M. Griffin, vice president; Mrs. William B. Sloan, recording secretary; Mrs. Walter Lalor, corresponding secretary; Mrs. Albert Meyer, treasurer; and Agnes MacDonald, auditor. Dr. Walter Abbott, president of the Mercy Hospital Medical Staff, gave a presentation about Mercy services. The meeting was held in the nurses home and vocal and instrumental musical numbers were provided by Mercy's student nurses. Mr. E. H. Mulock furnished $1,200 "seed" money for basic supplies.

An invitation was extended in the local newspapers to all women of Des Moines to join Mercy's new Guild at a general meeting on December 3, 1948. The early Guild meetings were held monthly, combined with programs of interest to women which were later designed to include student nurses. The first program featured Mrs. Kenneth MacGregor of the Des Moines Public Health Nurses' Association.

As more and more women began to take jobs outside the home, monthly Guild meetings stopped, and the Guild held two general meetings annually; one in May and another in October. Mrs. Northup determined that she would build the new Guild slowly. Through the leadership of a membership chairman, 300 members joined by the end of the first year's activities.

Mrs. Maurice (Mary) Northup, *above*, became the first Mercy Guild president in 1948. Mrs. Northup cheered the organization's progress until her death in 1990.

After a modest beginning, the Guild found themselves with an excess of about $100 in the treasury at the end of their first year. They asked the student nurses what they would most like to have. They said they would like toasters for quick breakfasts, and the Guild purchased two eight-slice toasters for use in the students' dining room.

Among the first hospital activities sponsored by Guild members were the flower delivery services, a Sewing Committee, and the service cart. The Guild did not involve themselves heavily with fund-raising the first year. "From our membership dues, we organized a 'silver tea' for the library to buy books." The teas continued as an annual event for several years, enabling the library to purchase $40 and $69 worth of library books for the first two years. The Guild also provided volunteers to staff the library for two evenings each week, allowing the students more access to the library. During the third year of Guild ventures, a total of $1,657.67 came back to Mercy in the form of: a formula refrigerator and a bottle warmer for the nursery, an incubator, landscaping, a patio, library expenses and other gifts.[2]

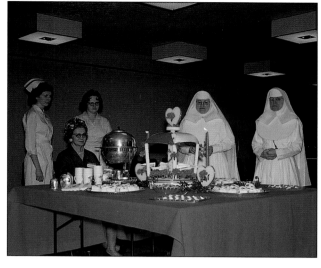

Part of the income for this year was the result of a new project begun by the Guild: baby pictures. New Mercy parents were offered the services of a professional photographer before the mother and baby went home from the hospital. The photographer came to Mercy on Tuesdays and Fridays, delivering the finished photographs on the following day. This Guild service began in 1950 and was generating $1,200 within four years. The Guild expanded this service in 1956 by offering birth announcements to accompany the first photographs. The money raised through this effort was turned back into the obstetrical department to purchase isolettes and other necessities. Color photo capabilities were added in the mid-1970s.

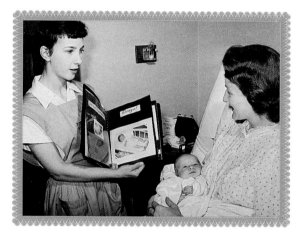

A valuable patient assistance program started by the Guild in the early 1950s began as a result of the many polio outbreaks that occurred in Des Moines at this time. Countless volunteer hours were donated by Guild workers to help care for convalescing children. As Guild workers provided services to these young patients, many found themselves pulled into the lives of their young charges. They were moved to do more for these children, some of whom came from poor families. The "Child Health Fund" grew out of generosity of the Guild members to help children who needed extraordinary care or treatment beyond their family's finances. A special committee to sponsor events to raise money for the new fund began with a card party that netted $500. Additional monies to continue this fund were generated by memorial cards.

As acceptance for this special project grew, another annual Guild-sponsored event began to provide monies to the Child Health Program. The first "Mercy Hospital Bazaar" was held in December 1954 at the Hotel Fort Des Moines. Net proceeds amounted to $1,900.

The Guild was encouraged by the good results from the bazaar because it also supported another purpose for the event: to promote good public relations for the hospital through a social gathering. The popularity

Mercy's Guild sponsored annual Valentine Day teas for employees and Sisters of Mercy, *top.* In 1950, the Guild began offering new Mercy parents, *above,* the services of a professional photographer. Countless hours were donated by Guild members and Candystripers, *below,* to help the children as they recuperated.

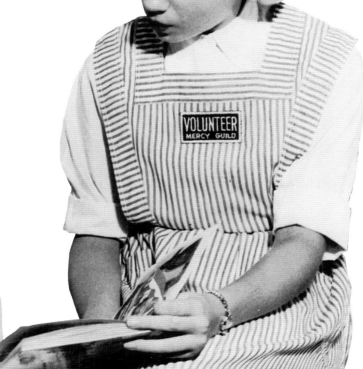

Marie Meyer and
Mary Northup, *right*,
evaluate merchandise
for one of the Guild's
annual spring rum-
mage sales. The
first Mercy Guild
Bazaar, *below*, was
held at the Hotel
Fort Des Moines in
December 1954.
❧ The Guild's travel-
ing "store on wheels,"
bottom, began on
May 29, 1952.

MERCY HOSPITAL GUILD BAZAAR
Benefit Child Welfare Fund

of the bazaar grew, and by 1956, income
amounted to $4,200.

As the fund-raising activities of the Guild
became an important source of additional
funding for Mercy, Guild members looked for
other ways to bring income into Mercy. One
suggestion turned into a good money-maker for
several years: an annual spring rummage sale.
This project proved to be enjoyable and
continued until the mid-1970s.

An early service offered by the Guild was its
traveling "store on wheels," the courtesy service cart
for patients. This project began on May 29, 1952, and 24
loyal cart volunteers and 12 substitutes soon staffed this
service. During 1953, this service cleared more than $1,600.
Two Guild volunteers wheeled the cart to every room on each
floor where visits were allowed, six days of the week.

The Guild spread cheer throughout the hospital and another
service evolved from volunteers delivering flowers to the
patients from the area floral shops. Mr. and Mrs. T. L. Boesen
donated a flower cart to aid these volunteers in 1952. Mercy
Guild members continue to deliver flowers in the 1990s.

As television captured the attention of the world, Mercy's
Guild established a working relationship with a local television
repair center to provide television sets to those patients who
wished the service. The repair center provided the televisions,
and the Guild took over the responsibility of keeping track of
them and collecting the $1.50 daily fee from patients who
wanted a television set for their room. This fee was split between the Guild and the
repair center. A satisfied patient commented:

*"I was very fortunate to secure
a bed in the largest ward in
the hospital with six beds. The
group rented a TV set from the
hospital, dividing the cost...at
25 cents each to pay daily."* [3]

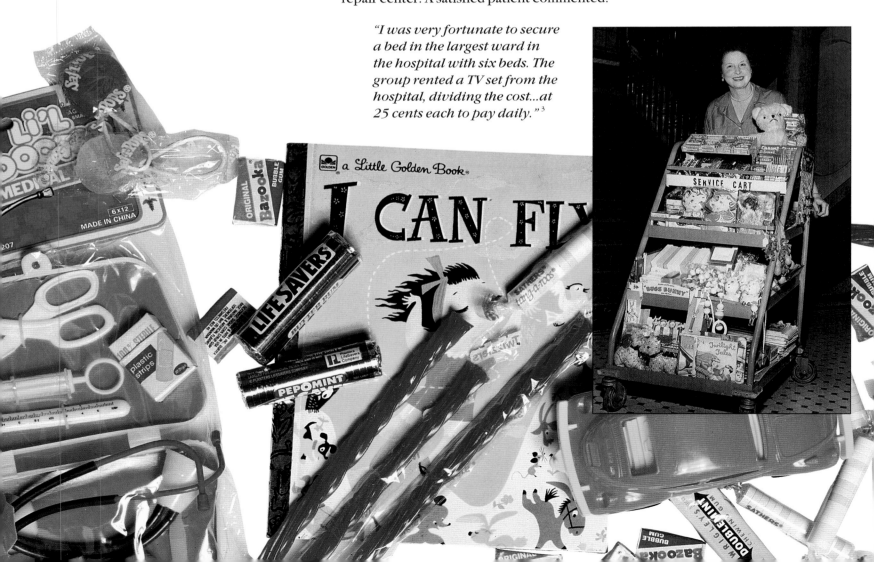

SERVICE CART

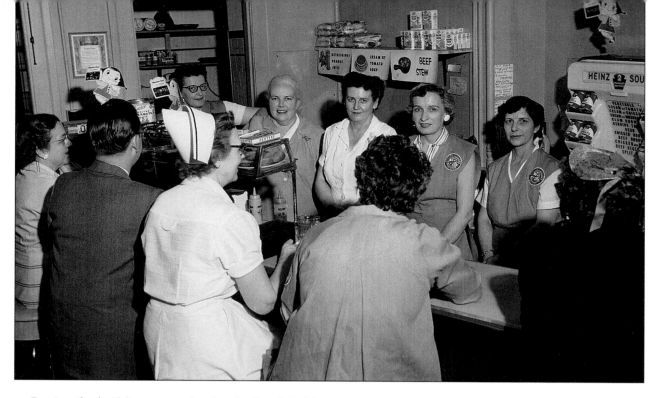

During the building campaign for the South Lobby expansion, the Guild was asked to donate $25,000. They pledged to give at least $5,000 annually. The Guild more than filled their pledge within three years.

The first Snack Shop was located on the ground floor of the Central Wing. Formerly the interns' dining room, this small space accommodated only 12 customers. Mrs. Al (Catherine) Bisignano became project chairman, planning for the Snack Shop to be open six days every week, from 8:00 A.M. to 8:00 P.M. Mrs. Bisignano was described as "so charming, so lovely."[4] Al (Babe) Bisignano recalled:

> *"Catherine planned everything. She made sure that the menus and the prices were all written out for the volunteers. In the beginning everyone was a volunteer. They had a special stew they called 'Murphy's Mess.'"*[5]

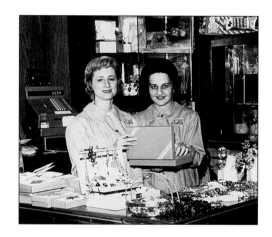

Babe Bisignano also became one of the Guild's "helpful husbands." He donated special equipment and meals prepared in his family restaurant, *Babe's.* Mrs. Bisignano usually worked every Tuesday, and arranged for the restaurant to prepare and deliver a special casserole or main dish. These dishes attracted quite a following: "Around 11:00 A.M. when the food was delivered, there would be a group of hungry employees and staff, applauding and cheering as the food was delivered."[6]

The Snack Shop filled a need. Without vending machines, this new eating area and the cafeteria were the only two places in the hospital where one could find food or drink. Rosemary Avise began her volunteer service in the Snack Shop: "I remember hamburgers and malted milks. And I smelled like hamburgers for the rest of the day."[7]

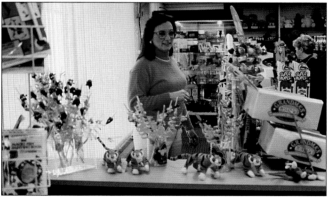

The Snack Shop operated in cramped quarters until the South Wing opened. A new eating area, complete with seating accommodations for 34 people, debuted across the hall from the new cafeteria. The menu became more varied, and the Guild hired a full-time cook. As the business increased, other paid staff were hired. Mabel Blanchard was the snack shop manager during the 1960s. The Guild operated in this location until the new cafeteria area opened during the tower expansion and the Snack Shop closed permanently.

A small corner of the first Snack Shop was converted to a gift counter. This modest beginning evolved into Mercy's spacious, lovely gift shop located today on the same floor as the main entrance to the hospital. In 1991, the shop provided more than $87,000 in revenues to Mercy Hospital.

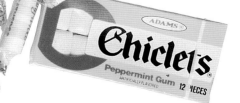

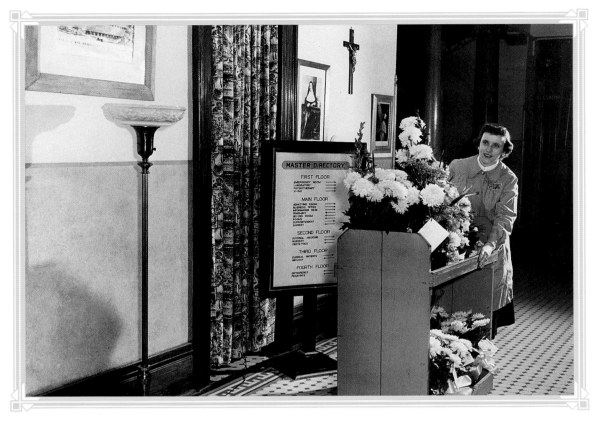

The Guild spread cheer throughout the hospital, *right*, delivering flowers from local shops to patients. ❧ In 1959, Mercy Guild volunteers began staffing the information desk, *below*, located just inside the front door of the South Wing.

One of Mercy's most faithful volunteers, Jo Northup, ran the Gift Shop Committee for many years, working 100 to 120 hours a month. As chairman of this important committee, Jo and other members were faced with the awesome task of "shopping" for gift items in other cities several times each year. Jo and her mother-in-law, Mary Northup, were invaluable assets to the growth and dynamism of Mercy's Guild.

During 1955, the Guild decided to supplement volunteers with teenager girls who worked in the Snack Shop during the summer. This was the beginning of the Candystriper Service, so-named for the red-and-white striped smocks the girls wore.

A special ceremony commemorating the tenth anniversary of the Mercy Guild was held in 1958. The past presidents were honored with special recognition. As each former president's name was called, a white candle was lighted and placed on a tall, white anniversary cake. Each received a past-president's pin. The Sisters of Mercy

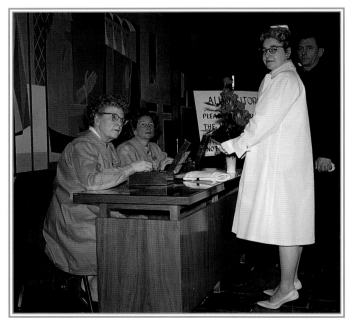

presented the Guild with a certificate "in appreciation for ten years of volunteer service and uncounted hours of valiant work by members of Mercy Hospital Guild." Mrs. Erwin Grask, as current president, listed the Guild's gifts to Mercy since 1947, totaling $67,476. Guild membership surpassed 2,000 women. The year 1958 also marked the beginning of a Guild award system, created to reward members for their service.

In 1959, Mercy's Guild volunteers began staffing the new information desk located just inside the front door of the South Wing. Thirty-five eager women arrived on a hot, muggy June day for the first orientation. Volunteers were trained to hand out visitor passes, route persons to the correct areas of the hospital, and greet all who entered Mercy's new doors with a smile. Mercy's first official gentleman Guild volunteer made his debut in this capacity. Mr. Adelbert Beem worked at the information desk with his wife in the evenings.

By 1960, the Mercy Guild raised $50,000 to remodel and create a new outpatient and emergency department in the old Central Wing. The Guild also actively sponsored their new nursing scholarship, donating more than $400 to the fund.

Mrs. J. J. Kelly became the first chairman of the special nursing recruitment project, and ten years later, when the Guild initiated a special scholarship, Mrs. Kelly's name was affixed to this award.

Without the tireless efforts of Guild members, Mercy may not have been able to purchase much-needed equipment as it became available. The Mercy Guild sponsored projects to pay for incubators, a heart resuscitator, a brain probe and rate meter, cardiac pulmonary laboratory, a cardioscope for surgery, hi-lo beds, the coronary care unit, a neuro-chair, heart pump, equipment for special procedures room, and a Bennett respirator. An early gift brought this response:

"May I also add a big thanks to all for the many wonderful things you have done for us—the chairs and footstools are wonderful and very much appreciated by the patients and personnel. Also the air conditioning in the nursery was such a great help this summer. No words of mine could express our thanks for adding so much comfort to both babies and personnel. May God bless you all for your great help to us." [8]

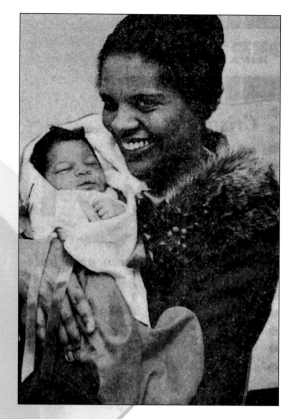

In December 1962, the Guild Sewing Committee began making red buntings, shaped like Santa's boot, for babies born at Christmas time. Mary Beth Bryant, pictured with her mother *left*, was the first baby wrapped in this labor of love. ❧ Through the tireless efforts of Guild members, Mercy was able to purchase much-needed equipment, such as cardiac monitoring and resuscitation devices, a pulmonary function lab, and the infant isolette shown *below*.

Guild members aided Mercy in many small ways that did not generate funds, but provided invaluable service. Patient mail delivery by Guild volunteers began in the late 1950s and continues today. Members of the Guild painted murals on the pediatrics department walls, adding cheer to a place which might otherwise appear frightening to a small child. Mary Northup remembered a time when the Guild wanted to redecorate one of the hospital waiting rooms. There was a telephone booth in one area which:

"was a grave distraction. So we went to the telephone company to Mr. Frank Carroll who was a good friend of ours. He gave us permission to paint this booth. We had this green paint...and we didn't reckon [that] when you got into the telephone booth and were painting, it would be difficult to get out...." [9]

The importance of helping Mercy's youngest patients was paramount to Guild activities. A new children's service began in December 1962. Members of the Guild Sewing Committee, began making red buntings shaped like "Santa's Boot" for newborns discharged during the Christmas season. Mary Bryant, a Mercy employee, was the first proud mother to take home her new infant, Mary Beth, wrapped in this cheery labor of love. [10]

Mercy Guild arranged for hospital visits by celebrities who performed in the Des Moines area. Stars of the annual ice shows, the circuses, Lawrence Welk, the Lennon Sisters, puppeteers, magicians, the Easter Bunny, and Santa Claus all spread cheer throughout Mercy.

Early in the 1960s, the Guild began staffing the surgery lounge. The cherry-smocked volunteers provided countless cups of coffee, and millions of hours of comfort to those waiting for loved ones in Mercy's surgical suites.

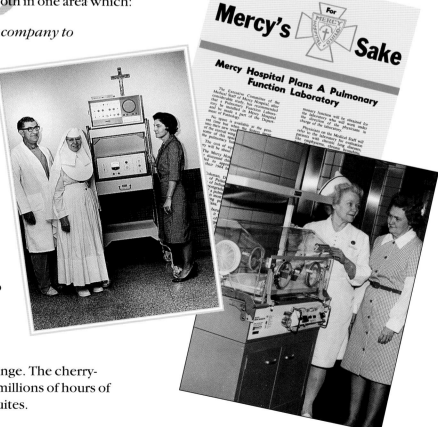

Mercy's For Sake

Mercy Hospital Plans A Pulmonary Function Laboratory

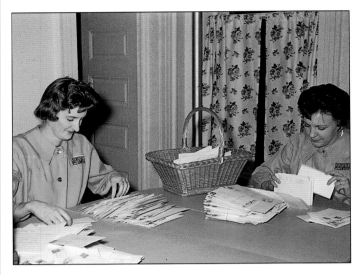

The need arose for a full-time Guild coordinator, and Vera McKeone was hired in 1960. Under Mrs. McKeone's leadership the volunteer program grew.

"It was quite a juggling act to make sure there were enough people to cover the numerous projects. The teenagers were outstanding. I called all the schools in Des Moines. Through their Future Nurse's Clubs the girls were invited to volunteer at Mercy. We spoke about it as a character-building project." [11]

Two volunteer coordinators have followed Mrs. McKeone: Dolores Hogan Roe in 1967 and Kaye Chabot in 1979, the current director.

During 1965, Guild members threw themselves into a new project to aid the Child Health Fund. In late March, a "Mod-Mad Musicale for Mercy" recruited local talent to present an afternoon of music to raise money for children referred by the Des Moines Health Center.

Mercy's Guild members extended their ever-open arms of comfort to stroke patients as Mercy initiated its stroke program in the late 1960s. Tuesdays were earmarked for Guild members to help recovering patients through occupational therapy, letter-writing, reading and friendly visits.

When Dolores Hogan Roe became "Guild Coordinator" after Vera McKeone retired in 1967, she recalled that her office was on the fifth floor in the old Central Wing.

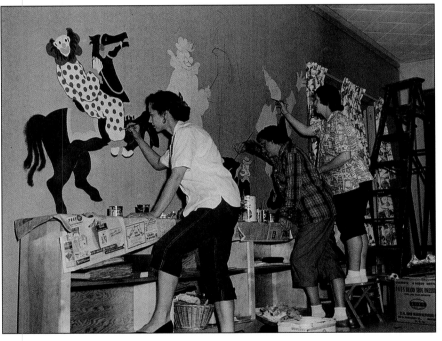

"I believe it was Sister Concepta's old room. I remember if we didn't keep the doors shut just right, the bats would come swooping in. We were all afraid of that." [12]

After the opening of the towers, Guild offices moved to the second floor near Mercy's administrative offices. During Dolores' term as coordinator, husbands joined their wives in providing service within Guild membership. Husband-and-wife teams helped with the mail, in the Gift Shop, as Snack Shop cashiers, at the reception desk, and on the Guild Board. In closing the books for 1968, the Mercy Guild proudly listed 20 years of service to the hospital. During that time, Guild volunteers unselfishly gave more than 260,000 hours of their time. Income-producing projects brought over $255,000 aiding the hospital, nurses, and the nurses' home.

Mercy Guild volunteers, *top,* sorted and readied patient mail for delivery. ☙ The Guild Art Committee of the 1950s, *above,* painted a mural on a wall of the West Wing pediatrics area. ☙ In 1976, 13 Guild Presidents gathered during the October meeting, *opposite top.* In February 1971, the Guild held a "Mod-Mad Musicale", *opposite,* and raised more than $4,600 to aid the hospital.

The annual Mercy Hospital Guild Nursing Scholarship was created in 1969. The Guild awarded a $1,000 for tuition and housing to an incoming freshman. Margaret Murphy from Jefferson, Iowa, was the first to receive this scholarship.

On October 14, 1973, more than 200 members and friends gathered to celebrate the Guild's 25th anniversary. A special champagne brunch was served at the Des Moines Golf and Country Club. Those who gathered to honor this event were applauded by Sister Gervase:

"Observing you almost daily going about your varied tasks throughout the hospital serves as a constant reminder to me of the true nature of our calling. Yours is truly a Christian service, given without thought of gain, reward or recognition." [13]

Guild activities during the 1970s included style shows, rummage and bake sales, art exhibits, and charity luncheons. The Guild's annual charity luncheon and style show began in 1972. Billed as the "major fund-raising event of the year," this occasion

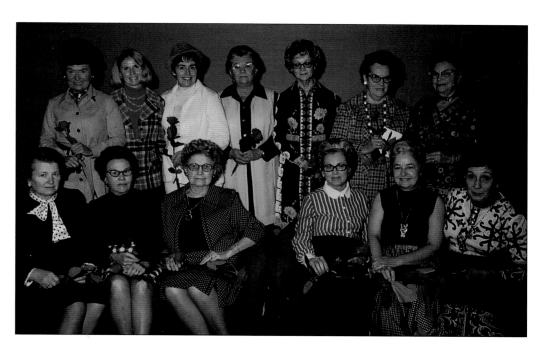

established monetary resources for the Mercy Angel Aid Fund in 1975. The proceeds were used by the social services department to help patients with personal or family emergencies which developed as a result of their hospitalization. Throughout the years, the Guild often sponsored teas to commemorate special days, such as Valentine's, or the annual Sisters of Mercy tea, or for Mercy employees, staff, and students in Mercy's School of Nursing.

In 1974, volunteers were cheered to hear that their hard work had pushed Mercy's Guild to achieve the status of "one of the most active and generous hospital auxiliaries in Iowa." During that year, Guild membership was the third largest in the state, second for number of service hours, and fourth in fund-raising.[14]

The first flower shop, the "Petal Pusher," opened in November 1976. Begun as a brain-child of Joyce Zelinsky, the Petal Pusher made Mercy the first Des Moines hospital to offer on-site preparation of fresh flowers. Rosemary Avise, Mercy's champion volunteer, was tapped by Joyce Zelinsky to be chairman of this new project. Rosemary had just finished her term as Guild president, and at first, she turned down the invitation. A few weeks later, she agreed to begin the project when another coordinator, Jo Northup, volunteered.

The flower shop began with a targeted profit of $60 per week. In 1991, the year's profits were $86,000. Through the efforts and talents of many dedicated volunteers, Mercy's Petal Pusher has expanded to include plants and silk arrangements, as well as fresh flowers.

As a result of the ambitious activities of Mercy's Guild members, the Clinical Pastoral Education program began in Mercy's pastoral care department in 1976. Betty Williams, Guild president in 1976, presented a $13,000 check to offset some of the anticipated expenses for beginning the program.

Another new Guild-sponsored service began at Mercy in September 1979. The Mercy Beauty and Barber Shop opened in its present location, which at that time was the former Guild flower delivery room. Employees, patients, and visitors could receive shampoos, haircuts, sets, and permanents. The Beauty Shop, a long-time dream of Mercy's Guild members, was made possible through a will bequest of Mrs. George P. Comfort and by a gift from Mr. and Mrs. E.T. Meredith III, in memory of Mr. and Mrs. George P. Comfort.

GUILD PRESIDENTS

Mary Northup, 1948
Cloe Van Rheenen, 1949
Virginia Chase, 1950
Genevieve Kelly, 1951-52
Marie Meyer, 1953
Ruth White, 1954
Jane Schiltz, 1955
Edna Ritz, 1956
Ruth Whalen, 1957
Florence Grask, 1958
Madge Hill, 1959
Edna Rubel, 1960
Elaine Crowley, 1961
Mary Cacciatore, 1962
Anne Dunn, 1963
Helen Taylor, 1964
Jean Thyberg, 1965
Jeanne Rowen, 1966
Dorsey Ewald, 1967
Bernice Kanke, 1968
Peg Friedman, 1969
Florence Irving, 1970
Virginia Mickunas, 1971
Jeannette Alberts, 1972
Barbara Cortesio, 1973
Rosemary Avise, 1974
Betty Williams, 1975
Joyce Zelinsky, 1976-77
Jo Northup, 1978
Florence Roth, 1979
Totty Thul, 1980
Lucille Knowles, 1981
Paula Bryant, 1982
Terri Schill, 1983
Jackie Gay, 1984
Dixie Harmeyer, 1985
Grace Jones, 1986
Catherine Ryan, 1987-88
Doris Welter, 1989
Marjorie Baum, 1990
Lucille Knowles, 1991-92

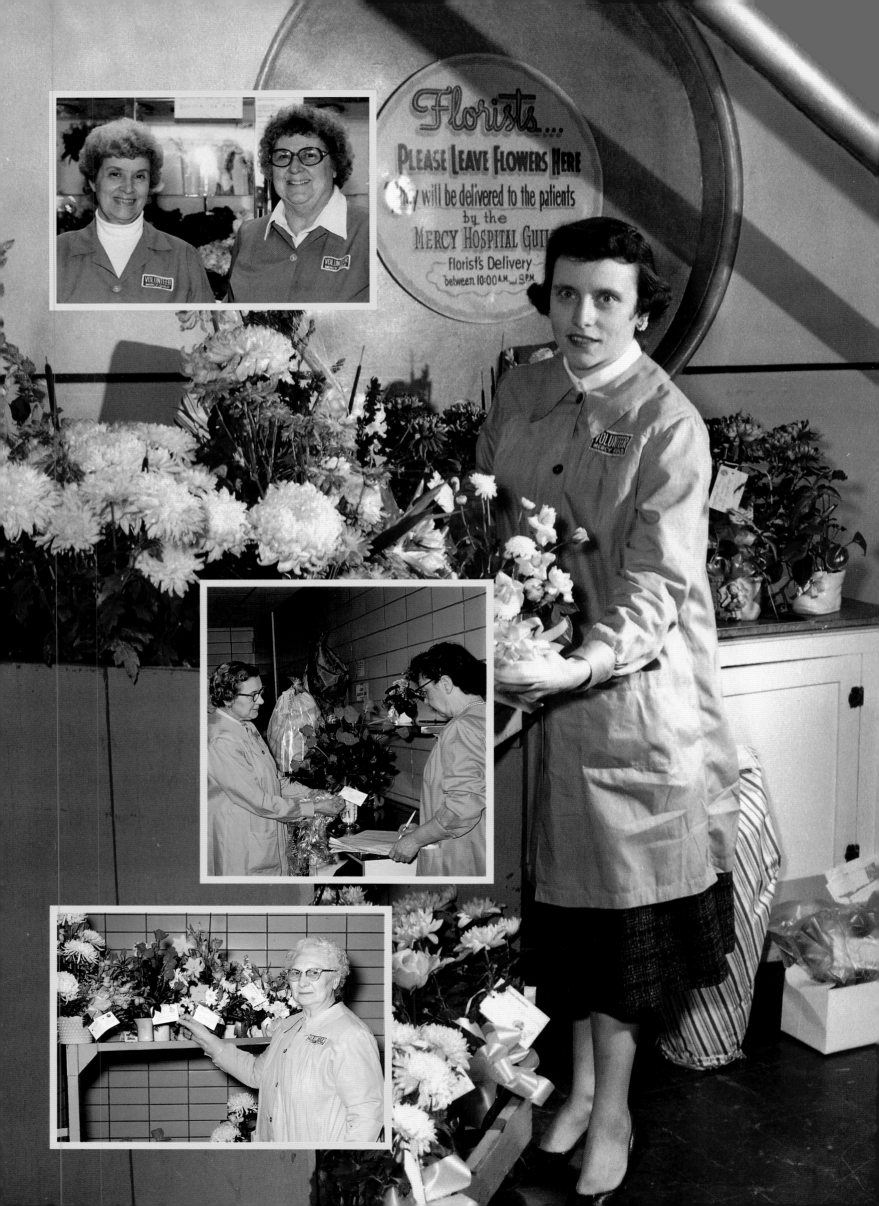

More than 300 volunteers, working 10 to 35 hours each week, continued services that provided growth at Mercy during the mid-1980s. In the Petal Pusher, Rosemary Avis and Becky Gernes used their special talents in a unique spirit of giving. Rosemary served as project chairman for the Guild's flower shop, and Becky provided artistic talent as the design chairman. Although somewhat different in personality, each woman felt a strong commitment to volunteer, and only at Mercy. Becky said:

"It's important to give something to somebody other than immediate family—to give something back to the community....I have had many friends who came here tell me that they could feel a different atmosphere at Mercy. They treat you like a person at Mercy." [15]

A new Guild service came about in 1985 as a result of changes in Iowa laws. New legislation required infants and children to be securely seat-belted while riding in cars. Through the Mercy Infant Car Seat Program, Guild volunteers kept track of 200 infant seats available to new parents. In 1992, Mercy's Auxiliary sponsors the complete program for this service, loaning more than 1,300 car seats to Central Iowa's young families.

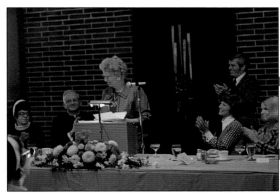

Mercy's Guild membership gathered in October 1988 to celebrate the Guild's 40th anniversary. A special brunch was held at the Des Moines Golf and Country Club. More than 125 members listened as Mary Northup, Mercy's first Guild president, recalled the beginnings of the organization's comforting service in 1948. Bishop William H. Bullock, the seventh bishop of Des Moines, gave the invocation and closing prayer.

In 1991, when she was awarded the Auxilian Award for contributing more than

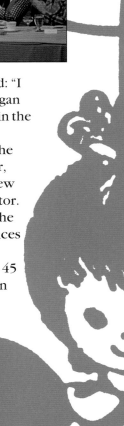

18,000 hours during her career as a Mercy Guild member, Rosemary Avise mused: "I just felt I had to be doing something. I came to Mercy on my own in 1956, and began frying hamburgers in the Snack Shop. I stayed there until they asked me to work in the flower shop." [16]

The 1990s marked five decades of Guild service to Mercy, and responding to the lead of the American Hospital Association, Mercy's Guild president, Doris Welter, moved to initiate renaming the Guild as the Mercy Auxiliary of Central Iowa. A new Mercy volunteer services was begun, with the former Guild coordinator as director. Volunteer services' staff include: the Gift Shop manager and three beauticians. The Auxiliary today has an active adult membership of 416 members. Volunteer services have begun an active campaign to bring more teenagers into the program.

The Mercy Auxiliary will join in the celebration of Mercy's centennial, touting 45 years of proud service begun by the first president who "had no idea the direction which the organization may take," but was guided constantly by the vision:

"There is a Destiny which makes us brothers,
No Man goes his way alone;
All that you give into the life of another
Always comes back into your own."

—John Donne

CHAPTER FIVE
BOUNTIFUL CARE: MOVING TOWARD THE FUTURE

Incredible technological growth occurred at Mercy Hospital in the 1980s and the early 1990s. Services expanded to meet the times, and the Mercy campus grew, pushing the hospital beyond previously delineated borders.

In 1980, Mercy contracted with John Graham to build a Medical Office Plaza with space for 40 physician offices at Fifth and Laurel Streets. Two skybridges connected the new building to Mercy's South Wing and the new Mercy parking ramp. Groundbreaking was celebrated on June 2, 1980. During the same year, an enclosed stairway was built in front of Mercy's main entrance to provide access between the lower and upper levels of parking. This entrance was updated in 1985, when a building with an extended canopy covered the walkway to Mercy's front door.

In 1981, the sixth floor of the towers was completed, and following the lead of a decade devoted to health consciousness, the hospital opened its Wellness Center, an extension between the West Wing and the cooling towers along Fifth Street. The facility offered exercise equipment, a whirlpool, racquetball court, and a swimming pool. The center was available for staff, employees, and patients alike.

Following the success of the Medical Office Plaza, Mercy decided to construct a second physicians' office building, as well as a 600-stall parking ramp, a Cardiac Rehabilitation Center, and larger space for the cath lab. A four-story, glass atrium connected all buildings, and a walking track was built for cardiac patients. Ground was broken on May 29, 1986, and the parking ramp opened on January 5, 1987.

In February 1988, an ambulatory surgical center was opened in the new Atrium Medical Plaza. Four suites accommodated patients who required simpler surgeries. The Mercy Nerve Block Center combined with this area.

A SPECIAL TOUCH Comfort suites opened in June 1986. The specially-designed rooms were made possible by long-time Mercy friend Marie Comfort. Eleven suites on Six South, Seven South, and Nine South, included regular hospital furnishings, a dining table, sofa-bed, and kitchenette. By the end of the first year, more than 950 patients had convalesced in these suites.

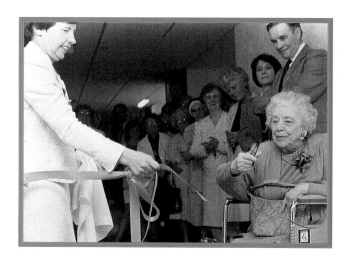

The growth in Mercy's surgery and outpatient services was a reflection of the overall growth experienced by the hospital during the 1980s. Sister Patricia Clare noted: "Mercy must meet the challenge to provide needed services and adequate care at competitive prices. Mercy must be prepared to continue to lead the way, as we have done in the past." Sister Patricia Clare highlighted future goals, including care for the indigent, financing care for the elderly, appropriate use of technology, and bioethical concerns.[1] With these goals in mind, Mercy expanded its unique comfort in increasingly creative and innovative ways.

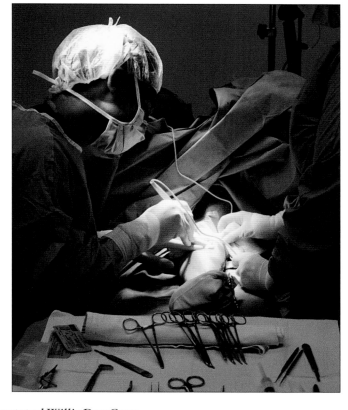

FOR THE ELDERLY AND INVALID

Many of Mercy's new programs specifically targeted the elderly, and some helped others as well: Willis Adult Day Care, Respite, Heritage, Home Care, Home Respiratory Care, and Lifeline.

Willis Adult Day Care was a premiere Mercy program that began as a result of a fire on May 30, 1980. The fire devastated Willis Day Care Center for the Elderly on Sixth Avenue, and the director, Natalie Reese, asked Sister Patricia Clare for a temporary meeting place. The center was unique in Des Moines, providing day care for senior citizens.

Another program called Mercy Respite expanded the services of Willis in 1983. The original program served those patients whose families needed elder-care services when they were going out of town, or for special care. Many persons were not strong after leaving the hospital and needed extra care before feeling comfortable about going home. Twenty beds were opened on West Two and were moved to Eight South in 1984.

Mercy Heritage was begun in October 1985 to provide special services to those 55 years and older. "Through Mercy Heritage we are providing programs and services to help [people] maintain their healthy lifestyles." [2] By the end of August 1992, more than 5,250 persons in Iowa were enrolled in Mercy's Heritage program.

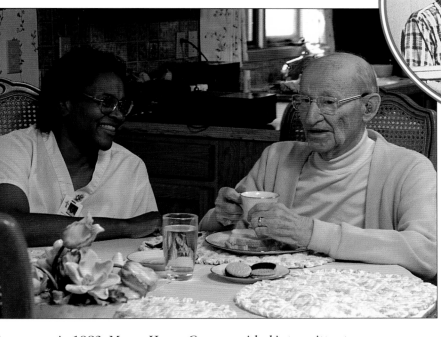

In 1982, Mercy planned to provide a continuation of some hospital services in the home. The program began in earnest in 1983. Mercy Home Care provided intermittent skilled nursing care and social worker visits to home-bound patients. It was the first of its kind to be offered by a Des Moines hospital.

Mercy opened Des Moines' first hospital-based Respiratory Home Care service in May 1983. The program expanded its services to patients when Mercy opened a home medical supply store in 1986.

Lifeline began in July 1985, designed to help persons live independently in their homes with 24-hour access to emergency assistance. This service was provided by Mercy's Social Services Department and continues today.

Sister Patricia Clare and John Graham, *opposite below,* broke ground in June 1980 for Mercy's Medical Office Plaza, the first of many collaborative projects, including the Atrium, *opposite top.* ❧ Long-time Mercy friend, Marie Comfort, *center,* cut the ribbon for the new Comfort Suites. ❧ Ambulatory surgery began in Mercy's second Office Plaza as Dr. Cass Franklin, *above,* performed the first procedure on May 16, 1988. ❧ Mercy reached out in new directions in the 1980s and 1990s with Willis Adult Day Care, *above,* and Private Care, *left.*

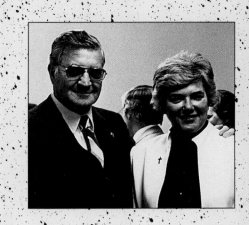

A CRY FOR HELP

Mercy reached out to chemically dependent persons and nutritionally needy clients during the 1980s in several ways: Mercy Alcohol and Drug Recovery Program (MADRP), Psychological Services, Nutritional Disorders, and Our Primary Purpose (OPP).

Mercy's Alcohol and Drug Recovery (MADRP) program began in the late 1970s as Mercy's West Suburban Center Substance Abuse and Alcohol Treatment Program. The first program started with an inpatient stay of three days, and extensive education and therapy sessions after discharge. In 1986, Mercy consolidated inpatient and outpatient alcohol and drug recovery programs.

In January 1987, Mercy's Psychological Services moved from the Mercy Medical Plaza to 73rd Street in Clive. The program was designed for patients who needed more than weekly therapy and less than 24-hour hospitalization. Today, Mercy does not offer a separate service for psychological needs, but counseling is available through many other hospital services.

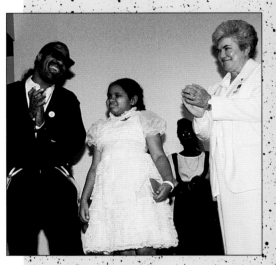

The MADRP and Nutritional Disorders Program evolved into the present-day First Step Mercy Recovery Center in June 1992. The programs moved to the office building previously occupied by the Arthritis Center.

Mercy first opened a nutrition disorders program in early 1984. The group therapy program focused on weight loss and management, eating disorders recovery, and counseling services. An inpatient treatment center opened in June 1987. In the summer of 1992, the program combined with Mercy's First Step Program.

Our Primary Purpose (OPP) began its affiliation with Mercy on the fifth floor of the South Wing in 1984. The inpatient adolescent chemical dependency treatment unit was dedicated to First Lady, Nancy Reagan, who attended the October 30, 1984, ribbon-cutting ceremony. Mercy's OPP program ended in 1991.

HOUSE OF MERCY

Continuing the nurturing mission of Catherine McAuley, Sister Patricia Clare envisioned a new program to provide a home for pregnant teenagers and low-income single mothers in early 1987. She asked Sister Mary Brigid

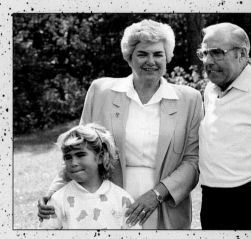

Condon to direct the program. Initial plans called for a portion of the former Bishop Drumm Home to be designated as the Clark Street House of Mercy, with plans for a free medical clinic, extensive education in job-training, parenting, financial management, nutrition, and a child development center.

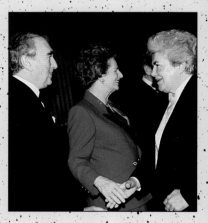

Sister Mary Brigid Condon, a Massachusetts native and a member of the Chicago Province of the Sisters of Mercy, received her master's and doctorate at the University of Iowa. She spent over 40 years building and strengthening Iowa nursing education programs. From 1973 to 1980, Sister Brigid served as vice president for nursing and health education for the Iowa Hospital Association. In 1987, she became director of the Clark Street House of Mercy.

Dedication ceremonies were held on May 16, 1987. Des Moines' new bishop, William Bullock, presided. A free, inner-city medical clinic opened at the House of Mercy in May 1989. At the same time, a $200,000 federal grant and numerous contributions from business, corporate, and private donors created tutoring areas, library, computer lab, craft room, classrooms, and additional living quarters. The Gannett Foundation gave $125,000 to begin a program for chemically dependent mothers, called Project Together. The funding enabled those mothers to receive inpatient treatment, knowing their children would be cared for and there would be a place for them after treatment.

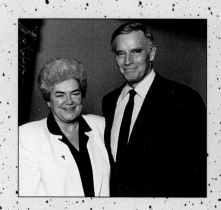

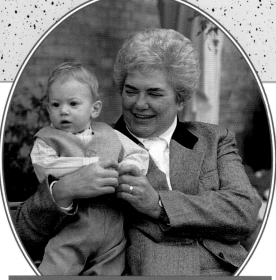

SISTER PATRICIA CLARE

Before Sister Gervase's death, the Mercy Board of Directors established the position of associate administrator, and Sister Patricia Clare (Timothea) Sullivan applied for that position. "It was really different for me because I had never applied for any position as a Sister of Mercy," recalls Sister Pat. "I wasn't used to saying: 'This is why you should hire me.' "

Sister Patricia Clare had spent two previous "tours of duty" at Mercy in Des Moines. From 1955 to 1958, Sister Pat (then, Timothea) supervised the pediatrics department. She remembers fondly: "Mercy was exciting for me because it was my very first assignment as a Sister of Mercy. My appointment card said: Pediatrics Supervisor of Mercy Hospital, Des Moines, August 1955. [On my first day,] I really thought God had me in the wrong place....Three children died...a very traumatic day." [3]

Those were the days of complete, "hands-on" nursing—no suction in the walls, only machines moved from place to place, and simple croup tents to treat the children.

In spite of the hard work, Sister Pat recalls that the 1950s were "happy times." On many evenings for recreation, she and the other sisters walked in twos through the neighborhood surrounding Mercy. "We [sisters] never had a day off...and being supervisors, we went back in the evenings when there wasn't enough help." [4] Sister Pat stayed at Mercy for three years, through the planning and most of the building for the South Wing.

Her next assignment was in Durango, Colorado. Sister Pat was in charge of obstetrics at Mercy Hospital there and instructor for public health nursing in a rural setting for the Denver school of nursing students. "Durango was marvelous." [5] In 1960, Sister Pat came back to Des Moines as director of Mercy's School of Nursing. She found nursing education was changing.

During her school of nursing years, Sister Pat served as president of the Iowa Nurses' Association. One of the students of that time remembered "how proud we all were to have our director be president." [6]

Sister Pat served as a panelist on the "Know Your Neighbor Panel," examining the issues of prejudice and emerging women's rights. In 1964, she was reassigned to Williston, North Dakota as director of nursing, and in 1965, Sister Pat was sent to Centerville, Iowa, to become administrator of St. Joseph's Mercy Hospital. She served there until 1969, enjoying the environment and feeling a spirit of ecumenism within the whole community.

Sister Pat received a master's in hospital administration in 1970. From 1971 to 1974, she worked as a member of the Renewal Team for the Sisters of Mercy. From 1974 to 1977, Sister Pat worked as community relations director of Bergan Mercy Hospital in Omaha.

Within a few months after Sister Pat's arrival back in Des Moines, Sister Gervase was dead, and Sister Patricia Clare interviewed again for the position of Mercy's administrator and president. She has remained at the helm of Mercy since that time. Thinking over her Mercy career, Sister Pat recalls more than 30 years of association with Des Moines:

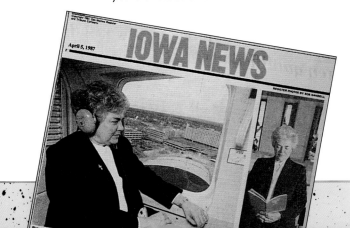

"I think Mercy is number one in human resources, technology, and education. Sister Gervase's and the board of directors' foresight in establishing the tower system was an innovative decision. Mercy's clinic and networking services have made a difference. We are providing services to rural hospitals which help them. Mercy's focus as a heart center—a center of excellence—has raised the prestige for the whole of Central Iowa." [7]

Sister Pat has received many honors: A Women of Vision Award from the Young Women's Resource Center, Distinguished Iowa Citizen from Mid-Iowa Boy Scouts of America, Iowa Women's Hall of Fame Award from the Iowa Commission on the Status of Women, People of Vision Award from the Iowa Society to Prevent Blindness, Administrator of the Year from the American Academy of Medical Administrators, and National Conference of Christians and Jews Leadership Award.

Presently, Sister Pat is vice president of the Greater Des Moines Committee of the Greater Des Moines Chamber of Commerce, president of the Hillside Neighborhood Development Corporation, a member of the board of directors of Boatmen's National Bank and the Catholic Health Association. She served as chair of the Iowa Caucus Project '88 and on the boards of directors for the: Convalescent Home for Children, Grand View College, and the American Academy of Medical Administrators.

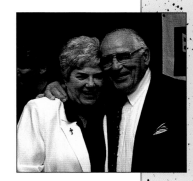

Although Sister Pat was born in Nebraska, her family grew pioneer roots in Iowa in the 1850s. Her great-great grandfather, Timothy Sullivan, migrated with his young wife and two sons, to the Cascade/Monticello, Iowa, area in the Irish exodus after the 1840s potato famine. The Sullivan family homesteaded in Jones County, Iowa, by 1850. In the 1860s, Daniel Sullivan married Elizabeth Cashen. They moved to Cortland, Nebraska, the birthplace of their great-granddaughter, Patricia Clare Sullivan.

When Sister Patricia Clare came back to Des Moines for the third time, she felt as though she was "really coming home." One of her favorite phrases is "commitment to the community, caring for people, through the help of the church and the Sisters of Mercy...what Mercy Hospital and my work as administrator are all about.... I have dedicated my whole life to healing, and I look at Mercy Hospital and I say 'What a Blessing,' and I would like everyone to see it that way." [8]

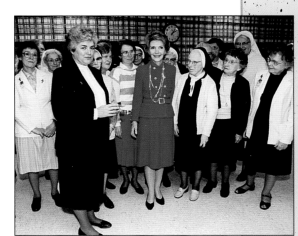

In 1992, the House of Mercy received an award at *right*, from the Catholic Health Association. ❧ Sister Mary Ann Burkhardt, *below*, director of Mercy Court, shares a cup of coffee with a resident. ❧ Mercy began its clinic system in August 1983 at Valley West Mall. Today there are fifteen facilities, including the Indianola Clinic, *bottom*.

An essential service was added to the House of Mercy in 1990 when an on-site child development center opened. Resident single mothers now had a place to take children while they spent daytime hours completing education, beginning new jobs, or attending counseling.

In 1992, the House of Mercy received national recognition from the Catholic Health Association for the center's commitment to outstanding healthcare services. Since 1988, three programs at the House of Mercy have helped many: Teen Pregnancy and Parenting Program (formerly The Bridge); Adult Transitional; and Project Together.[9]

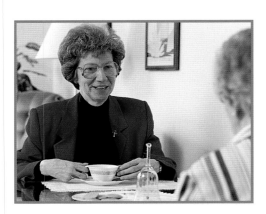

THE CAMPUS GROWS

Space for non-patient care areas prompted Mercy to purchase the former General Growth Building at 1055 Sixth Avenue in 1982. Mercy's financial, public relations, marketing, and other services moved into the building. In March 1983, the hospital acquired the Quality Care Building (renamed the Mercy Laurel Center), with plans to open 35 long-term beds, 15 for elderly patients requiring long-term care. Mercy's authorized bed-count grew to 535.

Also in 1983, Mercy bought the former Americana Park Apartments facing Third Street, across from Mercy. The hospital renamed the apartment building Mercy Park, and Ilene Borchert has been the director since June 1986. A new activity center was built in 1988 on the same site.

Mercy's education program received a boost in 1985 when the hospital purchased the former Charlie's Showplace dinner theater. Originally a Jewish synagogue, the building provided a home for Mercy's educational programs. In November 1985, as Mercy acquired other off-site facilities, a shuttle service made its debut.

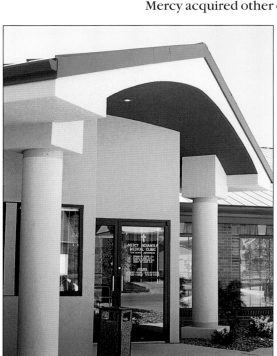

In January 1987, Mercy Hospital purchased the former Howard Johnson's Motel and converted it into 60 apartments for the elderly. Transportation, meals, housekeeping, activity center, and emergency services were provided. After extensive remodeling, the new facility was renamed Mercy Court. Mercy's Foundation moved to the ground floor in April 1987. During that year, Sister Mary Ann Burkhardt came from her position as a principal in Council Bluffs to be director of Mercy Court. In 1989, ten rooms were set aside for people needing additional support services.

MERCY CLINICS

Mercy began the clinic system in 1983 as a way to offer more convenient medical care. The hospital's first outpatient clinic opened at Valley West Mall in August 1983. By the 1990s, there were 15 Mercy clinics, affiliating with 55 area physicians. They were Mercy: Ankeny, Hilltop, Indianola, Urbandale, West, Geriatric, Arthritis, Central Pediatric, West Pediatric, Campus, Iowa Occupational Medicine, Clark Street, DMMG Medical, Multiple Sclerosis, and Rehabilitation and Physical Medicine.

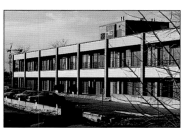

Mercy Office Plaza

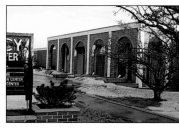

Mercy Laurel Center

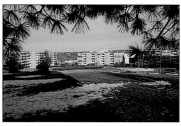

Mercy Park Apartments

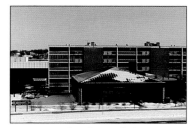

Mercy Geriatric Activity Center

Networking

Mercy began providing administrative services to county hospitals in 1985, when it signed agreements with Monroe County Hospital in Albia, Iowa. This important linkage enabled the smaller healthcare facilities to receive the benefit of the latest technology and training, ensuring the best care for their patients. Rural hospitals became affiliated with Mercy when the administrator was hired by Mercy or when the hospital contracted services. Speciality clinics also became available to the smaller hospitals, and educational programs, consultation, and physician liaison services were generously shared. By 1992, Mercy's talents and technology were linked with ten rural Iowa hospitals: Monroe County Hospital in Albia, St. Joseph's Mercy Hospital in Centerville, Hamilton County Public Hospital in Webster City, Ringgold County Hospital in Mount Ayr, Audubon County Memorial Hospital in Audubon, Manning General Hospital in Manning, Story County Hospital in Nevada, Davis County Hospital in Bloomfield, Adair County Hospital in Greenfield, St. Anthony's Regional Hospital in Carroll, and Wayne County Hospital in Corydon.

An air transport service flew physician specialists to many of Iowa's rural communities. This enabled patients to stay in their community whenever possible.

In 1989, Mercy was recognized in a United States Congressional Report for its superior resources, facilitating efforts to solve the broad range of problems facing rural hospitals. At the same time, the hospital was lauded for its commitment to respecting the autonomy of the hospitals it served. During the 1990s, Mercy Hospital and its affiliates were awarded two grants to study the incidents of cancer among Iowa farmers.

Old Friends, New Partners

Two institutions operated by the Sisters of Mercy became affiliates of Mercy in the summer of 1986: Bishop Drumm Retirement Center in Johnston, Iowa, and St. Joseph's Mercy Hospital in Centerville, Iowa.

St. Joseph's Mercy Hospital became a Mercy institution in 1910 when the Sisters of Mercy from Council Bluffs took over the administration of the community hospital. Sisters Mary Evangelista Claherty and Alacoque Lannon were the first sisters to arrive from Council Bluffs. Sister Evangelista was Centerville's first administrator, and in 1922 she became administrator in Des Moines. In 1965, Sister Patricia Clare Sullivan became administrator in Centerville, staying until 1969. St. Joseph's Mercy built a new $400,000, 60-bed hospital in 1979.

In the summer of 1986, the Bishop Drumm Retirement Center, below, and the St. Joseph's Mercy Hospital in Centerville, Iowa, bottom, became affiliates of Mercy Des Moines.

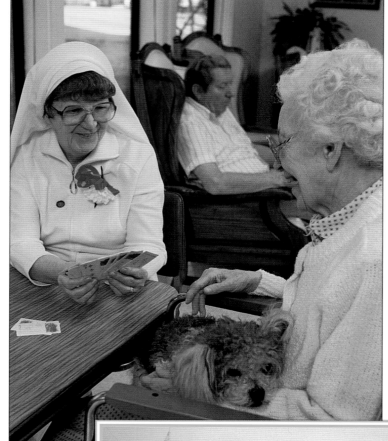

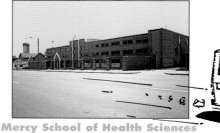
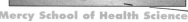

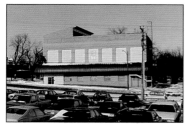

Mercy Educational Center

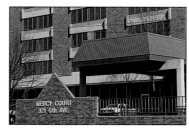

Mercy Court Apartments

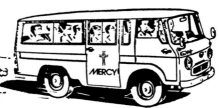

Mercy School of Health Sciences

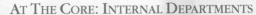

In January 1988, Mercy became the first Iowa hospital to open a hyperbaric oxygen unit, *below.* ❧ Changes in surgery and diagnostic technology reflected the dynamics of computerized imaging and state-of-the-art surgical assisting devices.

AT THE CORE: INTERNAL DEPARTMENTS

Internally, Mercy's many departments adjusted to meet the fast-paced 1980s. The housekeeping department became the department of environmental services in April 1980 and moved to West Four. The official opening of the newly located emergency department came in May 1980. Mercy's Emergency Department became the busiest in Iowa by the end of the 1980s.

After the demolition of the Central Wing, the technical services department moved several times throughout the 1970s and early 1980s. It finally came to its current location on the first floor of the West Wing in 1988.

The Mercy Sleep Disorders Center opened in 1982 to treat patients with sleep apnea problems. The hyperbaric oxygen unit brought recognition to Mercy in January 1988 when the hospital became the first in Iowa to offer this type of service. This highly-pressurized oxygen treatment chamber restored depleted oxygen levels in patients, hastening recovery. Patients with slow healing wounds and smoke induced or carbon monoxide respiratory problems benefited from the new treatment. In December 1988, a second chamber was added. Currently, the technical services department provides services in respiratory therapy, hyperbaric oxygen, sleep apnea, cardiac sonography, neuro diagnostics, and vascular studies.

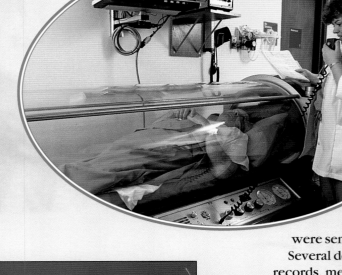

In 1985, nursing services realigned into three distinct areas: critical care, surgical care, and clinical care. And Mercy became the first hospital in the country to test a new drug delivery system in September 1985. As a Beta site for the Abbott Laboratories and the Eli Lilly Company, Mercy used the ADD-Vantage intermittent "piggyback" IV system. Vials containing drugs were packaged and connected to intravenous bags before the drugs were sent to nursing stations for patient use. This system continues today.

Several departments established new homes near the A-level entrance: medical records, medical staff, and quality assurance. Their vacated area became the new Mercy McDonald's in December 1988.

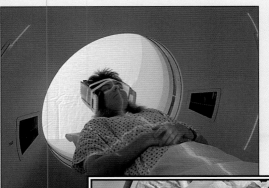

GROWTH IN THE WORLD OF MEDICINE

By the 1980s, tremendous growth in the medical field forced hospitals to implement new, state-of-the art equipment. Americans wanted instant solutions to their health problems. Malpractice insurance costs soared. To control the costs of Medicare and Medicaid, the Government set strict standards for inpatient and outpatient services. Businesses united to find less expensive ways of providing health insurance to their employees. All healthcare providers were challenged to control healthcare inflation. Mercy continued to seek every possible way of serving patients, while controlling the cost of those services.

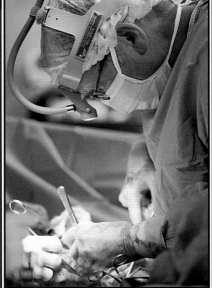

ANOTHER BABY BOOM

In August 1984, the nursery boomed with activity as labor and birthing recorded 208 births, the highest monthly total since July 1970. Outpatient testing procedures in the area set another record that month. To handle the booming baby business, Mercy added a Normal Newborn Nursery in the summer of 1986. Two large rooms for newborns, a charting area, and a physician-work area comprised the area set aside for newborns who did not need special care.

At the same time, Mercy's Nursery implemented mother-baby nursing. Having one nurse on a shift, caring for both mother and baby, provided for more continuity.

On March 27, 1987, Mercy's fourth-floor labor and birthing area was renamed The Brennan Family Center honoring Sister Mary Zita Brennan. This new area

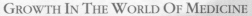

encompassed the former birthing center, nursery, special care nursery, postpartum area and gynecological care services.

The highest birth record at Mercy occurred in September 1989, when 281 babies were born. [10]

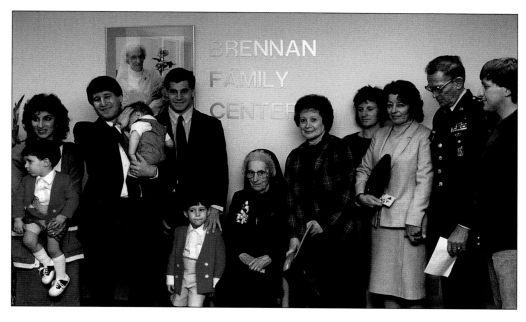

AID FOR THE CHRONICALLY ILL

Patients with kidney disease found new Mercy services during the 1980s: dialysis, stone dissolving, and kidney replacement.

In September 1985, Mercy was given the approval to begin a kidney dialysis center. Before this time, Mercy patients who needed dialysis were transported to Iowa Lutheran Hospital. Mercy opened the new treatment center on South One, and the program rapidly outgrew its facilities. From the original four dialysis stations, Mercy's unit expanded to 12 in 1987. In December 1992, the dialysis unit relocated to West Five with 20 stations. During fiscal year 1992, a total of 6,284 treatments were given. Mercy provides education and durable supplies to patients on home dialysis.

A new program for Mercy that became a successful joint venture with Iowa Methodist Medical Center was announced in May 1984. The two hospitals purchased a Dornier Kidney Lithotripter to dissolve kidney stones. In 1992, Iowa Lutheran Hospital became the third partner in this venture. A staff of seven assisted 18 urologists from five cities in treating 647 patients for Fiscal Year 1991-92. [11]

By 1986, Mercy had increased its help for those afflicted with kidney disease, and the hospital announced plans to begin a kidney transplant service. In December 1986, Mercy became the second Iowa hospital to begin the new procedure by performing two surgeries, two days apart. Andrew Peitzman was the first patient, receiving his new kidney from his brother. In October 1987, two kidneys were transplanted into an 8-year-old child after determining that the donor kidneys were too small. By early January 1993, Mercy had performed 63 kidney transplants.

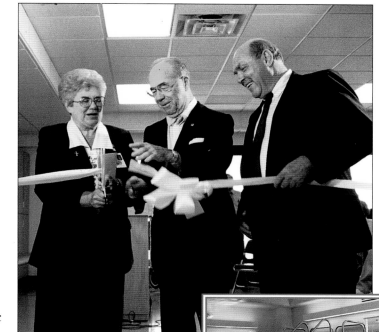

RUAN NEUROLOGICAL CENTER

In July 1988, Sister Patricia Clare and Des Moines businessman, John Ruan, announced the creation of a neurological disorders center. The Ruan Neurological Center was designed to emphasize care, treatment, and support of multiple sclerosis patients and their families. Patients suffering from head injuries or medical problems, Alzheimer's disease, Lou Gehrig's disease, and other neurologic problems would also receive help at the center. Ruan's interest in supporting this facility came as a result of family illness. Ruan's wife, Betty, and their daughter, Jayne Ruan Fletcher, both suffered from this disease. The center was located on the fifth and sixth floors of the east side of Mercy's service chassis.

On March 27, 1987, Mercy's fourth floor labor and birthing area was renamed the Brennan Family Center, honoring Sister Zita, seated *above*. Sister Patricia Clare, John Ruan, and Mel Straub, *left*, cut the ribbon on the Ruan Neurological Center, opened in the summer of 1989. A special cold-water pool facilitated exercise for multiple sclerosis patients.

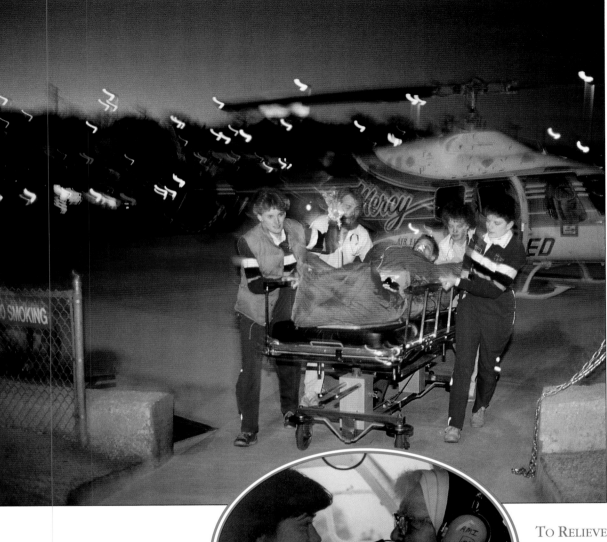

MERCY AIR LIFE

With the growth of Mercy's transplant services, and the critical need for air medical service to outlying areas, Mercy announced plans for its own helicopter service in 1986. The new service was called Mercy Air Life. A landing pad was built west of the emergency department entrance. Projections indicated there would be a need for 750 air-transport calls to Des Moines during 1987.

The helicopter was designed especially for Mercy in silver, burgundy and white. A 15-member Mercy Air Life team included flight nurses, flight paramedics, and dispatchers. Dedication ceremonies and an open house to acquaint hospital personnel with Mercy Air Life were held on October 20. Mercy initiated its first air transport service on November 2, 1986 rescuing a heart attack victim in Granger. During fiscal year 1992, Mercy Air Life flew 659 missions, transporting a total of 668 patients.

Mercy Air Life, began in November 1987. Sister Joseph, *right,* listened to chief flight nurse, Laurie Dickinson, while she explained the details of radio communications between the hospital and helicopter.

TO RELIEVE CHRONIC PAIN

Persons looking for relief from chronic pain were treated in a new program begun in February 1982. Mercy's Pain Center, under the medical direction of Dr. James Blessman, opened its doors on South Five. The first program consisted of short classes, testing, exercise, counseling sessions, and medical treatments as prescribed by the physician and staff. Hoptel rooms were available for those patients needing this service. In January 1984, the facility was given a three-year accreditation from the Commission on Accreditation of Rehabilitation Facilities. It was one of 14 programs in the country and the first in Iowa to meet the commission's standards. [12]

In 1992, the center celebrated its tenth anniversary. It has provided service to 1,821 clients since the program's inception. The center also offers outpatient services to patients suffering from multiple sclerosis.

A new approach to the treatment of arthritis began in early 1985. Dr. Ted Rooney, a rheumatologist, developed the Mercy Arthritis T.E.A.M.—Treatment and Education for Arthritis Management program. Dr. Rooney directed a team of healthcare professionals in the care of patients afflicted with arthritis. The arthritis program moved to Mercy West in September 1990.

EDUCATION IN THE 1980S

Mercy continued to offer superb education and training programs during the 1980s in: the health education department, nurses aides, security officers and surgical technicians training, and Mercy's School of Health Sciences. As a result of this breadth of commitment, Mercy was often the first in Des Moines to provide unique learning experiences.

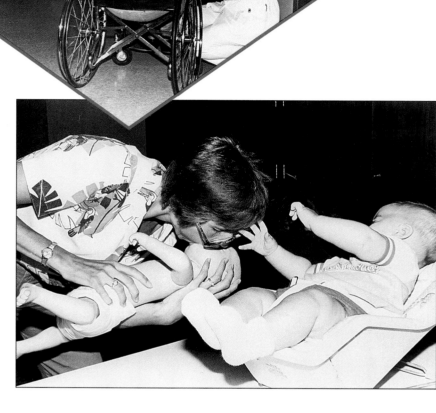

One "first" occurred in 1980 when Mercy was designated as the Des Moines area's Resource Hospital for Emergency Medical Services (EMS), meeting two criteria: education and medical control. This special designation was given to Mercy by the Central Iowa Emergency Medical Services Regional Council. [13]

The first criterion of educational commitment provided training of area pre-hospital advanced-care personnel. Other classes were offered to nurses, physicians, medical students, and others. Mercy was the first Des Moines hospital to offer advanced trauma life-support training. As part of the resource hospital, Mercy offered radio and telephone contact for emergency vehicles involved in the transportation of patients to Des Moines area hospitals. Erected late in 1982, a new 140-foot tower, with a geographical range of about 30 miles, improved Mercy's EMS communications. Simultaneous calls became an option. Matching funds from Mercy and the Central Iowa EMS Council brought the program to life. A first-level EMS training course was added in August 1984.

In April 1988, the Mercy Pre-Hospital Advanced Care Training Program became the Mercy Regional Emergency Training Center (MRETC). This staff became responsible for teaching first responder techniques to cadets from the Iowa Law Enforcement Academy. Mercy's program received a $99,701 grant from the Variety Club of Iowa in 1991 for the purpose of establishing the Variety Club Pediatric Emergency Services Training Center for Iowa. Since 1988, approximately 7,123 students have received training through MRETC. [14]

THE FIGHT AGAINST AIDS

Like all healthcare facilities during the past decade, Mercy has been waging a war against the growth of Acquired Immune Deficiency Syndrome (AIDS) within the community. The hospital began teaching staff about AIDS in November 1985. A community task force was designed to establish policies about the syndrome among the seven Des Moines hospitals.

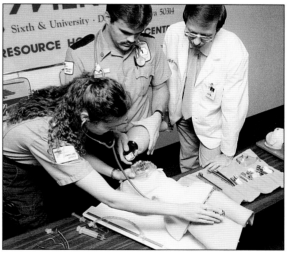

Guidelines provided by the Center for Disease Control and the American Hospital Association directed the activities of the 21-member task force. Four Mercy providers were part of this important policy group: Drs. Daniel Gervich and Donald Sweem, Cheryl Noyes and Connie Grout.

In October 1987, Mercy initiated a new needle disposal method. By March 1988, the task force developed a policy to address issues of confidentiality, discrimination, safety precautions, consent forms, employee educational programs, and testing of patients and healthcare workers. Mercy scheduled mandatory in-services for all employees.

Mercy began a training program for pre-hospital advanced-care personnel in 1980. This program was renamed the Mercy Regional Emergency Training Center in April 1988. Mercy continued to offer superb education and training throughout the 1980s.

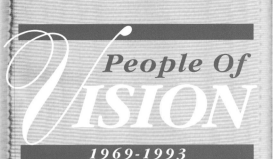

People Of VISION

1969-1993

CHIEFS OF STAFF

Austin Schill, 1969
Albert Clemens, 1970
John Polich, 1971
Paul From, 1972
James Kelso, 1973
Ralph Hines, 1974
Alfred Smith, 1975
M. Patricia Phelan, 1976
Marvin Silk, 1977
Byron Augspurger, 1978
Frederick Katzmann, 1979
Robert Jones, 1980
Joseph Song, 1981
Abraham Wolf, 1982
Donald Sweem, 1983
Stuart R. Winston, 1984
Ala Daghestani, 1985
James Caterine, 1986
John Gay, 1987
Kenneth Schultheis, 1988
John Ritzman, 1989
Stephen Eckstat, 1990
Thomas M. Brown, 1991
Steven Berry, 1992
Kenneth P. Anderson, 1993

LESS MONEY, MORE CARE

The 1980s saw new forces that impacted the growth of health care in unimaginable ways. As costs of medical technology and education skyrocketed, regulatory agencies forced healthcare providers to search for new modes of service. The federal government shifted a greater portion of the financial burden to other payers and forced hospitals to accept less money for more care.

Mercy continued, however, to be a creative innovator with new services and programs. By 1990, the hospital began the process of Continuous Quality Improvement (CQI) through a series of management seminars on total quality management. In 1991, this program evolved into a cohesive effort, emphasizing team efforts in addressing efficiency and cost-containment. At this time, the CQI process is coordinated by Annette Bair.

IN THE 1990s

Mercy met the 1990s facing exciting challenges and progress in American healthcare. As the decade began, Mercy physicians were the first in Iowa to implant a pacemaker and defibrillator. Another new specialized procedure was planned for kidney patients when conventional shock-wave therapy was not recommended.

In 1990, as the Des Moines population shifted westward, Mercy built a $15-million, three-story medical office building in Clive. This building in the 1600 block of N.W. 114th Street was developed by Graham Investment Co. Groundbreaking was held on July 25, 1989. Mercy West Health Center opened in Clive in September 1990. Three Mercy clinics moved to the new building immediately: Valley West Medical, Arthritis Center, and a satellite clinic of Mercy's Pediatric Clinic.

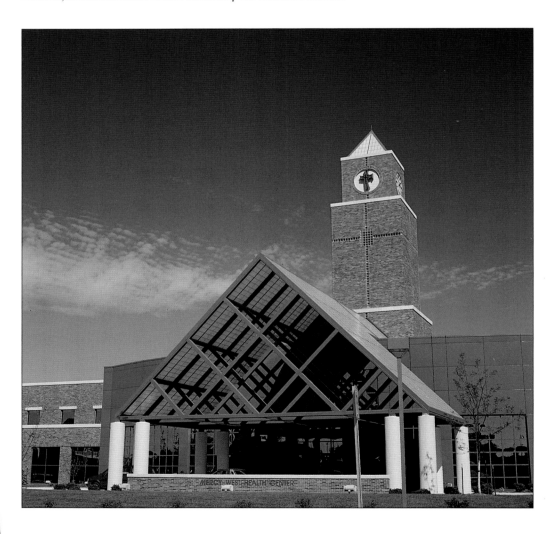

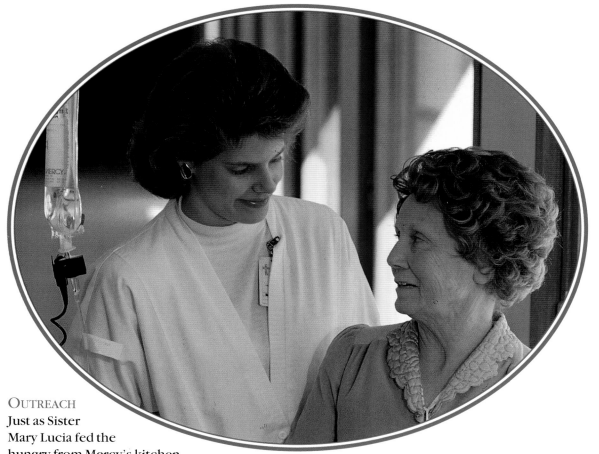

OUTREACH

Just as Sister Mary Lucia fed the hungry from Mercy's kitchen during the Depression, and Mercy's Meals on Wheels Program did the same in the late 1960s, Mercy reached out in the same way to the community in the 1990s. A special meal delivery service to the elderly began, and Mercy was one of only 17 hospitals in the country to receive grants from the National Health Care Foundation for this program.

In 1990, Mercy's outreach to corporate Des Moines was recognized when the Farmers Home Administration received a distinguished service award for health and safety from the U.S. Secretary of Agriculture in recognition for their Mercy wellness contract. Mercy has provided these programs to over 250 businesses, industries and governmental agencies in the Des Moines area. [15]

In June 1990, the Sisters of Mercy worldwide were honored by Variety Clubs International with a humanitarian award. Sister Patricia Clare Sullivan gave the invocation for the banquet. This award honored those who have shown unusual understanding, empathy, and devotion to mankind.

NURSING IN THE 1990s

To attract and retain nursing personnel, Mercy nurses on Seven South began an innovative staffing plan in the summer of 1990. Called the 7/70 plan, it allowed nurses to work 10-hour shifts for seven days in a row and receive the next seven days off. Two nursing teams worked alternative seven-day periods, with overlapping shifts, one of the best benefits of the new program.

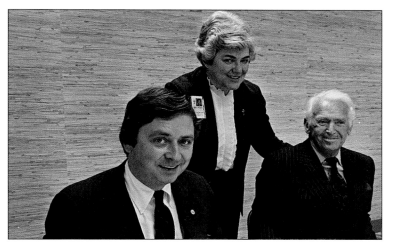

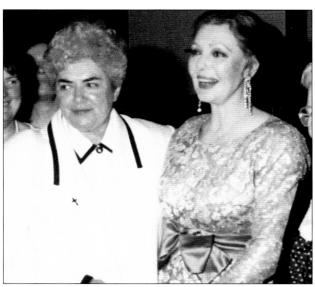

Mercy continued
its outstanding
commitment to
nursing education
during the 1980s
and 1990s. Deanne Remer,
bottom right,
became Mercy's
School of Nursing
director in 1989.

CHOOL OF NURSING: 1980S TO PRESENT

In May 1980, Grand View College and Mercy announced a new cooperative program in nursing education. Mercy continued with their three-year diploma program, and graduates were offered an option of continuing their studies for a bachelor's degree in nursing. Grand View was the only college in Central Iowa at that time to offer a BSN.

In 1981, the representatives of the National League for Nursing Board of Review praised Mercy as "a warm, hospitable, caring place. I don't know when I've been in an institution where I've had this feeling throughout the place." [16] Mercy was granted the maximum accreditation time of eight years. [17]

During the summer of 1986, the dormitory was moved into Mercy Park Apartments (formerly the Americana Apartments) which Mercy had recently purchased. In

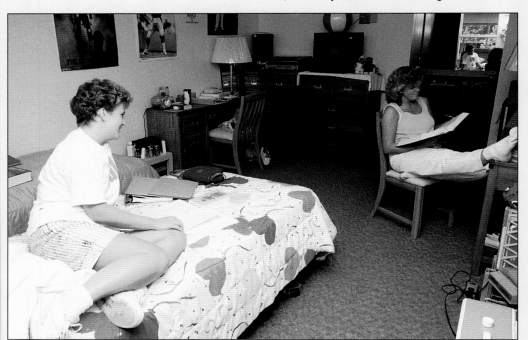

January 1987, the school's administrative offices were moved off-campus to the lower level of the former Howard Johnson Motel, renamed Mercy Court.

The smallest class in 20 years graduated from Mercy's school in May 1988. However, the situation reversed by 1989. Mercy's school enrollment increased for the third straight year when 47 students started classes in the fall. One reason for the added enrollment was a new half-time licensed practical nursing degree program (LPN) inaugurated in December 1987. [18]

A new director of Mercy's school began in November 1989. Deanne M. Remer, a Mercy employee for 13 years, became Mercy's ninth director since 1922. Suzanne Mains became the new counselor and manager of financial aid services for the nursing school.

There is an old saying: "What goes around, comes around," and this is true for Mercy students of the 1990s. During the late 1960s and early 1970s, the trend was to abandon the regimentation of wearing nursing caps and uniforms. The 1990 freshman class were required to wear uniforms. With easily recognizable clothing, the students are identified as "professionals-in-training." Students opted to return to the former blue-and-white striped uniform similar to the pioneer Mercy students of 1899.

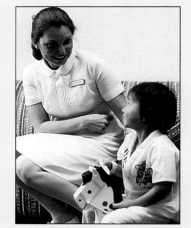

At the students' request, a capping ceremony similar to ceremonies of earlier times was begun again in 1991. Women students at the beginning of the second term received caps, and men were given a special pin. The ceremony utilized the candle and lamp symbols reminiscent of Florence Nightingale.

Beginning with the fall class in 1991, Mercy's school announced a revision of its three-year program into a two-year, five-semester educational track. This program, offered in conjunction with Des Moines Area Community College, allowed the student to graduate with an RN and an associate degree. Students have three options: an accelerated four-semester, plus one summer program (21 months) with a May

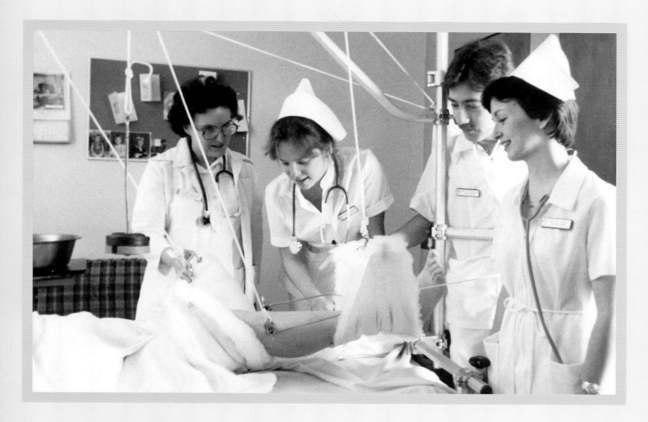

graduation; a traditional five-semester program with summers off (28 months) and a December graduation; or, a four-semester (three if challenge exams are successfully taken) advanced placement program for licensed practical nurses returning for completion of the RN program.

Mercy's total fall enrollment for 1992 reached 281 students, with three graduation ceremonies in 1993. Mercy's excellent record for passing state boards averaged 93.5 percent for the last five years, with two years at 100 percent. Attrition remains a high 91 percent, and for the last four years, all of Mercy's graduates found employment upon graduation. [19]

Over the years, Mercy's teachers blessed their students with the best educational guidance. One woman, M. Leona Sweeney, came to Mercy in 1944, and mentored Mercy's students for more than 40 years. A former student said of her: "Miss Sweeney...you could not ask for a more perfect role model. She was the epitome of what every nurse should be. She projected outstanding professionalism and caring." [20] Miss Sweeney, a Mercy graduate from Fort Dodge, Iowa, was given an honorary school of nursing diploma on the occasion of her retirement in 1986.

In June 1989, Mercy Hospital consolidated all of its educational training programs under the umbrella of the Mercy School of Health Sciences. The school of nursing joined with the schools of radiology, medical technology, perfusion, and the Mercy Regional Emergency Training Center. In addition to aiding the students and staff, a permanent location for the new school was selected, the former Midtown Motor Inn, across from the Mercy Court apartments at 928 Sixth Avenue.

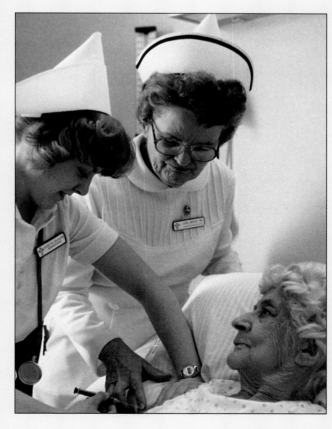

Students at Mercy's School of Nursing, *above*, benefit from the latest patient care technology. Leona Sweeney, *below*, an instructor in the school of nursing for over 40 years, was awarded with an honorary Mercy diploma upon her retirement in 1986.

Richard McCormick, SJ and Sister Seraphia, *below,* visit during a break in a medicine and ethics seminar held in September 1989. ☙ Sisters Concepta, Seraphia, and Therese share a happy moment on the occasion of Sister Concepta's 94th birthday, *below center.*

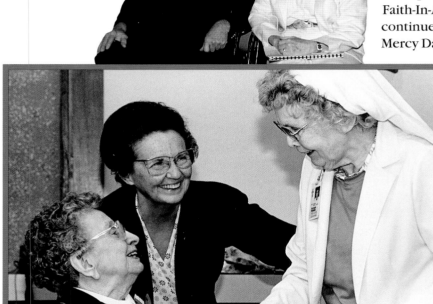

FOR THE DIGNITY OF LIFE AND DEATH

Mercy began addressing bioethical concerns during the late 1970s. The Sponsorship/Ethics Committee became the guidepost for creating Mercy's policies, under the direction of Sister Mary Seraphia McMahon. Sister Mary Seraphia McMahon was born Gertrude Marie McMahon in Chapman, Nebraska, where she and her two brothers and two sisters grew up on a farm.

When Gertrude graduated from high school, her parents wanted her to attend a Catholic college. She studied music education at the College of St. Mary in Omaha. There, she met the Sisters of Mercy: "happy, energetic women, who inspired me to join the order." She was given the name of Sister Mary Seraphia, and began teaching in Kansas City, Omaha, and Independence, Missouri. In 1966, she received a master's of music from Catholic University. In 1972, Sister Seraphia became head of the music department at the College of St. Mary. She came to Mercy in 1979 and worked in the public relations department.

In 1981, Sister Seraphia became Mercy's first sponsorship director. In this new role, she coordinated events and activities to influence the environment at Mercy and to support the mission and philosophy. Two new sponsorship committees evolved from the activities of the previous Faith-In-Action Committee: the Sponsorship Relational Committee continued former activities, such as the employee emergency relief fund, Mercy Day activities, and employee recognition celebrations; and the Sponsorship Ethics Committee examined the complex issues of formulating Mercy policies centered around moral choices in patient care.

The over-riding concern of the hospital to continue its quest for healing is rooted in its philosophy to "promote the dignity of persons and the right to quality life and death," says Sister Seraphia. Mercy believes that the decision to end a life must be in the hands of the patient, family and physicians, not the hospital. This works well for "the competent adult...but who speaks for the voiceless...[and] the newborn or the child? And who decides who shall speak?" [21] The total healthcare team is involved to help patients and their families make responsible, wise, and loving decisions."At Mercy the humanity of each individual is respected. Every decision for care and treatment is thoughtfully considered. We don't follow a 'cook book' recipe here. Each member of the patient's medical-care team has been sensitized to these bioethical considerations." [22]

A day-long Mercy conference was held in November 1991 to discuss critical issues regarding: fundamentals of ethical decision-making; resuscitation; legal issues relating to advance directives; trust as it relates to patients and healthcare providers; and balancing the benefits and burdens of technology. [23]

A few weeks after this conference, the Patient Self-Determination Act went into effect. This law required that hospital employees ask adult inpatients at the time of their admission if they have prepared documents outlining their healthcare wishes should they become unable to make their own decisions.

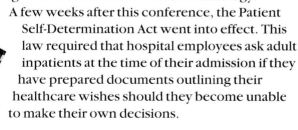

People Of VISION
1969-1993

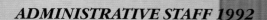

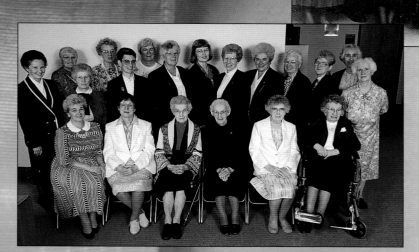

ADMINISTRATIVE STAFF 1992

Above, left to right:
Patricia McDermott
Richard Walsh
Sister Seraphia McMahon
Stephen Gleason, DO
Sara Drobnich
John Kolosky
Sister Patricia Clare Sullivan
William Bolin
Annette Bair
James Platt
Connie Brdicko
Carmela Brown

SISTERS SERVING MERCY HOSPITAL 1992

Above, standing left to right:
Seraphia McMahon, RSM
Mary Jane Hopkins, OSF
Alicia Gallagher, RSM
Peg O'Neill, OP
Valerie Natoli
Kathleen Doyle, OSB
Elaine Delaney, RSM
Carola Broderick, BVM
Mary Ann Burkhardt, RSM
Patricia Clare Sullivan, RSM
Joan LeBeau, CHM
Lucille Feehan, CHM
Mary Rocca, CHM
Kilian Clinton, RSM

Above, seated:
Carol Baum, BVM
Paula Radosevich, RSM
Mildred Ann Zaver, RSM
Zita Brennan, RSM
Therese Bannon, RSM
Concepta Mullins, RSM

Not pictured:
Josephine Collins, RSM
Carlotta Clinton, RSM
Monica Reichmuth, RSM
Genevieve Kordick, BVM

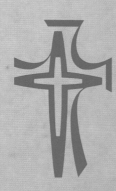

MERCY BOARD OF DIRECTORS, 1991 AND 1992 BOARD CHAIRS

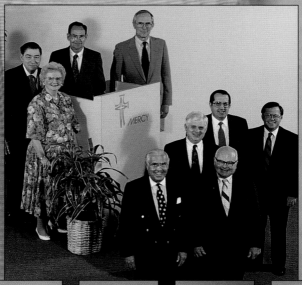

Stage left to right:
Paul From, MD
Lucille Knowles
Robert Drey
Charles Betts, Jr.

Front row floor:
Kenneth McCarthy
Gerald Jewett

Back row:
Clifford Swartz
Garland Carver
Stephen Southwick

Bottom left to right:
Dean Dutton
Robert Galligan
Thomas M. Brown, MD
William Krause
George Milligan
Dale Belknap
William Reed
Merlyn Johnson
Steven Berry, MD

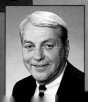
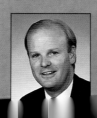
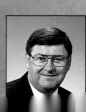

FROM THE SUN-KISSED HILL

Reflecting on Mercy Hospital's 100 years of healing service in Des Moines, there is no way to measure the bountiful nurturing and comforting care the Sisters of Mercy and their staff have unselfishly given. Day-by-day, they have reached out to help anyone in need. There is a specialness about this place, for an institution does not thrive or survive unless there are strong roots to support it. Imbedded deeply in healing soil, Mercy's roots were formed by a rare seed planted 185 years ago by Catherine McAuley. Sister Mary Frances Warde carried a tender branch of the fruits of that seed to America, and each Mercy founder who followed took a piece of the growth and planted it in countless missions throughout the United States. Mercy Hospital Medical Center in Des Moines is one of those special places, a blessing to Iowa. As we celebrate 100 years of healing, may God's grace continue to shine on "Those Who Come to Bless."

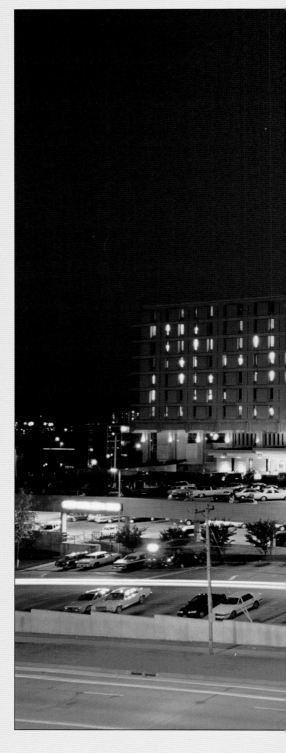

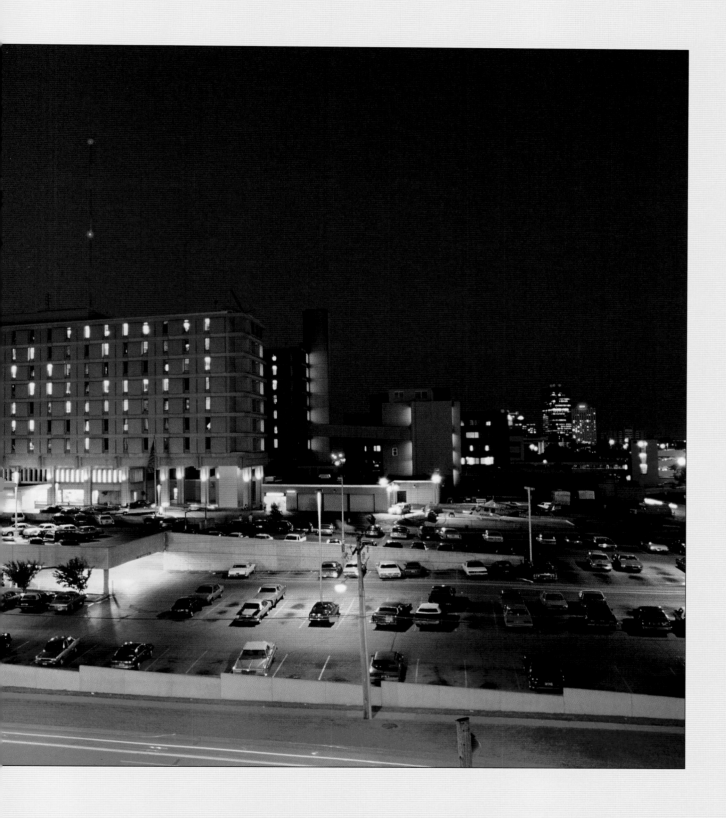

FOOTNOTES

SECTION I – Chapter 1 (pages 10-17)

1. The Union Historical Co., *The History of Polk County* (Des Moines: Iowa, Frank Mills & Co., 1880), 405.
2. Des Moines Mercy Hospital Abstracts. Thirty-eight years later Mercy began constructing its first building on this lot.
3. Jesse Griffith and Dwight Ogden, "St. Paul's Episcopal Church, One Hundredth Anniversary, 1854-1954," (n.p., 1954), 4.
4. Mercy Hospital Abstracts.
5. Certificate of Evidence, Polk County Circuit Court, 17 April 1885, 14.
6. Polk County Recorder's Office, Land Records, 106.13.
7. *Daily Iowa State Leader*, 13 February 1883, 4.
8. Polk County Recorder's Office, Land Records, 138.430.
9. *Daily Iowa State Leader*, 20 February 1883, 4.
10. Mercy Hospital Abstracts.

SECTION I – Chapter 2 (pages 18-21)

1. L. F. Andrews, *Pioneers of Polk County, Iowa and Reminiscences of Early Days*, vol. 1 (Des Moines: Baker-Trisler, Co., 1908), 39.
2. Ibid., 40.
3. Toner, Ex'r v. Collins et al., Brazill v. Toner et al (Iowa Supreme Court, October 1885).
4. *Daily State Leader*, 26 August 1885.
5. Ibid.
6. William L. Smith, "St. Mary's Church, 1867-1967," (Davenport, 1967), 48-9.
7. Madeleine M. Schmidt, CHM, *Seasons of Growth, History of the Diocese of Davenport, 1881-1981* (Davenport, Iowa: The Diocese of Davenport, 1981), 140.

SECTION I – Chapter 3 (pages 22-25)

1. M. Angela Bolster, RSM, *Catherine McAuley, Venerable for Mercy* (Dublin: Dominican Publications, 1990), 13.
2. Ibid.
3. *Letters of Catherine McAuley*, ed. M. Ignatia Neumann, RSM (Baltimore: Helicon Press, 1969), 18.
4. Bolster, 14.
5. Ibid, 28.
6. M. Beta Bauman, RSM, *A Way of Mercy* (New York: Vantage Press, 1958), 57.
7. Ibid., 7.
8. M. Joy Clough, RSM, *In Service to Chicago: The History of Mercy Hospital* (Chicago: Mercy Hospital and Medical Center, 1979), 15.
9. M. Magdalene Stransky, RSM, "Pioneers of Mercy in Iowa, Centennial History, 1869-1969, Mercy Hospital & Personnel", 1969, 2.
10. Board of Trustees and Historical Committee of the Iowa State Medical Society, *One Hundred Years of Iowa Medicine* (Iowa City, Iowa: Athens Press, 1950), 374.
11. Stransky, 65. The author documents other activities of the Sisters of Mercy in the Keokuk area at a later time. She writes that the Mercy sisters came to Keokuk again in 1896 to staff a hospital which was associated with the Keokuk College of Medicine.
12. M. Mark Kerin, RSM, *The Relief of Suffering Humanity, A Centennial History of Mercy Hospital, Davenport, Iowa* (Chicago: Saint Xavier College, 1969), 6-7.
13. Schmidt, 140.
14. Kerin, 5.
15. Ibid., 6-7.
16. *100 Years of Iowa Medicine*, 378.
17. M. Brigid Condon, RSM, "Obscurity to Distinction," (Iowa City, Iowa, 1993).
18. Kathleen O'Brien, RSM, *Journeys: A Pre-Amalgamation History of the Sisters of Mercy Omaha Province* (N.p., 1987), 404-08.
19. *Pioneer Healers: The History of Women Religious in American Health Care*, ed. Ursula Stepsis, CSA, and Dolores Liptak, RSM (New York: Crossroad, 1989), 8.

SECTION I – Chapter 4 (pages 26-29)

1. Robert Denny and LeRoy G. Pratt, "Highlights of Polk County History", 2nd section (Des Moines, Iowa: Polk County Historical Society, 1973), 4.
2. Ibid., 28.
3. Council of the Des Moines Academy of Medicine and Polk County Medical Society, *The History of Medicine of Polk County, Iowa* (N. p., 1951), 5.
4. *The History of Polk County*, 454-56.
5. *Daily State Register*, 17 September 1868, 1.
6. The site is near today's Midwest Energy Two Rivers Station.
7. *100 Years of Iowa Medicine*, 376.
8. Henry Hillaker, Iowa Climatologist, telephone interview 27 April 1989.
9. *Centennial History of Polk County, Iowa*, ed. J.M. Dixon (Des Moines, Iowa: State Register, 1876), 284.
10. *Daily Iowa State Register*, 12 January 1876, 4.
11. Ibid., 25 January 1876, 4.
12. Centennial History of Polk County, 284.
13. Bushnell's Des Moines City Directory, 1886-87, State Historical Society (SHS) microfilm, 100.
14. Polk County Office of the Assessor, land records.
15. *Daily State Leader*, 10 September 1877, 4.
16. *History of Medicine of Polk County*, 26.
17. St. Paul's Episcopal Church (Des Moines), Vestry Minutes, vol. 1.
18. Polk County Recorder's Office, Incorporations, 3.92.
19. *100 Years of Iowa Medicine*, 264.
20. Ibid., 383.
21. Edith M. Bjornstad, *Wings in Waiting* (Des Moines, Iowa: Des Moines Register and Tribune Co., 1952), 5.
22. *Des Moines Capital*, 18 June 1901, 7.
23. *Des Moines Daily News*, 11 September 1907.
24. Des Moines City Directory, 1892, SHS, microfilm, 56.

SECTION II – Chapter 1 (pages 30-37)

1. *Des Moines Leader*, 16 November 1893, 1.
2. O'Brien, 440-41.
3. *Des Moines Leader*, 18 November 1893, 8.
4. Iowa Department of Agriculture and Land Stewardship, State Climatologist Report, 8 December 1893.
5. Mercy Hospital Medical Staff Minutes, vol. 1, 2 December 1893.
6. *Des Moines Leader*, 16 November 1893, 1.
7. Schmidt, 140.
8. Kerin, 13.
9. *100 Years of Iowa Medicine*, 383.
10. *Des Moines Leader*, 28 November 1893.
11. M. Eulalia Herron, RSM, *The Sisters of Mercy in the United States, 1843-1928* (New York: MacMillan, 1929), 282.
12. Stransky, 48.
13. Iowa-Des Moines Community, box 4, Sisters of Mercy (SOM) Archives Omaha.
14. Mabel Trumm interview with the author, 2 October 1986.
15. Stransky, 73B.
16. Ibid.
17. Iowa Board of Nursing, Minutes 1907-30, State Archives of Iowa, box 1, vol. 1, 1.
18. Personnel file, SOM Archives Chicago.
19. Ibid.
20. Kerin, 15.
21. Personnel File, SOM Archives Chicago.
22. Necrology, SOM, Davenport, Iowa, Mercy Hospital, Davenport, Iowa.
23. DeWitt/Davenport Book of Chapters, box H11, SOM Archives Chicago.
24. Ibid.
25. *Des Moines Leader*, 11 February 1894, 8.
26. Personnel Records, SOM Archives Omaha.
27. O'Brien, 446.
28. Dorothy Smith interview for employee recognition, Des Moines, 1989.
29. Sister Anita Paul interview with the author, 26 June 1986.
30. Personnel file, Mercy Hospital Archives (MHA) Des Moines.
31. *Des Moines Sunday Register*, 30 November 1940.

SECTION II – Chapter 2 (pages 38-49)

1. *Iowa State Register*, 20 May 1894, 4.
2. Polk County Recorder's Office, Incorporations, 13.53.
3. Article of Agreement between Mercy Hospital Davenport and Mercy Hospital Des Moines, 30 June 1894, SOM Archives Chicago.
4. Isaac Hillis, Speech 23 April 1895, SOM Archives Omaha.
5. *Des Moines Leader*, 24 April 1895, 4.
6. *Iowa State Register*, 24 April 1895.
7. *Des Moines Leader*, 24 April 1895, 4.
8. Barclay, Daisie, Early history box, MHA.
9. *Daily Iowa Capital*, April 24 1895.
10. Annual Report of Mercy Hospital, Des Moines, January 1, 1896-January 1, 1897, MHA.
11. *Iowa State Register*, 24 April 1895.
12. Ibid.
13. Edwin B. Walson, "Progress and Reminiscences", Speech, 22 November 1949, MHA.
14. *Iowa State Register*, 24 April 1895, 6.
15. Corporation Book, Mercy Hospital, Davenport, 1898, SOM Archives Chicago.
16. Des Moines materials, 23 March 1898, f. 1., SOM Archives Chicago.
17. *Des Moines Daily News*, 15 November 1899.
18. Mercy Hospital Medical Staff Minutes, vol. 1, 8 April 1898.
19. Ibid.
20. *Des Moines Leader*, 18 June 1901, 5.
21. Mercy Hospital Medical Staff Minutes, vol. 1, 10 March 1901.
22. Barclay, Daisie.
23. Mercy Hospital Medical Staff Minutes, vol. 1, 12 January 1900.
24. Iowa Board of Nursing Minutes, vol. 1.
25. *Register and Leader*, 25 January 1908.
26. *100 Years of Iowa Medicine*, 466.
27. *Register and Leader*, 1 February 1914, 6.
28. *Evening Tribune*, 7 June 1918.
29. Ibid., 11 June 1918.
30. Ibid., 14 June 1918.
31. Ibid., 22 August 1918.
32. Ibid., 31 May 1918.
33. *Register*, 22 September 1918.
34. *Register*, 22 July 1920.
35. Ibid.
36. *Register*, 6 January 1921.
37. *Register*, 11 July 1921, 1.

SECTION II – Chapter 3 (pages 50-56)

1. Account journal, 1897-1903, MHA, 133.
2. Twelfth Census of the United States, Schedule No.1-Population, Polk County, Supervisor District 7, Ward 4, 13 June 1900, 156B-157A.
3. *Register and Leader*, 9 February, 3 March, 17 May, 29 August 1907.
4. *Des Moines Daily News*, 28 November 1902, 1.
5. Ibid., 16 December 1903, 1.
6. *Register and Leader*, 10 February 1905, 2.
7. Ibid., 5 February 1907, 6.
8. Ibid., 6, 8 and 11 February, 1907.
9. *Register and Leader*, 9 October 1907, 4.
10. Cosgrove to Flavin, 16 November 1900, Pre: 1912 Davenport papers, Catholic Diocesan Archives Des Moines.
11. Ibid., Kurtz to Cosgrove, 17 November 1900.
12. Mercy Hospital Medical Staff Minutes, 21 December 1900, 56.
13. Ibid., 58.
14. *Register and Leader*, 26 October 1907.
15. *Des Moines Tribune*, 25 January 1909, 3.
16. Charles J. Ritchey, *Drake University Through Seventy-five Years* (Des Moines: Drake University 1956), 78.
17. *Register and Leader*, 25 November 1909.
18. *100 Years of Iowa Medicine*, 390.

SECTION II – Chapter 4 (pages 57-65)

1. Barbara B. Long, *Des Moines and Polk County: Flag on the Prarie*, Windsor Publications, Inc., 1988, 71.
2. *Register and Leader*, 26 December 1909.
3. Ibid., 10 November 1912.
4. Ibid., 14 May 1912, 3.
5. Ibid., 8 May 1912, 10.
6. Polk County Recorder's Office, Land Records, 601.550 and 601.557-58.
7. *Register and Leader*, 15 December 1912.
8. Sister Dorothy Flaherty interview with the author, 12 June 1986.
9. *Register and Leader*, 21 August 1913.
10. Ibid., 23 January 1914.
11. Dr. Daniel A. Glomset interview with the author, 30 June 1986.
12. *Register and Leader*, 21 August 1913.
13. Ibid.
14. Ibid., 4 April 1913.
15. Polk Room Log Book, MHA.
16. *Register and Leader*, 8 October 1914.
17. Flaherty interview, 26 March 1986.
18. *Flag on the Prarie*, 71.
19. Sister Sebastian Geneser interview with the author, 5 February 1986.
20. *Des Moines Register*, 14 October 1918.
21. Flaherty interview, 12 June 1986.
22. Sister DeLourdes Hardiman interview with the author, 14 October 1987.
23. Flaherty interview, 26 March 1986.
24. "Brief Sketch of Connection between Mercy Hospital Davenport, Iowa and Mercy Hospital Des Moines, Iowa," enclosure with letter between Mercedes and Bonzano, 5 May 1915, Des Moines Community, SOM Archives Chicago.
25. Dowling to Bonzano, c.a. January 1916, SOM Archives Omaha.
26. "Brief Sketch."
27. Ibid.
28. Ibid.
29. Dowling to M. Aloysia McLaughlin, 23 April 1915, Des Moines Community, SOM Chicago.
30. Dowling to Bonzano, c.a. January 1916.
31. Ibid.
32. Bonzano to Aloysia, 16 July 1915, SOM Archives Chicago.
33. Dowling to Mercedes, 9 October 1915, SOM Archives Chicago.
34. Sharon to Sullivan, 11 November 1915, SOM Archives Chicago.
35. Sullivan to Sharon, 9 November 1915, SOM Archives Chicago.
36. Sharon to MacArthur, 11 November 1915, SOM Archives Chicago.
37. MacArthur to Sharon, 23 November 1915, SOM Archives Chicago.
38. Mercedes to Bonzano, 15 January 1916, SOM Archives Chicago.
39. Dowling to Mercedes, 16 February 1916, SOM Archives Chicago.
40. Dowling to Mercedes, 28 February 1916, SOM Archives Chicago.
41. Bonzano to Mercedes 30 March 1916, SOM Archives Chicago.
42. Dowling to Mercedes, 1 June 1916, SOM Archives Chicago.
43. Bank receipt, 8 November 1916, SOM Archives Chicago.

SECTION II – Chapter 5 (pages 66-69)

1. Personnel file, MHA, Des Moines.
2. Flaherty interview, 26 March 1986.
3. Sister Philomena Crock interview with Sister Cecelia Mary Barry, 4 October 1974, SOM Archives Omaha.
4. Sister Cecelia Mary Barry research notes on Iowa City transfers to Des Moines, SOM Archives Omaha.
5. Personnel files, SOM Archives Chicago.
6. Barry research notes.
7. Personnel files, SOM Archives Omaha.
8. Ibid.
9. Barry notes on Des Moines Community, Branch house to 1916, SOM Archives Omaha.
10. Index to St. Ambrose Cemetery, Des Moines, WPA project, State Archives.
11. Flaherty interview, 26 March 1986.

SECTION II – Chapter 6 (pages 70-73)

1. *Des Moines Tribune*, 28 December 1921.
2. Priestley to Drumm, telegram, 28 December 1921, Episcopal correspondence, Catholic Diocesan Archives Des Moines.
3. Drumm to Bonzano, 1 January 1922, Sister Cecelia Mary Barry notebook on research trip to Catholic Diocesan Archives Des Moines, 1 April 1969, SOM Archives Omaha.
4. Report on Investigation by John Mahony & Co., 1 January 1922 to 31 July 1922, Important Documents, MHA.
5. Drumm to Sisters of Mercy Convent, Des Moines, 12 January 1922, SOM Archives Omaha.
6. Des Moines, Sisters of Mercy Hospital, Internal Affairs, 1893-1924, SOM Archives Omaha.
7. Drumm to Sisters, 12 January 1922.
8. Ibid.
9. In a handwritten note in the letter referred to above, Drumm indicated there were eleven sisters in the room. There were twelve sisters in residence, so the bishop miscounted, or left someone out of the count.
10. Drumm to Sisters, 12 January 1922.
11. Eva Proulx to the author, 20 February 1988, MHA.
12. Proulx to Greiner, 6 March 1989, MHA.
13. Ibid.
14. Drumm to Bonzano, 20 February 1922, Barry notebook, SOM Archives Omaha.
15. Proulx, 20 February 1988.
16. Ibid.
17. *Journeys*, 465.
18. Ibid.
19. St. Gabriel's Monastery, Chronicle, 1914, vol. 1, 30, Passionist Order Community Archives Chicago.
20. Ibid.
21. Mother Bonaventure Carroll to Drumm, 3 June 1922, SOM Archives Omaha.

SECTION III – Chapter 1 (pages 74-83)

1. Important Documents, 1923, MHA.
2. Sister Concepta Mullins interview with the author 4 February 1986, MHA.
3. "The Push for Standardization, The Origins of the Catholic Hospital Association, 1914-1920," by Christopher J. Kauffman, *Health Progress*, January-February 1990, p. 57.
4. Mercy Hospital Medical Staff Minutes, vol. 2, 7 December 1920.
5. Ibid., 7 February 1922.
6. Sister Joseph Munch interview with the author 21 March 1986, MHA.
7. Ibid.
8. Lee Aldera interview with the author, 12 March 1991, MHA.
9. *Register and Leader*, 23 November 1923.
10. *Des Moines Tribune*, 2 April 1924.
11. "The Push for Standardization", 57.
12. Brochure printed in honor of National Hospital Day, Scrapbook collection, MHA.
13. *Des Moines Tribune*, 4 April 1929.
14. School of Nursing, Health Survery and Reports, 1927-1946, MHA.
15. Mercy Hospital Medical Staff Minutes, vol. 2, 6 October 1925.
16. Louise Brady interview with the author, 13 March 1991.
17. Personnel files, SOM Archives Omaha.
18. Mercy Hospital Medical Staff Minutes, vol. 2, 8 November and 6 December 1927.
19. Ibid., 6 December 1927.
20. *Des Moines Tribune*, 7 November 1924.
21. Ibid., 3 April 1925.
22. Mercy Hospital Medical Staff Minutes, vol. 2, 7 November 1928.
23. Peggy Albertson interview with the author 15 March 1991.
24. *Des Moines Tribune*, 4 April 1929.
25. School of Nursing, Miscellaneous reports, 1930s and 1940s, 11 January 1927, MHA.
26. Personnel files, SOM Archives Omaha.
27. Ibid.
28. Autobiography, Sister Joseph Munch, MHA.
29. Sister Joseph interview, 4 April 1986.
30. Tribute to Sister Joseph on the occasion of her 60th Jubilee as a Sister of Mercy, 28 August 1982, MHA.
31. Personnel files, MHA.
32. Remarks by Sister Patricia Clare at Sister Joseph's funeral, 25 September 1987, MHA.
33. "The Push for Standardization," 57.
34. *Des Moines Tribune*, 11 May 1926.
35. *Des Moines Register*, 12 May 1938, 9.
36. *Des Moines Tribune*, 13 October 1926.
37. "Sixth Annual Convention of the Iowa Hospital Association," 13-14 October 1926, Conference program, MHA.
38. *Flag on the Prarie*, 73.

SECTION III – Chapter 2 (pages 84-95)

1. *Pioneer Healers*, 139.
2. "The Push for Standardization", 31.
3. *Des Moines Register*, 26 January 1926.
4. Bishop Drumm Home for the Age thrived at this location until 1980 when the home was moved to Johnston, Iowa on the northwestern edge of Des Moines. This Clark Street facility was to have another life as the House of Mercy opened in 1987.
5. Dr. James Chambers interview with the author 28 November 1990.
6. Monsignor John McIlhon interview with the author 12 November 1990.
7. *Wings in Waiting*, 106.
8. Agnes Hardin interview with the author 21 February 1989.
9. Hardin interview, 23 February 1989.
10. *Des Moines Tribune*, 26 March 1930.
11. Ibid., 31 January 1930.
12. Ibid., 30 December 1930.
13. Sister Kevin O'Sullivan letter to the author 9 December 1990.
14. Chambers interview.
15. Kay Hardie interview with the author 24 February 1992.
16. Sister Concepta interview.
17. Ibid.
18. Hardin interview, 21 February 1989.
19. Ona Lorey interview with the author 11 March 1991.
20. *Mercy Hospital Bulletin*, 9 May 1975.

21. Sister Concepta interview.
22. Ibid.
23. Mercy Hospital statistics during those years, MHA.
24. *Des Moines Register*, 24 December 1935.
25. Mercy Medical Staff Minutes, 9 February 1937.
26. McIlhon interview.
27. James Heles interview with the author, 23 April 1991.
28. Executive Committee, Mercy Hospital Medical Staff, 4 April 1933.
29. Combined memories from interviews with Drs. Chambers, Crowley, and Monsignor Conley.
30. Monsignor Raymond Conley, "Bishop Drumm, a Man of Charity," *Jubilee of Faith, 75th Anniversary Diocese of Des Moines, 1911-1986*, 68.
31. Sister Joseph Munch interview with the author 21 March 1986.
32. *Jubilee of Faith*, 28.
33. *Des Moines Register*, 3-4-5 June 1935.
34. Ibid., 3-4-5 June 1936.
35. *Des Moines Tribune*, 2-3-June 1937-38.
36. *Des Moines Register*, 13 May 1938.
37. Ibid., 15 June 1937.
38. Ibid., 28 June 1937.
39. Ibid., 16 January 1938.
40. Unidentified newsclipping, c.a. November 1939, Scrapbook collection, Red scrapbook, 19, MHA.
41. Ibid., 18.
42. Albertson interview.
43. Kay Hardie letter to the author 24 February 1992.
44. Mercy Hospital Medical Staff Minutes 9 February 1937.
45. Alexander R. Griffin, *Out of Carnage*, (New York: Howell, Soskin), 1945, 110.
46. Chambers interview.
47. *Wings in Waiting*, 127.
48. *Des Moines Register*, 6 May 1937.
49. Lucy McLaughlin interview with the author 23 April 1991.
50. Dr. Daniel Crowley, Jr. interview with the author 11 November 1990.
51. McIlhon interview.
52. Sister Laurne Weinandt, St. Mary's Hospital, letter to the author 15 May 1991.
53. McIlhon interview.
54. Pete Markunas was honored in 1956 for forty years of Mercy service.
55. Mercy Hospital Medical Staff Minutes 7 November 1939.
56. Chambers interview.
57. "The Push for Standardization," 31.
58. Hardie interview.

SECTION III – Chapter 3 (pages 96-103)

1. *100 Years of Iowa Medicine*, 440.
2. Unidentified newsclipping, "The Ideal Scrapbook," 38, Scrapbook collection, MHA.
3. *100 Years of Iowa Medicine*, 441.
4. Dr. Frederick Katzmann interview with the author 10 December 1990.
5. Ibid.
6. Ibid.
7. *Des Moines Register*, 22 September 1943 and 11 January 1944.
8. Sister Sebastian interview 26 February 1986.
9. Mary McCoy interview with the author 27 June 1986.
10. *Des Moines Tribune*, 23 June 1942.
11. Unidentified newsclipping, c.a. 1942, Scrapbook collection, MHA.
12. Mercy Hospital Medical Staff Minutes, 4 March 1941.
13. Ibid., 18 December 1944.
14. Katzmann interview.
15. McCoy interview.
16. Sister Mary Anita Paul interview with the author 26 June 1986.
17. Barbara Paul, "Women in Administration," 1979, 3, Sister Anita file, MHA.
18. Ibid., 4.
19. Crowley interview.
20. *Des Moines Tribune*, 12 April 1959.
21. *Mercy Bulletin*, 11 May 1979.
22. *Des Moines Register*, 14 December 1944.
23. Administrative correspondence regarding the Nurses' Home, Administration files, 1940s, box 4 microfilm, MHA.
24. Ibid.
25. *Des Moines Register*, 2 July 1945.
26. *The Catholic Messenger*, 28 June 1946, sec. 2.
27. Ibid.
28. Ibid.
29. Mercy Medical Staff Minutes 6 June 1944.
30. Chambers interview.
31. Ibid.
32. Crowley interview.
33. Mercy Hospital 1956 Advisory Board, Iowa-Des Moines collection, folder 17, SOM Archives Omaha.

SECTION III – Chapter 4 (pages 104-117)

1. Aldera interview
2. Ibid.
3. Report of Survey, Mercy Hospital Des Moines, 11 January 1927, School of Nursing Miscellaneous reports, 1930s and 1940s, MHA.
4. Mildred Walker interview with the author 12 March 1991.
5. Aldera interview
6. Ibid.
7. Walker interview.
8. Aldera interview.
9. Ona Lorey interview with the author 11 March 1991.
10. Lucille Glas interview with the author 15 March 1991.
11. Aldera interview.
12. Ibid.
13. *Journeys*, 425-26.
14. Marie Bloomquist interview with the author 18 April 1991.
15. Walker interview.
16. Bloomquist interview.
17. Brady interview.
18. Class Roll Log 1932, School of Nursing Log Books, MHA.
19. Glas interview.
20. Ibid.
21. Bloomquist interview.
22. Eveyln Tidrick telephone interview with the author 26 April 1991.
23. Student files, School of Nursing, MHA.
24. Chambers interview.
25. Bloomquist interview.
26. Teresina Bartolomei telephone interview with the author 2 May 1991.
27. Albertson interview.
28. Bloomquist interview.
29. Unidentified newsclipping, c.a. 1943, "The Ideal Scrapbook," 50B, Scrapbook collection, MHA.
30. Albertson interview.
31. *The Catholic Messenger*, 28 June 1946.
32. Sister Sebastian Geneser telephone interview 2 May 1991.
33. *The Catholic Messenger*, 28 June 1946.
34. Ibid., 1.
35. Ibid., 5.
36. "The Ideal Scrapbook," 13, Scrapbook collection, MHA.
37. *The Catholic Messenger*, 28 June 1946.
38. Ibid.
39. Brady interview.
40. Ibid.

SECTION III – Chapter 5 (pages 118-121)

1. Conley interview.
2. Mary Northup interview with the author 6 October 1986.
3. Katzmann interview.
4. Northup interview.
5. Brady interview.
6. Betty Hammes telephone interview with the author 10 May 1991.
7. Molly Hewitt interview with the author 8 May 1991.
8. Hammes interview.
9. Frieda Steele telephone interview with the author September 1992.
10. Chambers interview.
11. Ibid.
12. Crowley interview.
13. Personnel files, SOM Archives Omaha.

SECTION IV – Chapter 1 (pages 122-133)

1. *Mercy News*, 15 December 1947.
2. Ibid., September 1959.
3. Mercy Hospital Advisory Board Minutes, 18 February 1964.
4. Dr. Roy Overton interview with the author 8 October 1991.
5. Sister Kieran Harney letter to the author 18 September 1991.
6. Ibid.
7. Ibid.
8. *Mercy News*, May 1956.
9. Ibid., September 1956.
10. Ibid., December 1956.
11. Sister Patricia Clare Sullivan interview with the author 27 December 1991.
12. Hardie interview.
13. Dr. Noble Irving letter to the author November 1991.
14. Lucie Kelly, *Dimensions of Professional Nursing*, Macmillan Publishing Co., 1985, 63.
15. Sister Kieran letter.
16. *Des Moines Register*, 9 February 1964.
17. Overton interview.
18. Ibid.
19. Hardie interview.
20. Dr. Julius Conner interview with the author 26 November 1991.
21. Evelyn McClure interview with the author August 1992.
22. Mercy Hospital Advisory Board Minutes, 24 March 1954.
23. Ibid., 22 September 1953.
24. Ibid., 19 January 1954.
25. These statistics were accurate from 1921. Records from before then are nonexistent.
26. Facts and Statistical Information for Mercy Hospital Building Fund, Public Relation 1950s information, MHA.
27. Mercy Hospital Advisory Board Minutes, 16 February 1954.
28. Sister Zita Brennan interview with the author May 1992.
29. *Mercy News*, December–January 1958.
30. *Mercy Bulletin*, 16 July 1965.
31. *Des Moines Tribune*, 15 November 1960.
32. Dr. Conner interview.
33. Dr. John Bakody interview with the author 15 October 1991.
34. Mercy Hospital Advisory Board Minutes, 23 February 1956.
35. *Mercy News*, September 1959.

SECTION IV – Chapter 2 (pages 134-147)

1. Bishop Edward Daly letter to Arthur Gormley April 1955, MHA.
2. *Mercy News*, January 1956.
3. Final Service Report to Advisory Board and Sisters of Mercy, 14 June 1955, Public Relations 1950s information, MHA.
4. *Mercy News*, Special Dedication Issue, April 1959.
5. *Des Moines Register*, 11 April 1959.
6. Mercy Hospital Advisory Board Minutes, 15 September 1959.
7. *Mercy News*, April 1959.
8. *Des Moines Tribune*, Saturday edition, 12 January 1963.
9. Betsey Schoeller telephone interview with the author 22 April 1992.
10. Bakody interview.
11. Barbara Walters telephone interview with the author 21 April 1992.
12. Personnel File, MHA
13. *Mercy News*, September 1959.
14. *Des Moines Tribune*, 23 May 1962.
15. *Mercy News*, April 1959.
16. *Mercy Bulletin*, 11 March 1960.
17. Ibid., 22 April 1960.
18. Report of the operation of Mercy Hospital, Des Moines, 1 May 1959-30 April 1960, to the Board of Directors of the corporation of the Sisters of Mercy of Council Bluffs, Iowa, microfilm, Administration 1960s and 1970s, MHA.
19. *Mercy Bulletin*, 11 June 1965.
20. Convent archives, black scrapbook dated to 1962, 5, MHA.
21. Eileen Lex interview with the author September 1992.
22. *Mercy News*, July 1959.
23. *Des Moines Reigster*, editorial, 25 November 1964.

SECTION IV – Chapter 3 (pages 148-155)

1. *History and Trends of Professional Nursing*, Seventh Edition, Gerald J. Griffin and Joanne Griffin, St. Louis: C.V. Mosby Company, 1973, 143-44.
2. Mercy Hospital Advisory Board Minutes, 11 August 1948.
3. National League for Nursing Accreditation Reports, 10, School of Nursing, MHA.
4. *Des Moines Register*, 20 November 1949.
5. Barbara Paul letter to the author 16 June 1992.
6. Judy Eldredge interview with the author 12 December 1991.
7. Ronald Caulk letter to the author 20 January 1991.
8. Eldredge interview.
9. Caulk interview.
10. State Board of Nurse Examiners, State Office Building, Des Moines, 13 January 1954, Report of visit to Mercy Hospital, SHS Archives.
11. Report of a survey of Mercy Hospital School of Nursing, Des Moines, Iowa, 5-7 April 1954, 5, SHS Archives.
12. Broadlawns Hospital was the other.
13. Judy Eldredge interview.
14. *Mercy News*, December 1964.
15. Mary Pearce telephone interview with the author 2 January 1992.
16. Pat Spurlock telephone interview with the author 30 December 1991.

SECTION IV – Chapter 4 (pages 156-167)

1. *Des Moines Register*, 3 December 1961.
2. Don Conroy letter to Mother Mary Baptista, 16 April 1962, microfilm, Administration 1960s and 1970s, MHA.
3. *Des Moines Tribune*, 17 April 1965.
4. *The Catholic Messenger*, 24 June 1960, sec. 2, 7.
5. *Mercy Bulletin*, 30 September 1960.
6. Sister Francis Hunt, paper presented to the Health Division of the Council of Social Agencies, 11 December 1962, MHA.
7. *Mercy News*, June 1965.
8. Ibid., March 1965.
9. Convent archives, Scrapbook, December 1962- 25 March 1964, 44, MHA.
10. Molly Hewitt interview with the author 16 August 1991.
11. Karen Goodman telephone interview with the author 19 May 1992.
12. Generalate quarterly, 29-2, 1960, 39.
13. Sister Francis Hunt presentation.
14. *Des Moines Sunday Register*, 11 August 1963, 21.
15. Ibid., 27 September 1964.
16. The Sisters of Mercy of the Des Moines Diocese, booklet, c.a. 1928, SOM booklets box, MHA.
17. Sister Eileen Moore interview with the author 1 March 1992.
18. Ibid.
19. *The Catholic Messenger*, 1 September 1966.
20. Convent archives, Items of Interest to Mercy Hospital Scrapbook, 1912-1963, 141.
21. *Mercy News*, March 1960.
22. Convent archives, Scrapbook 1963-25 March 1964, 14 May 1962, 151.
23. *Mercy Bulletin*, 13 December 1968.
24. *Des Moines Register*, 14 April 1968, 3-W.
25. *Mercy News*, March 1969.

SECTION V – Chapter 1 (pages 168-183)

1. *Des Moines Register*, 30 March 1971.
2. *Mercy Bulletin*, 10 September 1976.
3. Ibid., 5 March 1976.
4. *Mercy Journal*, 11 October 1978.
5. Administrative group interview with the author 13 August 1992.
6. Robert Williams, Kay Wright, and Evelyn McClure, "Mercy Our Computer Center, An Integrated Service," February 1974, MHA.
7. *Mercy Annual Report* January 1974.
8. Sara Drobnich interview with the author 13 August 1992.
9. *Mercy Bulletin* 1 April 1977.
10. *Mercy News*, September 1970.
11. Eulogy of Sister Charles by Sister Patricia Clare 19 December 1990.
12. Sister Charles Keane interview with the author 14 April 1986.
13. *Mercy Bulletin* 22 May 1970.
14. Ibid., Special Report, 2 April 1976.
15. Dr. Paul From interview with the author 4 December 1991.
16. *Mercy Bulletin*, 10 September 1976.
17. Pat Meintel letter to the author 3 March 1992.
18. Sandy Caligiuri interview with the author 4 August 1992.
19. *Mercy Bulletin* 22 April 1977.

SECTION V – Chapter 2 (pages 184-191)

1. *Register and Leader* 25 June 1905.
2. Ibid., 17 September 1924.
3. Mercy Medical Staff Minutes, 1933-1947.
4. Chambers interview.
5. *Mercy News*, December 1967.
6. *Mercy Journal*, February and March 1982.
7. Ibid., August-September 1982.
8. *Mercy Bulletin*, 18 December 1986.
9. Ibid., 11 February 1983.
10. Sister Patricia Clare interview with the author 13 August 1992.
11. *Mercy Bulletin* 20 May 1983.
12. Ibid., 18 January 1990.
13. Ibid., 26 May 1988.

SECTION V – Chapter 3 (pages 192-195)

1. *Mercy News* April 1956.
2. Ibid., December 1956.
3. *Mercy Bulletin* 17 December 1965.
4. *Mercy News*, October 1968.
5. Ibid., January-February 1973.
6. Dr. Harrison Pratt telephone interview 19 August 1992.
7. *Mercy Bulletin*, 10 May 1974.
8. Ibid., 26 March 1976.
9. *Mercy Journal*, October 1988.
10. *Mercy Bulletin*, 23 January 1986.
11. *Mercy Journal*, January 1987.
12. *Mercy Bulletin* 22 November 1985.

SECTION V – Chapter 4 (pages 206-215)

1. Mercy Guild Twentieth anniversary brochure, Guild 40 years of History box, MHA.
2. Mercy Guild Third Annual Report, 1951-52, Guild 40 years of History box, MHA.
3. *South Des Moines Messenger and News*, 2 March 1961, 2, Convent Archives, 1948-62.
4. Mary Pearce interview with the author 17 October 1991.
5. Al (Babe) Bisignano interview with the author 22 April 1991.
6. Mary Pearce interview.
7. Rosemary Avise interview with the author 26 November 1991.
8. Sister Zita Brennan letter undated c.a. 1955, Guild Scrapbook, 1953-54, MHA.
9. Mary Northup interview.
10. Mary Bryant telephone interview 10 November 1991.
11. Vera McKeone telephone interview 21 May 1992.
12. Dolores Hogan (Roe) interview with the author 6 May 1992.
13. *Mercy Bulletin*, 19 October 1973.
14. Ibid., 27 June 1975.
15. *Mercy Annual Report*, 1981.
16. Rosemary Avise interview.

SECTION V – Chapter 5 (pages 206- 233)

1. *Mercy Bulletin*, 12 October 1984.
2. Ibid., 18 October 1985.
3. Sister Patricia Clare Sullivan interview with the author 27 December 1991.
4. Ibid.
5. Ibid.
6. Sandy Caliguiri interview with the author 20 April 1992.
7. Sister Patricia Clare interview.
8. Ibid.
9. Joe Burke interview with the author 16 September 1992.
10. Comparative Analysis Report, Mercy Hospital Medical Center, Medical Records Department.
11. Connie McFarlin telephone interview with the author 24 August 1992.
12. *Mercy Bulletin*, 6 January 1984.
13. Ibid., 2 July 1981.
14. Mary Jones telephone interview with the author 14 September 1992.
15. *Mercy Bulletin*, 7 June 1990.
16. Ibid., 20 February 1981.
17. Ibid., 2 July 1981.
18. Ibid., 30 April 1987.
19. Program Data, Mercy School of Nursing, August 1992.
20. Sara Drobnich telephone interview with the author 17 August 1992.
21. Dr. John Bakody, *Mercy Journal*, October 1984.
22. Ibid.
23. *Mercy Bulletin*, 27 November 1991.
24. Ibid., 12 December 1991.

LEGEND

State Historical Society of Iowa (SHS)

Sisters of Mercy (SOM)

Mercy Hospital Archives (MHA)

INDEX

A

Abbott's Alley, 125
Abbott, Walter, 91, 115, 124-26, 140, 155, 164, 206
Abricka, Veronica, 129,
Accreditation, 93-94, 147
Adventureland Park, 181
Aggers, Ruby, 167
AIDS, 225
Air-conditioning, 140, 153, 159
Akaydin, Vicean, 133
Alberts, Jeannette, 211, 213
Alberts, M.E., 155, 166
Albertson, Margaret, 92
Albia, IA,
  Monroe County Hospital, 221
Aldera, Lee, 105
Alvarado, Virginia, 133
Amalgamation, 71, 73, 76-77, 83
American Cancer Society, 148, 192-93
American College of Surgeons, 80, 85, 93-94, 193, 195
American Heart Association, 184
American Hospital Association, 95, 146, 215
American Journal of Nursing, 107
American Legion Auxiliary, 148
American Medical Association, 85, 91, 131, 183
American Red Cross, 48, 49, 73, 97
American Registry of Radiologic Technologists, 162
American Society of Clinical Pathologists, 146
Amphitheater, 42-43, 45
Ancient Order of Hibernians, 40
Anderson, H. N., 91-92, 102, 115
Anderson, Kenneth, P., 226
Anesthetics, 41, 89, 91, 102, 125
Appelquist, Mrs. F.G., 167
Archbishop Bergan Mercy Hospital.
  See Bergan Mercy Hospital
Ascension Street, 130, 137
Atomic Energy Commission, 127
Augspurger, Byron, 226
Avertin, 91
Avise, Rosemary, 209, 213, 215

B

Baby boom, 127, 130-31, 223,
Baggot Street, 23-24
Bahamas, 188
Bair, Annette, 176, 226, 231
Bakody, John, 132, 155, 177
Banker's Trust Company, 98
Barclay, Dasie, 47-48
Barnard, Christiaan, 187
Barnes, Bernard, 89, 91, 115, 124, 155
Barnum, P.T., 28
Baum, Carol, 231
Baum, Marjorie, 213
Beem, Adelbert, 210
Belknap, Dale, 231
Benedict Home, 85
Bennett, M. Magdalen, 27
Bergan, Bp. Gerald, 83, 89, 99, 101-02, 114-15, 127, 167
Bergan Mercy Hospital, 144, 163, 178, 219
Berry, Steven, 226
Betensky, Nathan, 181
Betts, Charles, Jr., 231
Bierring, Walter, 91, 184
Biondi, Angela, 104
Biopsy, 193
Bishop Drumm Home, 55, 84, 95, 157
Bishop Drumm Retirement Center, 150, 221
Bisignano, Babe, 121, 209
Bisignano, Catherine, 209
Biskup, Bp. George J., 146-47, 166
Blackmer, Margaret, 112
Blanchard, Mabel, 209
Bleadorn, Perry, 177
Blessman, James, 22,
Blood bank, 81, 98, 144
Blood transfusion, 79, 91
Bloomquist, Marie (Jones), 111, 133, 172
Blue Cross, 89, 178
Boatmen's National Bank, 219
Boesen, Mr. and Mrs. T.L., 208
Bolin, William, 231
Bolton Act, 99
Bolton, Frances, 112
Bonaventure Carroll. See Carroll, M. Bonaventure
Bonzano, Archbp. John, 64, 65, 70-71
Borromeo Johnson. See Johnson, M. Borromeo
Boss, E.A., 166
Brady, Louise, 78, 164, 173
Brain surgery, 91
Brandstetter, Rosemary, 176
Branton, G.Ralph, 101-03, 127, 206
Brazill, Rev. John F., 12, 14-15, 18-21, 25, 27, 32, 42, 64
Brdicko, Connie, 231
Brennan Family Center, 222
Brien family, 89
Broadlawns Hospital, 55, 83, 85, 99, 107
Broderick, Carola, 231
Broekens, Douwe, 133
Brooks, Borg, and Skiles, 130, 161
Brooks, J.Woolson, 102-03, 130, 166
Brooks, Thomas K., 26
Brown, Carmela, 231
Brown, Thomas M., 226, 231
Bryant, Mary, 211
Bryant, Paula, 213
Buckley, E.F., 102-03
Bucknell, Earl, 166
Bullock, Bp, William, 215, 218
Burch, Mabel, 140
Burcham, Thomas, 126
Byrnie, Kathryn, 111

C

Cacciatore, Mary, 213
Cadet Nursing Program, 99, 112-114
Caesareans, 91
Calingasan, Eufrocina, 133
Callaghan, William, 23
Callahan, Catherine, 149-50
Callanan College, 54
Cameron, Leah C., 94
Camp Dodge, 62
Campbell, Robert, 176
Cancer, 57, 77, 85, 192-95
Candystripers, 127, 164, 210
Cantwell, A.W., 40
Capital City Brick & Pipe Company, 42, 60
Cardiac, 184-191
Carroll, Frank, 211
Carroll, M. Bonaventure, 73, 76, 118
Carver, Garland, 231
Cataracts, 91
Caterine, James, 226
Catgut, 125
Catheterizations, cardiac, 186-87
Catholic Charities, 116
Catholic Health Corperation, 179
Catholic Hospital Association, 68, 83, 95, 146, 163, 219-220
Catholic University, 154,178, 180, 230
Catholic Women's League, 84
Caulk, Ronald, 151
Cavanaugh, Jackie, 209
Centerville, IA,
  St. Joseph's Mercy Hospital, 25, 77, 81, 87, 106, 110, 119, 157, 178, 219, 221
    Central Wing, 42-43, 45, 49, 54, 57-59, 100, 120, 130, 139-40, 142, 145, 151, 158-61, 170-71, 184-85, 109, 222
Chabot, Kaye, 212
Chambers, James, 93, 124-25, 155, 166, 184
Chandramouli, B., 191
Chaplains, 41, 56, 89, 103, 141, 146, 157, 166, 173
Chase, Virginia, 213
Chemotherapy, 195
Chicago & Great Western Railroad, 40
Chicago & Northwestern Railroad, 51
Chicago, IL,
  Sisters of Mercy, 24
Chiropractors, 85
Chloroform, 41
Cholera, 24, 26, 34
Christ Child Home, 116
Civil War, 24, 34
Clark, M. Maura, 171
Clark, Miss, 106
Clark Street House of Mercy, 55, 218, 220,
Clarkson Memorial Hospital, 118
Clarkson, J.S., 14-15, 19, 27
Clausen, Leila, 112-13
Clemens, Albert, 226
Clifford, M. Clare, 163
Clinton, M. Xavier, 106, 163
Coal mining, 19, 50, 51
Codeine, 47
Cokenower, James W., 33, 40
Coleman, Frank, 98, 101, 125, 132-33, 146, 155, 192, 206
College of Osteopathic Medicine and Surgery, 178, 183
College of St. Mary, Omaha, NE, 178, 180, 230
Collins, Harry, 102, 115, 184
Collins, Lizzie, 14, 19
Collins, Myles, 14
Colombia, 189
Comfort, Frank, 64
Comfort, George P., 213
Comfort, Marie, 213, 216-17
Comfort, Mrs. George, 166
Condon, J.R., 115
Conkling, W.S., 51, 184
Conley, Rev. Raymond, 89, 103
Connell, John, 125
Connelly, Rev. Paul, 146
Conner, Julius, 132-33
Connolly, John, Jr., 157
Connolly, Patricia, 127,
Connolly, Rev. Lloyd, 137, 166
Conroy, Donald, 134, 163
Consumption. See Tuberculosis
Convalescent Home for Children, 219
Coonan, M.F., 166
Coos Bay, OR, 127, 150, 152
Coramine, 78
Cornerstone, 42, 101
Coronary angiography, 186-87
Coronary bypass, 186
Cortesio, Barbara, 213
Cosgrove, Bp. Henry, 15, 18-20, 40, 53, 63-64
Cottage Hospital, 17, 19, 28, 29, 54
Council Bluffs, IA,
  St. Bernard's Hospital, 25, 104, 106-07, 116, 157, 180,
  Sisters of Mercy, 17, 25, 71-73, 76-77, 83, 104, 106, 111, 118-21, 140, 144, 149, 157, 163, 180
Court,
  Polk County Circuit, 14
  Iowa Supreme, 14-15, 19
Cownie, Charles T., 157, 166
Crawford, J. B., 40
Creighton University, 110, 141, 149, 180
Crivaro, Peter, 218
Crogan, Rev. Damian, 158
Crowley, Daniel F., Sr., 94, 115
Crowley, Daniel F., Jr., 94, 102, 133, 155, 166, 183
Crowley, Elaine, 213
Cyclural sodium, 91

D

Daghestani, Ala, 226
Dahl, Harry, 126
Daily Iowa State Leader, 15
Daily Iowa State Register, 17, 27
Daly, Bp. Edward C., 127, 134, 146-47, 157
Darling, J.N. "Ding", 61, 90
Daughters of Isabella, 40
Davenport, IA,
  Catholic Diocese, 17-19, 39, 147
  St. Mary's Parish, 20
  Sisters of Mercy, 20, 24-25, 32-33, 35, 39, 42, 63-66
Davis, Bp. James, 63, 66
Davis, Theresa, 133
De Witt, IA, 24
Decker, Henry, 86
Defibrillator, 190-91
Denser, Clarence H., Jr., 146
Depression, 84-85, 88-89, 95, 107, 124, 126
DePuydt, Frank, 189
Des Moines,
  Area Community College, 228
  Catholic diocease, 57-58, 63-65, 89, 127, 134, 141, 147, 173
  Chamber of Commerce, Greater Des Moines Committee, 219
  Diocesan Council of Catholic Nurses, 127
  Health Center, 212
  Police, 57, 92
  Population, 57
  Rotary Club, 188
  United Campaign, 134
  YMCA, 134
Des Moines & Kansas City Railroad, 40
Des Moines Daily News, 29
Des Moines Insurance Company, 40
Des Moines Lions Club, 98
Des Moines Mandolin Club, 40
Diabetes, 83
Dickinson, Laurie, 224
Dietetics, 83
Digitalis, 47, 184
Dingman, Bp. Maurice J., 146-47, 167, 170-72
Diphtheria, 19, 26, 28, 57, 77
Directional coronary arthrectomy, 190
Dooley, John, 124
Dowling Junior College, 107
Dowling, Bp. Austin, 58, 62-66, 69-70, 73
Doyle, Kathleen, 231
Doyle, Rachel, 86
Drake University, 29, 45, 55, 146, 148, 153, 192
  Medical School, 54, 57
  Relays parade, 151
Dressler, Art, 176
Drey, Robert, 231
Drobnich, Sara, 189, 231
Drumm, Bp. Thomas W., 37, 68, 70-73, 89
Dubansky, Marvin H., 155
Dubuque, IA
  Catholic Diocese, 19, 21,
  Hospital, 24
  St. Mary's Catholic Church, 34
Duhigg, Thomas, 60
Dulin, Lucille, 48
Dunn, Anne, 213
Dutton, Dean, 231

E

Eagle Iron Works, 42
East Wing, 14, 39, 41-42, 91, 99, 101, 105, 130, 136-37, 147
Eastern Cooperative Oncology Group, 193
Echemendia, M., 117
Echocardiograms, 186
  fetal, 188
Echoencephalography, 186, 193
Eckstat, Stephen, 226
Education, 46-49, 104-16, 146, 148-154, 162, 182, 207, 228-29,
EENT, 86, 91, 144
Eisenhower, Dwight, 184
Eldredge, Judy, 153
Electrocardiograms, 81, 93, 184
Electron microscope, 193
Elefson, Don, 133, 167
Ellis, Howard, 155, 162
Epivol Soluble, 91
Ether, 41, 91, 120
Ethylene, 125
Ewald, Dorsey, 213

F

Fagan, Rodney, 77
Fairbanks, Douglas, Jr., 227
Fay, Oliver J., 59
Federal Works Agency, 99
Feehan, Lucille, 231
Fee-splitting, 85, 93-94
Feinberg, Milton, 102
Field, Archeleus G., 26-27
Finn, M. Concilli, 178
Firestone, E.C., 40
Fischer, Rev. Harold, 166
Fisher, S.R., 166
Flannagan, Mary, 47
Flavin, Rev. Maurice, 34
Flavin, Rev. Michael, 15, 18-20, 25, 27, 32, 34-35, 40, 42, 53, 60, 76
Fletcher, Jayne Ruan, 223
Flynn, Frank, 40
Ford Foundation, 134
Ford Motor Company, 85
Fort Des Moines, 111
Foster, Ella, 114
Foulk, Frank E., 115, 124-25
Four-Mile Railroad Wreck, 28
Franklin, Cass, 217
Friedman, Peg, 171, 213
Friedman, S.L., 166
Friesen plan, 160-61
From, Paul, 185, 188, 226, 231

G

Gaass, Louise, 48
Galligan, Rev. John, 62
Galligan, Robert, 231
Gannett Foundation, 218
Gatchel, Theodore, 54
Gay, Jackie, 213
Gay, John, 187-88, 191, 226
Geiger counter, 127
Geneser, John W., 27
Gernes, Becky, 215
Gervich, Daniel, 225
Gifford, C.W., 103
Gift of Life, Inc., 188
Gleason, Stephen, 231
Glomset, Daniel A., 59
Glomset, Daniel J., 59-60
Glomset, Mrs. Daniel (Anna), 59
Goldburg, Rabbi Jay, 171
Goodman, Karen, 163
Gordon, David, 186, 188
Gordon Friesen Associates. See Friesen plan
Gormley, Arthur T., 103, 130, 138, 166
Graham Investment Company, 226
Graham, John, 216
Grand View College, 219, 228
Grask, Mrs. E.S. (Florence), 166, 210, 213
Gray Ladies, 97
Gray, Howard D., 115
Green, Jack, 189
Griffin, John M., 115
Griffin, John S., 26
Griffin, Mrs. John, 206
Griffin, Milt, 176
Griffith, Sallie, 28
Gross, Harold, 133
Groundbreaking, 38, 137, 162, 170, 216
Grout, Connie, 225
Grubb, John R., 191
Guam, 112
Gubbels, Rev. Richard, 173

H

Haley, E.R., 166
Hall, Brothers, 12
Hall's Addition, 12, 14-15, 17, 19, 39
Hammes, Betty, 120, 176-77
Hammes, John, 120
Hardesty, William, 98
Hardie, Kay, 86, 93
Hardin, Agnes, 85
Hardin, Robert, 162
Harding, William L., 61
Harmeyer, Dixie, 213
Hart, Mrs. J., 48
Hawkinson, John, 157
Hay, Merle, 61
Hayden, Clarence, 146
Hayes, Lucretia, 48
Hayne, W.W., 125
Health System of Mercy, 179
Health Planning Council, 161, 171, 179, 181, 186
Heart disease, 77, 184-91
Heles, Jimmy, 81, 88
Hennessy, Bp. John, 21
Herndon Hall, 58
Hess, Stan, 141
Hewitt (Hammes), Molly, 120, 162
Hickner, Lawrence, 124
Hill-Burton Act, 130, 136
Hill, Madge, 213
Hillis, Isaac, 40
Hillside Neighborhood Development Corporation, 219
Hines, Ralph, 127, 226
Hip-pinning, 92-93
Hoffman, Christine, 48, 149
Hogan, Dolores, 167, 212
Hollander, Erich, 96
Hollenkamp Interior Decorating , 102
Holy Trinity School, 71
Home for Friendless Children, 28-29
Hopkins, Mary Jane, 231
Hospital Association of Greater Des Moines, 178
Hospital Progress, 107
House of Mercy. *See Baggot Street: and Clark Street*
Houts, Sandra, 176
Hubbard tank. See Hydrotherapy tank
Hubbell, James W., Jr., 166
Hughes, John, 15
Hummer, John W., 166
Hydrotherapy tank, 92

I

Iannone, Liberato, 188, 190
Ichioka, Tsutayo N., 97
Immigrants, 19, 27
Incubator, 78, 91, 130, 211
Infant mortality, 85
Influenza, 26, 62, 69,
Ingham, Harvey, 60
Interns, 83, 86, 94-96, 117, 132, 146, 183
Iowa Catholic Hospital Association, 83, 91
Iowa Caucus Project '88, 219
Iowa Commission on the Status of Women, 219
Iowa Conference of Catholic Hospitals, 144, 146
Iowa Congregational Hospital, 84
Iowa Division of Nursing Education, 105
Iowa Heart Association, 184, 186
Iowa Hospital Association, 146, 218
Iowa Lutheran Hospital, 85, 181, 223
Iowa Lutheran Maternity Hospital, 84-85, 93, 107
Iowa Medical Society, 183
Iowa Methodist Hospital, 29, 54-55, 85, 92-93, 99, 130, 181, 223
Iowa Nurses' Association, 146, 219
Iowa Nursing Board, 48, 85
Iowa Oncology Research Association, 193
Iowa Public Health Department, 130, 144
  Board of Nurse Examiners, 151
  Nurses' Examining Committee, 35, 151
Iowa Sheet Metal Company, 162
Iowa Society to Prevent Blindness, 219
Iowa State, Capitol Building, 19, 38, 40
Iowa State Fair, 81
Iowa State League of Nursing Education, 110
Iowa State Medical Society,
  Women's Auxiliary, 149
Iowa State Register, 14, 27
Iowa State Traveling Men's Association, 53
Iowa State University, 127
Iowa Women's Hall of Fame, 219
Ireland,
  Dublin, 23-24
  Sisters of Mercy, 23-24, 58
Iron Lung, 92
Irving, Florence, 213
Irving, Noble, 126-27, 132-33, 155, 162, 181, 186, 192,

J

Jackson, Arnold, 133
Jackson, Frank, 40
Jackson, Lovrene, 217
Jacobson, Regina, 150
Japanese, 97
Jarvik-7, 189
Jaundice, 125
Jewett, G.A., 166,
Jewett, Gerald, 231
Jewett, Thomas D., 12
Jewish Community Center, 116
John Deere Company, 88
Johnson, Charles, 133
Johnson, M. Borromeo, 24, 27, 34
Johnson, Merlyn, 231
Johnston, Iowa, 62
Jones, Grace, 213
Jones, Robert, 226

K

Kanke, Bernice, 213
Kansas City Public Health Service, 99
Kantrowitz, Adrian, 187
Katzmann, Frederick, 96, 226
Kavanaugh, Marcus, 60
Kelleher, T.F., 33, 54
Kellen, Don, 181, 192
Kelley, E.J., 115
Kelly, Anna C., 48
Kelly, Genevieve, 102-03, 166, 211, 213
Kelso, James, 226
Kennedy, John F., 147
Kenney, Mrs. M., 40
Keokuk, IA, 24, 54
Kessell, J.E., 115
Kieler, Madeline, 150
King, M.H., 15, 27
Klein, Harold, 102-03, 157, 166, 179, 206
Knowles, Lucille, 213, 231
Kolosky, John, 231
Kongtahworn, Cham, 187, 189
Kordick, Genevieve, 217, 231
Korea, 188
Krause, William, 231
KRNT, 98
Ku Klux Klan, 61
Kurtz, Bernard D., 166
Kurtz, L.C., 53

L

L'Estrange, James, 66
Lalor, Mrs. Walter, 206
Lalor, W.L., 166, 217
Lanham Act, 98
Laser, 193
LeBeau, Joan, 231
Lengh, Franz, 98
Levitt, Ellis, 157, 162, 166, 183
Levitt, Mrs. Ellis (Nellie), 162
Levy, Lou, 102
Lex, Eileen, 146
Liddle, Estella, 47
Lier, N.O., 59
Lithotripter, 223
Lobectomy, 126
Loras, Bp. Mathias, 18, 24
Losh, Clifford, Jr., 155
Losh, Clifford, Sr., 53, 79, 102, 115, 120, 124-25
Lovison, Natalie, 133
Ludwig, Sam, 215
Lynch, Robert J., 65, 115

M

MacDonald, Agnes, 206
MacGregor, Mrs. Kenneth, 206
Magnetic Resonance Imaging, 190, 193
Mahoney, Rose, 48
Mains, Suzanne, 153, 182, 228
Maksem, John, 195
Malone, Rev. Henry V., 89
Manning, Paul T., 166
Markunas, Peter, 94-95
Marquisville Coal Mine, 184
Martin, Ellen, 34
Martin, M. Evangelist, 34
Mathaison, Emmett, 96,
Matthews, Alexander, 186, 188
Matthews, Robert O., 48
Maynard, James, 124
Mayo, Charles, 133
Mayo Clinic, 181
McAuley, Catherine, 5, 21-25, 40, 171, 232
McCarthy, Nellie, 48
McCarthy, Kenneth, 179, 231

McCarthy, Wilton, 50, 51, 59,77
McClean, Earl D., 115
McClure, Evelyn (Savage), 129, 176
McConnell, Mrs. 40
McCormick, Richard, SJ, 230
McDermott, M. Vincent, 27
McDermott, Patricia, 231
McDonnell, Rev. Joseph, 173
McGarvey, Neil, 133, 155
McGinn, S.F., 166
McGorrisk, J.B., 15, 27, 40, 60
McGregor, Jeanne, 150
McGuire, Ed, 40
McIlhon, John, 85, 94-95
McKeone, Vera, 212
McKinney, Harold E., 102
McLaughlin, Jimmy, 94
McLaughlin, John, 157, 166
McLaughlin, Lucy, 139
McLaughlin, Mother M. Aloysius, 63
McLaughlin, Stacia, 95
McMahon, Rev. William, 89
McMullen, Bp. John, 15, 18
McNab, James, 195
McNamee, Jesse, 86, 124, 155
Medicare, 160, 222
Medicaid, 222
Meiggs, Isabel, 114
Meintel, Patricia, 181
Mercy (Des Moines)
administrator, 36, 53, 77, 83, 95, 99, 125, 144, 157, 162, 178-79, 219
admitting, 176
Advisory Board, 102-03, 125, 127, 130, 134, 140, 148, 157, 160-61, 163, 165-66, 206
Air Life, 224
Alcohol and Drug Recovery, 218
Alzheimer care, 223
Articles of Incorporation, 179
assistant administrator, 177, 179,
Atrium, 190, 216
awards, 98, 142, 227
Auxiliary, 215
bacteriology, 144
Beauty shop, 213
beds, 40, 43, 80, 85, 101, 136, 146, 160 61, 170, 172
Beh auditorium, 144
blood bank, 144
boiler, 101, 136, 162, 170
Board of Directors, 177-79, 183, 219
Board of Trustees, 27
bridge, 171
Bulletin, 133, 176,
cafeteria, 139, 171
cancer, 192-195
registry, 192
cardiac care, 177-78, 184-91
Cardiac Rehabilitation Center, 216
Cardiac Risk Identification and Modification Program, 190
cardiac sonography, 222
Cardiac Surgical Intensive Care Unit, 189-90
cardiovascular care, 170
cashier, 176-77
catheterization laboratory, 187, 189-91, 216
CAT scanner. See CT scanner
census, 41, 50, 80, 88, 99, 101, 127, 130-31, 133, 160
central supply, 137, 144, 177
Channel Two, 183
chapel, 41, 99, 130, 137, 144, 147, 158-59, 171
charity care, 50, 51, 58, 60,130
chemotherapy, 193-94,
chemistry, 101, 144
chief executive officer, 179
chief of staff, 56, 115, 155
Child Development Center, 177
clinics, 220
Comfort suites, 216
continuous quality improvement, 226
convent, 144, 159-60, 176, 186
courier, 176
Court Apartments, 220, 228-29
credit, 176-77
Credit Union, 176
CT scanner, 177, 181, 193
cystoscopy, 144
cytology, 144, 146
data processing, 17, 173, 176
delivery rooms, 130, 137, 139, 171-73
department heads, 177
dietary, 137, 139, 142, 147, 176
Drive, 173
Educational Center, 220
electro-therapeutic.
See physical therapy
emergency, 129, 144-45, 161, 172-73, 186, 222
Emergency Medical Services, 225
employee health, 177
Employee recognition, 164, 181
Employee Recreation Committee.
See Recreation Committee
employees, 146
environmental service, 222
First Step Recovery, 218
Foundation, 173, 181, 220
front door, 137, 161, 171
general information meetings, 181
Gold Coast, 37
grants, 99
Guild, 126-8, 137, 145, 147, 150, 164, 181, 185, 206-215
fireprevention, 176
Hall, 171
health education, 177, 183, 224
Heart Day, 187
helicopter, 224
helioport, 17,
hematology, 144
Heritage, 217
histology, 146
Home Care, 217
Home Respiratory care, 217
hoptel, 224
Hospice, 195
hospital, 25, 33-35
housekeeping, 176
hyperbaric, 222
infection control, 173
intern apartments, 144, 159-60
isotope laboratory, 192
Journal, 176
kidney care, 223
kitchen, 59, 130, 142, 171
laboratory, 42, 59, 60, 76-77, 81, 86, 91, 98, 101, 125, 133, 144-46, 172,176-77
laundry, 59, 136, 162, 170
Laurel Center, 220
library, 79, 80, 107, 124, 162, 183
Lifeline, 217
linear accelerator, 195
locksmith, 176
Major Diseases Committee, 185
mail delivery, 177
maintenance, 173, 177
materials management, 173, 177
McDonald's, 222
Medical Day, 133, 185
medical education, 183
Medical Office Plaza, 216
Medical Records, 140, 176, 222
Medical Staff, 33, 46, 58, 86, 96, 101-02, 124, 132, 149, 157, 176, 187, 193, 206, 222
MedLab, 176
Mercy Hall, 158, 167, 171
microbiology, 144
milk laboratory, 100, 130-31
motherhouse, 63-73
MRI, 190, 193
mural, 141
neonatal intensive care, 173
Nerve Block Center, 216
Networking, 221
News, 133
nursery, 78, 91, 130, 137, 150,171, 222-23
nursing services, 222
nutritional disorders, 218
obstetrics, 78-80, 91, 99-100, 130, 158-59
Office Plaza, 220
oncology, 193
operating room, 41, 43, 45, 59-60, 86, 130, 133
orthopedics, 91
outpatient, 129, 144-45
Pain Center, 224
parasitology, 144
Park Apartments, 220, 228
parking lot, 17,161, 170, 173, 216
pastoral care, 87, 173, 180, 213
pathology department, 144, 192
patient accounts, 173, 176-77
Pediatric Intensive Care Unit, 191
pediatrics, 78, 91, 99, 126, 128, 130, 144-45, 153, 180
personnel, 173, 177
Petal Pusher, 213, 215
pharmacy, 91, 94, 143, 222
physical plant, 173
physical therapy, 59, 60, 79, 80, 81, 92, 144
picnic, 158
pneumatic tube, 137, 140
power plant, 162
pre-hospital advanced-care, 225
Progressive Cardiac Recovery Unit, 189
Psych Services, 218
public relations, 87, 173, 176, 180
purchasing, 177
quality assurance, 222
radiation therapy, 195
radiology, 126, 133, 144, 146, 170, 172, 186, 189
recovery, 137, 144
Recreation Committee, 158, 181
Regional Emergency Training Center, 225, 229
respiratory therapy, 222
Respite, 217
retreat, 158
room rates, 139
safety, 176
School of Health Sciences, 221-24, 229
School of Medical Technology, 146, 229
School of Perfusion, 229
School of Radiology, 120, 162, 229
security, 173, 224
serology, 144
shuttle, 176
shrine, 159-60
Sisters' Council, 177
Sisters' Governing Board, 161
Sleep Disorders Center, 222
Snack Shop, 142, 209, 215
social services, 173, 176, 180, 195, 217
Sponsorship Ethics Committee, 230
Sponsorship Relational Committee, 230
stockroom, 177
Stroke Study Center, 177
surgery, 177
surgery rooms, 137, 144, 172
surgical pathology, 144
surgical residency, 162
surgical technician, 163, 224
TEAM program, 224
technical services, 185, 222
tonsil ward, 129
towers, 100, 127, 161, 170-183, 186
townhouses, 159
tumor registry, 192
urinalysis, 144
urology, 79,80,91
utilization review, 173, 176
valet, 176
Variety Club Children's Lifeline Yucatan Program, 187-88
wellness center, 216
West Health Center, 224, 226-27
Willis Adult Day Care, 217
x-ray, 42, 59,76,81,86,91,92,93,137
see also radiology
Mercy Hospital,
Algona, IA, 25
Anamosa, IA, 25
Cedar Rapids, IA, 25
Chicago, IL, 21, 24-25
Clinton, IA, 25
Council Bluffs, IA, 25, 87, 100, 125, 134, 140, 147, 161, 163, 180
Cresco, IA, 25
Davenport, IA, 17, 24, 27, 33-34, 39, 62-66, 147
Denver, CO, 144, 180
Devil's Lake, ND, 178
Dubuque, IA, 25
Durango, CO, 144
Fort Dodge, IA, 25
Iowa City, IA, 25, 66-68
Joplin, MO, 141
Marshalltown, IA, 25, 35
Mason City, IA, 25
Oelwein, IA, 25
Pittsburgh, PA, 21, 24-26
Sioux City, IA, 25
Valley City, ND 140-41
Waverly, IA, 25
Webster City, IA, 25
Meredith, Mrs. E.T., Jr., 166, 213
Merle Hay Mall, 73
Meyer, Mrs. Albert (Marie), 206-08, 213
Mikunas, Virginia, 213
Miller, Jerry, 146
Milligan, George, 231
Mills, Pleas J., 60
Milwaukee Overland Limited Railroad, 51
Mitchell, Abbie, 28
Mitchell, Arnold, 176
Moeller, A. Diane, 179
Monholland, M. Francis, 24
Moore, Loretta, 112
Morden, Richard, 96
Morphine, 47
Morrissey, William J., 155
Mosca, CO, 144
Mount Loretto, 81, 83, 100, 119, 125
Muelhaupt, Carl, 166
Mulock, E.H., 102-03, 206
Mulroney, Margaret, 48
Multiple sclerosis, 223
Murphy, J.H., 93
Murphy, Margaret, 212
Murray, Sarah, 48
Myers, Merrill, 184

N
National Conference of Christians and Jews, 100, 178, 219
National Council of Catholic Nurses, 146
National Health Care Foundation, 227
National Hospital Day, 83, 91
National League for Nursing, 152, 228
Natoli, Valerie, 231
Naughton, John, 181
Nebraska Methodist Hospital, 192
Neumann Brothers, Inc., 162
Neumann, Walter H., Jr., 162
New Deal legislation, 98
Nightingale, Florence, 83, 228
Nimbus hemopump, 190
Normile, Florence, 102-03
Norris, Louis, 166, 179
North Central Cancer Treatment Group, 193
North Wing, 58-61, 78, 137, 171
Northup, Jo, 210, 213
Northup, Mary, 102-03, 166, 206-08, 210-13,
Nourse, L.M., 115,
Noyes, Cheryl, 225
Nugent, Rev. Joseph, 40
Nugent, W.B., 166
Nurse Training Act, 153
Nurses,
aides, 97, 153, 163-64, 182, 224
registration, 35, 37
wages, 49, 127, 151, 153
Nursing,
assistants, 153
caps, 116, 152-53
education, 83, 148-55, 182
funding, 153-54
practical, 100
shortage, 127, 148, 150, 153, 163
staffing, 22
Nye, Jo, 172

O
O'Connor, M. Isidore, 25
O'Gorman, Bp. James, 20
O'Neill, Mary, 47
O'Neill, Peg, 231
Oberg, Marvin F., 166
Olson, J.E., 166
Olson, Phyllis, 176
Olson, Robert, 154
Omaha, Regional Community of, 46, 77, 179
Operation-77, 186
Operation Shape-Up, 186-87
Order of the Eastern Star of Iowa, 149
Orthopedic procedures, 91
Osteopaths, 85, 178, 183
Ostercamp, Barbara, 191
Ottumwa, IA, J.B. Sax Charity Fund, 149
Our Primary Purpose, 218
Overton, Roy, 133
Overton, Roy, II, 125

P
Pacemaker, 188, 190-91
Page, A.C., 184
Passionist Fathers, 73
Pasteurization of milk, 59
Patchin, R. A., 40
Patient Self-Determination Act, 230
Paul, Barbara, 150
Pearlman, Leo R., 155
Peasley, Harold, 98, 115
Peck, J.H., 184
Peet, Rev. Edward, 12
Penicillin, 93, 102
P.E.O. Sisterhood, 149
People of Vision, 21, 27, 56, 89, 103, 115, 119, 121, 155, 166, 179, 213, 226, 231
Peppers, T.D., 93
Pfaff, R.O., 93
Phelan, M. Patricia, 124, 226
Phenylketonuria, 144
Phillips, Steven, 187-89,
Plasma, 125
Plastic surgeries, 89
Platt, James, 231
Pleural Effusions, 102
Plowman, E.T., 93
Pneumonia, 47, 57, 77
Pocuruell, Joseph, 117
Polich, John, 226
Polio, 92, 128, 207
Polk County, IA., 61
healthcare, 26
insane asylum, 29
poorhouse, 26, 29
tuberculosis association, 149
Polk, Harry H., 60
Polk, Jefferson S., 58
Polk, Julia H., 58
Polyclinic, 85
Poorman, William, 166
Pope Pius X, 57
Portel, Gertrude, 49
Powell, Lester, 155
Priestley, James T., 60, 70,
Priests, 18-19
Project Together, 218,
Protestant Hospital Association, 95,
PTCA, 188,
Public Health Nursing, 83,

R
Radio frequency catheter ablation, 190-91
Radioisotopes, 127, 144
Radium, 57, 192
Railroads, 19, 51
Rande, Joanne, 150
Rawson, C.D., 54
Ray, Gov. Robert, 171-72
Ray, Hal S., 60
Raymond Blank Memorial Hospital, 128
Reagan, Nancy, 218
Red Wing, 58-60
Reed's Ice Cream, 106
Reed, Rev. J. Sanders, 28
Reed, William, 231
Reese, Natalie, 217
Regan, J.C., 15, 27
Reiff, Mary, 167
Remer, Deanne, 228
Renihan, Rev. J.H., 41
Residency, 132, 162
Residents, 146
Retreat, 85
Reynolds, Stan, 227
Rh factor, 81
Richards, William G., 192
Ringland, John, 166
Ritz, Edna, 166, 213,
Ritzman, John, 226
River Hills Urban Renewal Project, 156-160
Riverview Park, 158, 181
Rocca, Mary, 231
Rockafellow, John C., 51, 59, 115
Rome project, 188-89
Rooney, Ted, 224
Rosenblatt, Max, 102
Rotary Club, 149
Roth, Florence, 213
Rourke, Jeri, 167, 176
Rowen, Mrs. J.R., 166, 213
Ruan, Betty, 223
Ruan, John, 223
Ruan Neurological Center, 223
Rubel, Edna, 213
Russell, John, 184
Rutherford Chapel, 12, 15, 17, 19, 39
Ryan, Catherine, 213
Ryan, Granville, 51
Ryan, Kelly, 176
Ryan, Norah, 107

S
St. Ambrose Catholic Church, 12, 14, 19, 20-21, 27, 33, 35, 99, 109, 115, 149, 153
St. Ambrose School, 157, 177
St. Augustin Catholic Church, 97
St. Camillus Guild, 127
St. Catherine's Hall for Business Women, 71, 83, 95, 99
St. Gabriel's Monastery, 73
St. James Orphanage, Omaha, NE, 144, 180
St. Joseph Academy, 149
St. Louis University, 144, 178, 180
St. Paul's Episcopal Church, 12, 17, 19, 28-29
St. Peter's School, Des Moines, IA, 71, 140
St. Vincent's Home, Omaha NE, 163, 180
Salk, Jonas, 128
Salt Lake City, UT, 69
Salvation Army Retreat and Maternity Home, 85
Samaritan Hospital, 55
Sams, Janet, 146
Sandler, Nate, 102
Sargent, F.W., 60
Sarnecki, Paul, 189, 218
Savery, Mrs. J.C., 28
Sawtelle, W.W., 124
Scales, E.Thomas, 155, 157
Scarlet Fever, 26, 47
Schaeffer, Lillian, 81
Schick Test, 77
Schill, Austin, 155, 185, 226
Schill, Teri, 213
Schiltz, Jane, 213
Schiltz, Miralda, 112
Schiltz, N.C., 33, 192
Schmitz, Herbert, 115, 133
Schneider, Ray, 177
Schnellar, Rev. Bernard, 89
School of Nursing, 46-49, 59, 94, 104-117, 120, 141, 148-154, 182, 207, 228-29
accreditation, 147, 151-52
Alumni Association, 48, 106-07
capes, 112
capping, 97
caps, 47, 116, 228
curfew, 49, 106, 110, 151, 153
curriculum, 152
director, 56, 104, 106, 110-11, 115, 149, 152, 154-55, 178, 182, 228
dormitory, 91, 99, 101-02, 105, 114, 173, 175, 228
CEU, 182
faculty, 151-52, 228
graduation, 46, 153, 228
late permit, 106
male students, 151, 228
married students, 154
probationers, 46
scholarship, 148, 182, 228
stipend, 107, 112
tuition, 153
uniforms, 46, 107, 149, 228
Schropp, R.C., 124
Schultheis, Kenneth, 226
Schumacher, George H., 50
Scott, Eva, 47
Seiler, Barbara, 47
Selective Service, 96
Seventh Day Adventist Sanatorium, 55
Seventh District Iowa Nurses' Association, 100, 107
Seventh Street Hospital
See Cottage Hospital
Sharon, Emmett, 40, 64
Sherman, Hoyt, 32-33
Place, 20, 32-33, 36, 39-40
Shore, F.E.V., 33, 115
Silk, Marvin, 226
Silverio, Raymunda, 177
Sisters of Mercy Des Moines, 18, 39, 43, 49, 50, 56, 84,119, 121, 155, 179-80, 219, 230-31, 238
Skin-grafts, 89
Skinner, James, 189
Slattery, M. Catherine, 36
Sloan, Mr. William B., 206
Small pox, 26
Smith, Alfred, 226
Smith, Gerald, 189
Smith, Oliver O., 42
Smith, Victoria, 195
Smyth, Bp. Clement, 21
Snodgrass, Ralph, 96
Sohm, Herbert A., 115
Solomia, Rev. Paul, 81, 173
Sondag, Rev. Joseph, 147
Song, Joseph, 192, 226
Sostrin, Morey, 102, 103
Southwick, Stephen, 231
South Wing, 100, 127, 130-31, 133-48, 156, 158, 160, 172, 176, 209, 216
Specht, Bernice, 112
Springer, Floyd, 126-27
Spurlock, Patricia, 154
Stapelton, Veronica, 48
State Journal, 14
Steele, Frieda, 120, 176
Stefani, Louise, 150,
Still Osteopathic College, 55
Stoll, Rev. Vitus, 80, 83, 89, 99
Stolte, A.G., 102
Stransky, M. Magdalene, 35
Straub, Mel, 223
Streptokinase, 188
Strikes, 94
Stumbo, Florence, 128
Sulfa, 93
Sullivan, John, 64
Surgery, 41, 89, 91, 102, 104-05, 125-26
Surgical clinics, 89, 91
Surgical instruments, 86, 124
Swartz, Clifford, 231
Swedish Lutheran Church, 55
Sweem, Donald, 225-26
Sweeney, M.Leona, 229

T
Taft, David, 133
Tang, Paul, 48
Taylor, Helen, 213
Thailand, 189
Thatcher, Margaret, 219
Thoracotemies, 102
Throckmorton, J.Fred, 155
Thul, Totty, 213
Thyberg, Jean, 213,
Tobago, 188
Tometich, Sierra, 218
Toner, Kate, 14
Toner, Peter, 14
Toney, William, 102
Tonsi, Irene, 139
Tonsillectomy, 88, 91, 129
Toon, Richard, 189
Torrence, Mildred, 139
Torruella, Joseph, 186
Tracy, Annie B., 17, 28-29
Tracy Home Hospital, 29
Trained Nurse, 107
Transplantation,
cardiac, 189-91
kidney, 223
Trephining, 51
Tribromethanol, 91
Trinidad, 188,
Trumm, Mabel, 35
Tuberculosis, 14, 47, 66, 77, 89, 102
Typhoid fever, 26, 47, 53, 57, 78
Hospital, 27
Tyrell, Emma (Shackelford), 47, 149

U
Union Hospital, 19, 28

Unions, 94
University of Iowa Hospital, 127
University of Iowa Medical School, 132, 162
United Food Markets Foundation, 149
Urban Renewal, 156-57, 160

V
Val-Air Ballroom, 167
Valley West Mall, 220
Van Driel, Catherine, 177,
Van Rheenen, Cloe, 213
VanWerden, William, 33, 54
Variety Club, 102, 187-88, 191, 225, 227
Veiock, T.I., 166
Veterans Hospital, 162, 193,
Vollmer, Henry, 40
Volunteers, 96-97, 127, 133, 206-215
Voight, Adolf, 127
Voss, Milo, 127

W
Wakonda Village, 132
Walker, Mildred, 181
Wallace, Henry, 40
Walsh, Richard, 231
Walston, Edwin B., 41-42, 149
Walter, Dennis, 155
Warde, M. Frances, 21, 24, 231
Weather, 33, 98
Weiland, Rev. Duane, 141
Weingart, Julius, 77
Weingart, Rabbi Irving A., 139
Welch, W.H., 15
Wellehan, M. Mercedes, 64-66
Wells, F. L., 33, 54
Welter, Doris, 213, 215
West Wing, 54-55, 60, 78, 91-92, 100, 126, 137, 139-40, 144-46, 170-72, 185-86, 193, 216, 222
Weston, R.A., 79, 115
Whalen, Ruth, 213
Whiskey, 78
White, Mary, 48
White, Ruth, 213
Williams, Betty, 213
Williams, Bob, 133
Wilson, Al, 176
Wilson, Joe, 177
Winston, Stuart R., 226
Wintermantel, Cathy (Barton), 146
Wirtz, D.C., 91
Wolf, Abraham, 226
Woodard, Floyd, 132-33
Wonderlin, F.Marcellus, 167
Woods, J.W., 164
Works Progress Administration, 69
World War I, 48, 55, 61, 62, 65, 67, 69, 72, 76-78, 152
World War II, 96-99, 101-03, 112, 124-27, 133, 147-48, 154, 184
Wren, Mae, 164
Wurst, Ronald, 133

X,Y,Z
Yellow fever, 26,
Young, Loretta, 227
Younker Brothers, 40
Younker's Tea Room, 149
Yucatan, 187-88
Zaletel, Joe, 125
Zeff, Robert, 189
Zelinsky, Joyce, 213

Sisters of Mercy
M.(Mary) Adelaide Lynch, 35
M. Agnes Klein, 140, 155
M. Agnita Dutton, 155
M. Alacoque Lannan, 76, 106, 119, 221
M. Alicia Gallagher, 179
M. Aloysius Byrne, 68-69
M. Aloysius McGuire, 79, 104, 118-19, 121
M. Ambrose Schaub, 119
M. Angela Gilmore, 155
M. Anita Paul, 35, 77, 98-99, 101-03, 119, 125, 130, 134, 136-38, 147, 166, 176
Anne Mary Kelly, 155, 179
M. Anthony Bonen, 155
M. Anthony Reilly, 37, 64-66
M. Antoinette Hill, 72
M. Anton Lucius, 155
M. Augustine O'Flaherty, 66-68, 71-73, 76
M. Austine O'Donohoe, 79, 119
M. Baptist L'Estrange, 67-69
M. Baptist Martin, 20, 24-25, 32-33, 36, 53
M. Basil (Agnes Marie) Smith, 119
M. Benedicta McCarten, 80, 83, 91, 119
M. Bernadette Mulroney, 179
M. Bertha O'Brien, 66-68
M. Brian Harty. See, Helen Harty
M. Brigid Condon, 179, 218
M. Carlotta Clinton, 179-80
M. Carmelita Manning, 119
M. Catherine Carroll, 115, 119
M. Cecelia Zaver 179
M. Charles Keane, 176, 179-80
M. Christina Weil, 155
M. Clare Clifford, 79, 104, 106-07, 110, 115, 119
M. Claudia Robinson, 179
M. Concepta Mullins, 87, 119, 141, 146, 151, 172-73, 176, 212, 230-31
M. Consilii Finn, 66-67
M. Consolata Wagner, 119
M. Damian Novak, 119
M. del Rey Ekler, 155
M. DeLellis Hotz, 155
M. DeLourdes Hardiman, 62
M. dePaul Collins, 80, 119
Dolores Preisinger, 179
M. Donata Landkamer, 179
M. Dorothy Flaherty, 61, 62, 69
M. Eileen Moore, 155, 157, 161-63, 166-67, 178, 180
Elaine Delaney, 179
M. Elizabeth Ann Paul, 176, 179
M. Elizabeth Butler, 35, 41
M. Eugene Dunleavy, 68
M. Eustace Wondrask, 79
M. Evangelist L'Estrange, 67-69
M. Evangelista Claherty, 68, 76-77, 80, 83, 119, 221
M. Francene Summers, 179-80
M. Francis Hunt, 144, 147, 155, 157, 163-64
M. Francita O'Meara, 155
M. Gabriel Bruce, 119
M. Gabriel Mulcrone, 35
M. Genevieve Reed, 71-73
M. Geraldine Gleeson, 106, 118-19
M. Gertrude, 41
M. Gervase Northup, 154-55, 170-183, 186, 193, 212, 219
M. Gloria Heese, 179,
M. Gonzaga McGuire, 79, 98, 111, 118-19, 121
Helen Harty, 179
M. Helen Mackenzie, 102, 111-12, 115, 121, 125, 133-34, 148-49, 206
M. Herbert Kaufmann, 129, 155
M. Immaculata Striegel, 110, 115, 119
M. Innocentia Zaver.
See M. Mildred Ann Zaver
M. Isabel Stack, 155
M. James McDonald, 76, 119
M. Jane Reichmuth, 179
M. Janel Sawatzki, 179
M. Jean Marie (Richard) Gardiner, 155.
M. Jeanette Brennan, 155
Jeanine Salak, 179
Jeanne Marie Christensen, 179
M. Jerome Burns, 86, 115, 119, 162
M. Joachim Dutton, 119
M. John O'Leary, 115, 119
M. Joseph Byrne, 68-69
M. Joseph Munch, 77, 79, 81, 89, 98, 106, 119, 171, 184, 224
M. Joseph Rogge, 39, 41
M. Josephine, 41
M. Josephine Collins, 104, 179-80
M. Josephine Curran, 67-8, 72
M. Julia McKee, 155
M. Kevin O'Sullivan, 97, 119
M. Kieran Harney, 126, 148, 155, 179, 183
M. Kilian Clinton, 155, 179-80
M. Leona Weil, 86, 119
M. Lois Castelein, 179
M. Loretta Laughlin, 121
M. Lorraine (Eleanor) Daniels, 121, 152
M. Louise Owens, 118-19, 121, 140
M. Loyola Kelleher, 121
M. Lucia Endres, 89, 95, 110, 119-20, 139, 227
M. Margaret Ann White, 179
Marie Elena Maldonado, 179
M. Marla Heman, 155
M. Martina Woulfe, 155
Mary Ann Bintner.
See M. Ricarda Bintner
Mary Ann Burkhardt, 179, 220, 231
M. Mary Anne Curran, 155
M. Regina Selenke, 179
M. Maureen Tracy, 155
M. Mechtildes Hogan, 35, 37, 48
M. Mercedes Reed, 71-73
M. Michael Huban, 121
M. Michaele McGuire, 179
M. Mildred Ann Zaver, 155, 173
Monica Marie Reichmuth, 179
M. Natalie Senecal, 121
M. Nolasco O'Connor, 127, 133, 155
M. Patrice Phelan, 155, 157, 161
Patricia Clare Sullivan, 5, 126, 128, 145, 152-53, 171, 178-79, 182-83, 187, 217-219, 221, 223, 227, 231
Patricia (Kurt) Forret, 155.
Patricia Scanlon.
See M. Rosine Scanlon
M. Paula Radosevich, 179
M. Pauline Hammes, 80, 86, 96, 120-21, 124, 130, 132, 134, 151, 159, 163, 170
M. Philomena Keating, 36, 39, 41, 53-54, 60-61, 63-66, 68-71
M. Pierre Brennan, 121
M. Raphael Murphy, 140, 155
M. Ricarda Bintner, 155, 163
Rita Mary O'Brien, 179,
M. Rosaire Keairnes, 80, 121
M. Rosalin Keane, 179-80
M. Rosalita Culjat, 121
M. Rosine (Patricia) Scanlon, 155, 182
M. Rosita Goebel, 155
Sally Smolen, 179
M. Salome Grimes, 119-21
M. Sarto McMahon, 145, 155, 159
M. Scholastica Kerns, 35
M. Sean Crimmins, 155
M. Sebastian Geneser, 61, 97, 115, 121, 148-50, 152, 171, 206
M. Seraphia McMahon, 179, 230-31
M. Stella Lillie, 179
M. Teresa Connell, 73, 76, 95, 98, 121
M. Tersita Zaver.
See Cecelia Zaver
M. Terrence (Terese) Tracy, 155, 179
M. Therese Bannon, 138, 140, 155, 173, 176, 230-31
M. Theresa McDermott, 73
M. Thomas Wilson, 73, 76, 86, 104-6, 115, 121
M. Timothea Sullivan,
See also Patricia Clare Sullivan
126, 128, 152-55, 159, 178, 219
M. Vera O'Connor, 154-55, 179
M. Veronica Ryan, 121
M. Vidette (Regina Marie) Jacobson, 155, 179
Virginia Marie Kendrick, 179
M. Visitation Faherty, 53-4
M. Winifred Leusen, 76, 79, 86, 121
M. Xavier Clinton, 121,
M. Xavier Malloy, 36, 39, 41-2, 53-4, 63-66, 69-73
M. Zita Brennan, 79, 100, 102, 107, 121, 131, 150, 164, 182, 222-23

CREDITS

Many thanks to the following for the use of their time, talents, and treasures, in the visual portion of this volume:

Mercy Archives:
Sisters of Mercy, Omaha: Sister Dorothea Turner, Archivist—p.25 St. Bernard's Hospital, postcard; p.43 Central Wing; p.56 Mercy cross pin; p.69 Letter; p.76 Mother Bonaventure Carroll; p.77 Mother Evangelista Claherty; p.83 Sister Benedicta McCarten; p.95 Sister Teresa Connell; p.106 Sister Clare Clifford; p.110 Sister Immaculata Striegel; p.121 Sister Salome Grimes; ❧ Sisters of Mercy, Chicago: Srs. M. Noreen Mahon and Pat Illing, Archivists—p.27 and 34 Sisters Borromeo Johnson and Baptist Martin, photos ❧ p.21 Mother Frances Warde, Sisters of Mercy of the Americas, Silver Spring, MD; ❧ p.25 Chicago Mercy Hospital, postcard, Mercy Hospital and Medical Center, Chicago; ❧ p.25 Pittsburgh Mercy Hospital, postcard, Mercy Hospital Pittsburgh.

State Historical Society of Iowa, Archives, Des Moines and Iowa City:
p.11 Hawkeye Insurance Atlas; p.12 Chapel; p.13 Family; p.14 J.S. Clarkson; p.17 Cottage Hospital; p.19 Father Brazill; p.24 Steamboat; p.24 Union Letter; p.26 Wagon train; p.27 Scandanavian Boardinghouse; p 28 Train wreck; p.29 Tracy Home Hospital; p.32 Hoyt Sherman and his home; p.51 South Park Mine; p.52 Sixth Avenue streetcar; p.54 Sixth Avenue postcard; p.62 Soldiers; p.72 St. Gabriel's Monastery; p.85 Congregational Hospital.

State Historical Society of Iowa, Microfilm Newspaper Library, Des Moines:
p.14 *The Iowa State Register*; p.15 Lizzie Collins Will; p.28 Barnum Ad, *The Daily State Leader*, 6 September 1877; p.33 New City Hospital, *The Iowa State Register* 16 November 1893; and Many People There, *The Des Moines Leader* 29 November 1893; p.53 Medical Ads; p.59 Glomset Attacks City Milk Supply, *Des Moines Register and Leader*, 14 January 1914.

Diocesan Archives:
p.20 Father Flavin, detail, Annual priests retreat at St.Ambrose College, c.a. 1903-05, Davenport Catholic Diocesan Archives; ❧ p.147 Bishop Edward Daly, Des Moines Catholic Diocesan Archives.

Special Archives:
p.13 Brazill warranty deed and plat map, Polk County Recorder's office; ❧ p.14 St. Ambrose churches, St. Ambrose Cathedral, Des Moines; ❧ p.16-17 Des Moines panoramic view from the existing courthouse of Des Moines, c.a. 1872-74, Polk County Archives, Misc records of the Auditor; ❧ p.35 Hoyt Sherman home interior, Des Moines Women's Club, David Penney, photographer; ❧ p.57 Policemen, detail, 29 June 1906, Des Moines Police Department; ❧ p.58 Jefferson and Julia Polk and Hearndon Hall, Better Homes and Gardens Real Estate Division; ❧ p.61 "One Year's Work," and "Bringing the Truth Home to Us," and p.90 "Why We Have A National Hospital Day," cartoons by J.N. "Ding" Darling, reprinted with permission of the *Des Moines Register*; ❧ p.68 Second Annual meeting of the Catholic Hospital Association, June 1916, Catholic Health Association; ❧ p.72 Passionist emblem, Passionist order, Chicago; ❧ p.84 "White Angel Bread Line, San Francisco, 1932," Dorothea Lange Collection, detail, reprinted with permission of the City of Oakland, Oakland Museum 1992; ❧ p.124 Scene from Guadalcanal Diary, *The Des Moines Sunday Register*, 15 August 1943, reprinted with permission of the *Des Moines Register*.

Family Archives:
p.16 Plan of Des Moines, Terry O'Connor; ❧ p.18 Bible, Eric Groves; ❧ p.23 Belleek teacup, harp pattern, and p.118 Peat harp, Sister Seraphia McMahon; ❧ p.41 Microscope, Jeff Jutting; ❧ p.56 Watch chain award for interns, Dr. Daniel Crowley, Jr.; ❧ p.57 Farm scene, c.a. 1905, Charles Greiner; ❧ p.59 Mrs. Daniel J. Glomset, Dr. Daniel A. Glomset; ❧ p.59 Baby with bottle, Dr. Marion Alberts; ❧ p. 5 picture frame and p. 63-65 Stamps, Sally Cooper Smith; ❧ p.66 Irish Postcards, Sister Zita Brennan; ❧ p.67 L'Estrange sisters, Kieran Moran; ❧ p.78-79 Quilt, Nancy Fandel; ❧ p.79 Bead identification band, Chris Conyers; ❧ p.85 and 95 John McIlhon and McIlhon children, Monsignor John McIlhon; ❧ p.93 Hip-pinning photo, Kay Hardie; ❧ p.100 Sister Zita in backhoe, Louise Brady; ❧ p.113 Cadet certificate, pins, badge, Helen Southard; ❧ p.121 Sisters Aloysius and Gonzaga, Sister Michaele McGuire and Mary Bryson; ❧ p.184 Electrocardiograph machine, Harold Gross; ❧ p.19 Piety Hill; p.25 Davenport Mercy Hospital; p.53 St. Catherine's Hall; p.71 Bitters bottle; p. 180 embroidery, Loretta Greiner; ❧ p. 187 Drs. Kantrowitz with pipe, Christiaan Barnard seated, Phillips at right, courtesy of Dr. Steven Phillips.

Reprinted with permission from:
p.66 *Our Sunday Visitor*, 17 March 1917; p.80 *Des Moines Tribune-Capital*, 11 July 1927, 4; p.84 *Des Moines Register*, 13 May 1938; p.87 *Des Moines Tribune*, 7 September 1943;p.90 *Des Moines Register*, 5 June 1936; p.90 *Des Moines Register*, 13 May 1938; p.97 *Des Moines Register* 25 January 1943; p.98 *Des Moines Tribune*, 23 June 1942; p. 98 *Des Moines Register*, 24 January 1943; p.101 *Des Moines Register*, 2 July 1945; p. 127 *Des Moines Register*, 30 March 1948; p. 128 *Des Moines Register*, 29 August 1952; p.128-129 *Des Moines Register*, 24 September 1952; p.131 *Des Moines Register*, 13 April 1956; p.134 *The Messenger*, 23 December 1955 and 13 January 1956; p.138 *Des Moines Register*, 11 April 1959; p.147 *Des Moines Tribune*, 23 November 1963; p.147 *Des Moines Register*, 24 November 1964; p.149 *Des Moines Register*, 20 November 1949; p.156 *Des Moines Tribune*, special section, 23 July 1958; p.162 *Des Moines Register*, 20 October 1968; p.170 *The Catholic Mirror*, 28 April 1971, 8; p.173 *Des Moines Tribune*, 14 May 1970; p. 182 *Des Moines Tribune*, 29 May 1970, 3; p. 185 *Des Moines Tribune*, 18 January 1957, 7; p. 186 *Des Moines Register* 14 February 1968; p. 192 *The Evening Tribune*, 2 July 1917, 1; p. 210 *Des Moines Register*, 22 December 1962, 7; p. 219 *Des Moines Sunday Register*, 15 April 1987, Iowa Section.

Bibliographic Sources:
p.20 Current St. Ambrose Cathedral, p.27 Dr. Brooks, and p.29 Dr. Cannon's Office, Des Moines Illustrated Souvenir, Iowa Historical Illustrative Co., Des Moines: Iowa Printing Company, 1895; ❧ p.22 Catherine McAuley's desk, Fr. William Breault, The Lady From Dublin, Sacramento, CA: Landmark Publishing Group, 1986, 120; ❧ p.27 Dr. Achelaus Field, Portrait and Biographical Album of Polk County, Iowa, Chicago: Lake City Publishing Co., 1890, 780; ❧ p.124 Dr. Barnes, and p.184 from top clockwise, Drs. Conkling, Page, Peck and Bierring, Council of the Des Moines Academy of Medicine and Polk County Medical Society, The History of Medicine of Polk County, Iowa, 1951, p.116-17.

Photographic Assistance:
New photography:
David Penney, p.5, 18, 21, 23-24, 33, 36, 41, 46-47, 49, 53, 56, 73, 78-79, 100, 112-13, 116-18, 132-33, 140, 155, 161, 164, 166, 180, 184, 208, 211, 220, 230, 231–1992 board chairs ❧ Sister Seraphia McMahon, p.81 Raggedy dolls; p.160 Our Lady of Fatima Shrine; p.180 Sr. Kilian; p.209 gift shop; p.218 Sr. Pat with Charlton Heston; p. 227 Sr. Pat with Stan Reynolds and Douglas Fairbanks, Jr.; ❧ Loretta Greiner, p. 15 and 73 Grave markers; p.220 Mercy Activity Center and Mercy Ed Center, ❧ Sue Moravec, p.182 Suzanne Mains, p. 228 Deanne Remer; ❧ Kyle Phillips, p. 179 Stained glass, p. 190 Walking track; p.231 administrative staff.

Existing photography:
Mark Baldwin: p.185 The Heart Center billboard, p.187 cardiac rehab, p.188 Dr. Chandramouli and Dr. Gay and family, p.189 cath lab, transplant, picnic, Jarvik procedure, p.190 perfusion, p.194 cancer hotline, p.216 Comfort suite, p. 217 Dr. Franklin, p.218 and cover-Sr. Pat with transplant patients, p.220 Laurel Center, p.223 Ruan ribbon cutting and pool, p.225 MRECT, p. 228 Dormitory, p.230 Sr. Concepta birthday; ❧ Kyle Phillips: p.191 Grubb ribbon-cutting; p.215 Infant car seat; p.219 Sr. Pat and Babe Bisignano; p.221 School of Health Sciences; p. 223 Brennan Family Center; p.224 Laurie and Sr. Joseph; ❧ Jim Heemstra: p.9 Atrium; p.187 cath lab control room; p. 189 cath Lab through fisheye lens; p.190 cath Lab, monitor; p.191 electrophysiology, second miracle, Dr. Iannone and Msgr. Holden; p.194 MRI; p.195 laser, linear accelerator, cancer coordinator; p.217 home care; p.218 House of Mercy; p.219 Sr. Pat with child; p.220 Sr. Mary Ann; p.220 Mercy Park; p.221 Sr. Martina, Mercy Court; p.222 Hyperbaric, CT, Surgery; p.224 Air Life; p.226 Mercy West; p.227 Mercy care; p.231 Sisters, 1991 Annual Report; p.232 Mercy at Night; ❧ David Penney: p.189 transplant going home; ❧ Sister Seraphia: p.219 Bishop Bullock; ❧ Andy Lyons: p.218 Stevie Wonder visit; ❧ Candy Foster: p.220 Indianola Clinic; ❧ Busby Productions: cover, Pioneer sisters in buggy and back cover, sister with doctor and patient.

Special Photographic Effects:
David Penney, photographer, copying; ❧ Tom Sargent, retouching; ❧ Lynn Neymeyer, colorization; ❧ Chris Conyers, Nancy Fandel, styling

Special Effects:
p.196-204 Bill Stirler and Ryan Hawkins, who drew the past and present architecture; ❧ Staff of Allied Business Consultants, Inc.; Designgroup, Inc.; Watt/Peterson, Inc.; and Busby Productions, Inc., who worked diligently to aid in the creation of this volume.

Special Assistance:
Staff of Mercy's Records Management and Archives Department, Public Relations Department, Communications Department, Maintenance Department, Security Department, Library, Data Processing Department, Medical Records Department, Sponsorship/Relational Committee, Centennial Committee, Linda Montet,and Karen Low, talented individuals who gave help in many ways throughout the project.

Mercy Hospital Medical Center Archives:
Special thanks to all the known and unknown who preserved and donated artifacts and photographs which portray the corporate memory in a richness that is uniquely Mercy in Des Moines.